DRUGS
AND
BEHAVIOR

FRED LEAVITT

California State University
Hayward

1974

W. B. SAUNDERS COMPANY

Philadelphia   London   Toronto

W. B. Saunders Company: West Washington Square
Philadelphia, Pa. 19105

12 Dyott Street
London, WC1A   1DB

833 Oxford Street
Toronto, Ontario M8Z 5T9, Canada

Drugs and Behavior

ISBN 0-7216-5695-1

Last digit is the print number: 9   8   7   6   5   4   3   2   1

This book is dedicated to the women in my life.
In chronological order

GOLDIE

DIANE

JESSICA

MELANIE

Introduction

WHAT IS PSYCHOPHARMACOLOGY?

Psychopharmacology is the science which deals with the effects of drugs on behavior. A drug is any chemical agent which has an effect on living protoplasm. Behavior has been variously defined; a definition which is adequate for most purposes is that it is any observable response of an organism. Such a definition is sufficiently broad so as to encompass drug-induced changes in perception, mood, thinking, and so forth.

WHY STUDY PSYCHOPHARMACOLOGY?

Works of fiction, and some literature which is not labeled fiction, abound in descriptions of fascinating drug effects. Travelers through Hades sipped from the river Lethe and became oblivious to all which went before. *Time* Magazine reported in 1966 that man might some-day have memory pills which would enable him to instantaneously assimilate large bodies of knowledge. Ponce de Leon was unsuccess-ful in his attempts to find a fountain of youth, although he did dis-cover Florida; but Brown-Sequard, a French physician and modern day Ponce de Leon, reported self-rejuvenation at the age of 72 after he injected himself with a special extract of dog testes. (For an ex-planation of the Brown-Sequard effect see Chapter 13.) Kindly Dr. Jekyll swallowed a blood-red potion and became transmogrified into the evil Mr. Hyde. The inhabitants of Brave New World used soma, and were content. Rosemary drank a special brew and her baby grew strong.

Man does not yet have at his disposal drugs which will produce blissful oblivion or instant knowledge. The fountain of youth still awaits discovery. Many substances are capable of reducing our inhibitions, but none transform man to beast. Soma-like drugs are available, but none are completely free of annoying side effects. And, although many people believe that certain drugs exist primarily to provide nourishment for the devil, the claim is disputed. Nevertheless, drugs may someday be available which will accomplish most of the above-named ends. And that is the lure of psychopharmacology.

There are at least three general reasons for studying psychopharmacology:

1. The understanding of a phenomenon—in this case, all aspects of human behavior—is usually greatly facilitated by the development of reliable means for producing the phenomenon. Drugs can be powerful tools to this end. For example, the physiological mechanisms underlying sleep and dreaming have been clarified by investigations with drugs which promote or reduce the need for sleep (see Chapter 15).

2. Drugs can be used to elicit or suppress various behaviors. The phenothiazines are highly effective in suppressing psychotic agitation; marijuana is used, outside the doctor's office, for its euphoric properties. One aspect of the psychopharmacologist's job is to find drugs which are of value in modifying behavior; equally important is work toward the development of congeners (related drugs) which produce even more powerful effects than the original compound, yet which have fewer undesirable side effects.

2. Man is a drug-taking animal. Anthropologists have reported the use of various drugs in virtually every culture studied. The ancient Sumerians of 4000 B.C. had a name for the poppy—"joy plant." In America, physicians and unsavory characters on dimly lit streetcorners are not the only sources of substances which affect behavior. Any supermarket will do. Caffeine, nicotine, and many vitamins and spices have powerful mind-altering effects. Only through well-controlled experimentation will these effects become sufficiently well understood so that users will be able to derive maximum benefit from them. For example, most coffee drinkers probably know that caffeine may produce insomnia, so they take their last cup of the day well before bedtime. But probably very few people who eat citrus fruits are aware of the postulated effects of vitamin C, which is found in great abundance in citrus fruits, on mood and affect.

GOALS OF THE BOOK

I have attempted to give a methodologically oriented, comprehensive, but concise introduction to the very exciting field of psychopharmacology. My aim has been to make the book suitable for home study as well as the classroom. Therefore, I have assumed no prior knowledge of actions of drugs or of psychological principles. Instructors of psychopharmacology may find it a useful text for a one semester course. It may also be helpful as a supplementary text for courses in physiological psychology, sociology, experimental design and methodology, and pharmacy.

ACKNOWLEDGMENTS

Whatever the merits of this book, it is vastly better than it would have been had I written it without any help. Baxter Venable, the Psychology editor at Saunders, and three of his reviewers did a tremendous job of adding, deleting, reorganizing, and of making unclear writing comprehensible. The book profited because of several valuable discussions I had with colleagues, and because they called many important references to my attention. For that, I wish to thank Norm Livson, Roy Matsumoto, Jordan Rosenberg, Bill Sawrey, Howie Willer, and Stephen Winokur. The typing was shared by several people. My thanks to Norene Avakian, Sharon Cosgrove, Julie Daugherty, Jo Jorgenson, Wanda Kiger, and Sally Mladinich. Finally, I wish to thank Diane, for being there.

Contents

CHAPTER 1

CLASSIFICATION
OF DRUGS

No two drugs are identical in all respects, but many have qualitatively similar actions on a great many physiological and psychological systems. Thus, when a pharmacologist is told that a particular drug is antimuscarinic, he knows that it dilates the pupils of the eyes, speeds up heart rate, slows up secretions from sweat and salivary glands, and reduces activity in the stomach and intestines. Placebos, another class of drugs (see Chap. 2), may differ in color, size, shape, and effectiveness (9); nevertheless, considerable information is conveyed by the statement that a particular drug is a placebo.

Drugs may be ordered along many different dimensions. Since the purpose of classifying is to provide a convenient framework around which to organize information and thinking about drugs, the particular system chosen should reflect the interests of the users. Thus, the purposes of lawyers might best be served simply by classifying drugs as licit or illicit (or, for sophisticated lawyers, the illicit drugs may be further subdivided into those punishable as misdemeanor or felony). Some drug users make do with a simple two-factor system: uppers and downers. For serious scientists, more descriptive categories are needed. Most pharmacologists classify drugs according to molecular structure, which enables them to best understand structure-activity relationships. Chemists do the same, so that they can most efficiently direct research aimed at synthesizing new drugs. However, classification according to molecular structure is not always satisfactory for researchers who are interested

1

in behavior; it results, for example, in the placement of LSD, one of the strongest of all drugs which affect the central nervous system (CNS), with 2-bromo-LSD, which has weak CNS actions (2). Still, drugs of the same family do tend to have similar actions. The difference between LSD and 2-bromo-LSD is explained by the failure of the latter to penetrate the blood-brain barrier. Attention to chemical structure can lead to valuable ideas about directions for research. For example, when a clinically useful drug has some undesirable properties, a program for synthesizing structurally similar compounds can be instituted. This strategy probably maximizes the probability of finding a new drug with a more favorable therapeutic index.

Because classification systems are useful but arbitrary, several different ones are described below. No attempt has been made to single one out as being superior to the rest. Before describing the various systems, two points should be emphasized. First, all drugs have many actions; chlorpromazine may be classified as a major tranquilizer, but it is also an antiadrenergic and acts to depress activity within the CNS. Secondly, drugs do not act in vacuo. Their effects depend on the resultant of their interactions with the four sets of variables (organismic, drug, environmental, and task) listed in Chapter 2. A drug which activates behavior under some circumstances may depress it under others.

CLASSIFICATION ACCORDING TO CLINICAL UTILITY

Balter and Levine (1) classified psychoactive drugs primarily on the basis of clinical use, and secondarily on their chemical structure. They stressed six actions: major tranquilization, minor tranquilization, antidepressant, stimulant, sedative, and hypnotic. A much more extensive classification system, which includes hallucinogenics, has been arranged by Usdin (12).

Balter and Levine called those drugs which are used primarily in the treatment of psychoses the major tranquilizers. The major tranquilizers reduce hallucinations, delusions, and disordered thought. The most common side effects are drowsiness, parkinsonism (characterized by rigidity, tremor, and weakness, which are similar to the symptoms of Parkinson's disease), and postural hypotension. Major tranquilizers are not physiologically addictive. They are rarely abused, i.e., people do not self-administer them except when directed to do so by a physician. Other names for major tranquilizers are neuroleptics and antipsychotics. Examples are chlorpromazine and reserpine.

Minor tranquilizers relieve anxiety without producing drowsiness. More prescriptions are filled for the minor tranquilizers than

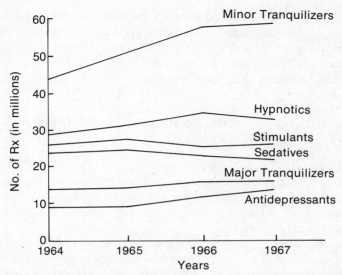

Figure 1-1 Analysis of psychotropic drug use in the United States (1964–1967), by number of new and refill prescriptions. In 1964, 149.1 million prescriptions for psychotropic drugs were filled. In 1967, the total number had reached 173.6 million. The breakdown of the psychotropics into the six classes shown clearly indicates the predominance of the use of minor tranquilizers. (From Balter, M., and Levine, J. The nature and extent of psychotropic drug usage in the United States. Psychopharmacol. Bull., 1969, Vol. 5, 4: p. 9.)

for any other class of psychoactive drugs; in 1967 there were 59.7 million new prescriptions. (See Fig. 1–1.) These drugs can lead to physiological dependence. Some workers use the term anxiolytic in place of minor tranquilizer, and the term ataractic to describe both major and minor tranquilizers. Examples are diazepam, chlordiazepoxide, and meprobamate (Librium and Miltown are well-known brand names of the latter two).

Antidepressants are used to combat depression. Some may be more effective against depressions which originate in (and can be traced to) well-defined external events; others may work better against endogenous depressions. The antidepressants do not have physiological addiction liability. Antidepressants have also been called psychic energizers and thymoleptics. Examples are imipramine and the various monoamine oxidase inhibitors (isocarboxazid, tranylcypromine).

Stimulants are used to reduce fatigue and to treat depression. Many have powerful anorexic (appetite suppressing) effects, and so are often prescribed for obese patients. Stimulant drugs are often abused, and may produce physiological dependence. The amphetamines and methylphenidate are the best known stimulants.

Sedatives are not used as extensively as they once were. Their major clinical property, sedation or calming, is achieved equally well with the tranquilizers. The latter produce less drowsiness and are less likely to be abused. The long-acting barbiturates, such as phenobarbital, are classed as sedatives.

Hypnotic drugs shall be discussed in detail in Chapter 15.

EXPANDED CLASSIFICATIONS, TO INCLUDE DRUGS WHICH DO NOT HAVE CLINICAL UTILITY

WORLD HEALTH ORGANIZATION CLASSIFICATION. The World Health Organization recognizes five categories of psychoactive drugs, and expects to create new categories as drugs with unique mechanisms of action or therapeutic importance are developed. The present categories are:

I.	Neuroleptics	antipsychotic action; effective in the treatment of some psychiatric disorders which are accompanied by neurological signs (chlorpromazine)
II.	Anxiolytic sedatives	reduce anxiety without affecting perception or cognition (chlordiazepoxide)
III.	Antidepressants	combat depression (imipramine)
IV.	Psychostimulants	increase level of alertness (amphetamine)
V.	Psychodysleptics	produce abnormal mental phenomena, particularly of perception and cognition (LSD)

JARVIK'S CLASSIFICATION. Murray Jarvik, in *Psychology Today* (8), gives a very useful classification system. It includes most drugs likely to be of interest to the behavioral pharmacologist.

I. Psychotherapeutic drugs: These are used in the treatment of psychological and psychiatric disorders.
  A. Antipsychotics
  B. Antianxiety Drugs
  C. Antidepressants
  D. Stimulants

II. Psychotogenic drugs: These produce changes in mood, thinking, and behavior. Representative psychotogenics are LSD, marijuana, mescaline, and psilocybin.

III. Stimulants: These rate a separate class, in addition to having occasional therapeutic use. They elevate mood, increase confidence and alertness, and prevent fatigue. Many diverse drugs may serve as stimulants, including amphetamine, caffeine, nicotine, and LSD.

IV. Sedatives and hypnotics: These produce general depression (sedation) in low doses, and sleep (hypnosis) in larger doses. They are used clinically to treat stress, anxiety, and insomnia. The barbiturates are the best known representatives of this class.

V. Anesthetics, analgesics, and paralytics: General anesthesia, such as is produced by diethyl ether, chloroform, and nitrous oxide, is a total loss of consciousness. Local anesthetics, including cocaine, procaine, and lidocaine, block nerve conduction near the site of action. Analgesics relieve pain (see pp. 234–241 for a discussion of analgesic actions of drugs). Well-known analgesics are acetylsalicylic acid (aspirin) and other salicylates; acetanilid; and morphine and related drugs. Paralytic drugs produce muscular paralysis (see below). The best known paralytic drug is curare; others include gallamine and succinylcholine.

VI. Neurohumors (neurotransmitters): See later discussion.

CLASSIFICATION BY MEANS OF THE ELECTROENCEPHALOGRAPH

The electroencephalograph (EEG) is a sensitive machine which is used to measure electrical activity of the brain. It consists of recording electrodes which are placed on the scalp, and which carry the small electrical oscillations of the brain into an amplifier. The amplified waves are generally displayed visually on an oscilloscope. They vary in frequency from about 3 to 40 cycles per second, depending on state of arousal and the place in the brain from where they are recorded.

When a person rests quietly with eyes closed, the dominant wave form is called an alpha wave; it is of high amplitude and low frequency (about 10 cycles per second). As the level of arousal increases, the waves shift to lower amplitudes and faster frequencies. During deep sleep the waves are of very high amplitude and slow frequency. Interestingly, when a person dreams, the waves resemble those seen during arousal. Figure 1–1 diagrams the changes in EEG which are associated with changes in the level of arousal.

Fink (3) has recently summarized research which shows that the EEG is very sensitive to drugs. He developed a system for classifying drugs based on patterns of EEG frequency and amplitude changes. A shortened version is given in Table 1.1. Table 1.2 lists representative drugs in each class.

Fink has described the behaviors which are associated with types of EEG changes:

1. Shifts toward EEG slowing are associated with sedation, drowsiness, relaxation, inhibition of psychomotor activity, confusion, memory loss, and, in psychotics, fewer illusions, hallucinations, and delusions.

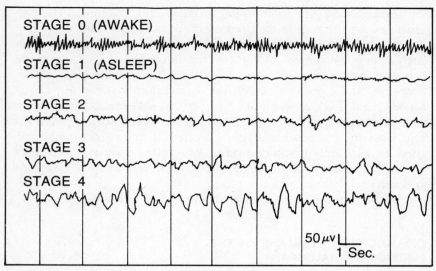

Figure 1–2 Changes in the electroencephalogram which occur with different degrees of alertness, ranging from deep sleep to wakefulness. During stage 1 rem (discussed in Chap. 15), the subject is making rapid eye movements and probably is dreaming. (From W. Webb, *Sleep: An Experimental Approach,* New York, Macmillan, 1968.)

TABLE 1.1   EEG Changes Associated With Different Classes of Drugs*

I. INCREASED SLOWING OF FREQUENCIES
Drugs in class I slow the alpha frequency, and at the same time reduce the abundance of faster frequencies. There are three sub-types.
A. alpha occurrence is more frequent, amplitudes of all frequencies are increased
B. alpha occurs less frequently, seizure activity is common
C. increased seizure activity

II. INCREASED FAST ACTIVITY
Frequencies greater than 13/sec are considered fast. Class II drugs make these frequencies more common.
A. amplitudes increase, the frequencies become very rhythmic, and alpha may become more abundant
B. rhythmic activity and alpha are both less common, amplitudes decrease

III. INCREASED SLOW AND FAST FREQUENCIES
Class III drugs increase both slow and fast frequencies.
A. least rhythmic activity, low amplitudes

IV. ALPHA VARIATION
Class IV drugs modify the total proportion of waves that are alpha waves.
A. increased abundance, often with slowing of frequency
B. decreased abundance

*Adapted from Fink, M. EEG classification of psychoactive compounds in man: a review and theory of behavioral associations. *In* Efron, D. (Ed.) *Psychopharmacology,* U.S. PHS Pub. No. 1836, 1968.

TABLE 1.2 Classification of Drugs by EEG Criteria*

CLASS: I—INCREASED SLOWING OF EEG FREQUENCIES

Ia.	Ib. Increased Alpha	Ic. Increased Seizure Activity
chlorpromazine	butaperazine	reserpine
chlorprothixene	fluphenazine	
(fluphenazine)	perphenazine	(amitriptyline)
haloperidol	thioproperazine	(bemegride)
pinoxepin	trifluoperazine	cycloserine
thioridazine		diphenhydramine
thiothixene		prochlorperazine
trifluperidol		promazine
triflupromazine		(promethazine)
(bromides)		
(lithium)		

II.—INCREASED FAST ACTIVITY

IIa. Increased Amplitude	IIb. Decreased Amplitude
amobarbital	amphetamine
chlordiazepoxide	bemegride
diazepam	dimethyltryptamine
ethchlorvynol	di-ethyltryptamine
fenfluramine	epinephrine
glutethimide	lysergide (LSD-25)
meprobamate	mescaline
methylpentynol	methamphetamine
pentobarbital	methylpenidate
phenobarbital	phenmetrazine
secobarbital	psilocybin
thiopental	

III.—INCREASED SLOW AND FAST ACTIVITY

IIIa. Maximum Amplitude Decrease	IIIb. Little Amplitude Decrease
atropine	amitriptyline
benactyzine	cyclazocine
diethazine	imipramine
Ditran	levomepromazine
(phencyclidine)	nalorphine
scopolamine	promethazine

IV.—ALPHA VARIATION

IVa. Alpha Variation, Increase	IVb. Alpha Variation, Decrease
alcohol (ethyl)	(azacyclonol)
	benactyzine
heroin	(deanol)
(hydroxyzine)	iproniazid
morphine	(isocarboxazid)
methadone	(isoniazid)
(sulthiame)	(nialamide)
	pipradol
	(tranylcypromine)

*From Fink, M. EEG classification of psychoactive compounds in man: a review and theory of behavioral associations. *In* Efron, D. (Ed.) *Psychopharmacology.* U.S. PHS Pub. No. 1836, 1968, p. 500.

2. Increased abundance of fast activity and increased rhythmicity are associated with sedation, drowsiness, and relaxation.

3. Increased abundance of alpha waves, and increased rhythmicity are associated with euphoria, relaxation, sedation, decreased psychomotor activity, and fewer illusions, hallucinations, and delusions in psychotics.

4. Increases in frequencies of both fast and slow activity, usually with increased variability of frequencies and amplitudes, are associated with confusion, memory defect, illusions and thought disorder, and delirium. The increase in slow wave activity increases stupor, and increased fast wave activity increases psychomotor activity and irritability.

5. Decreased alpha activity and increased fast frequencies and amplitudes are associated with illusions, fantasies, hallucinations, anxiety, and motor restlessness or increased speech production.

More detailed analyses of EEG effects of several classes of drugs can be found in Fink (4, 5). A different technique for classifying drugs according to EEG responses has been developed by Goldstein and Beck (6). It involves the use of an electronic integrator, from which values can be obtained for the average amplitude and variability of populations of electrical events. Their technique is sensitive to changes produced by a wide variety of experimental conditions.

NEUROHUMORAL TRANSMISSION

The functional unit of the CNS is the nerve cell, or neuron. Although they vary greatly in size and shape, all neurons have three principal parts (see Fig. 1–2): in common with all cells, each neuron has a cell body; there are one or more slender dendrites, which most frequently carry nerve impulses into the cell body; and there is one relatively thick axon which carries impulses away from the cell body.

Neurons transmit information to each other at junctions called synapses. Electrical transmission has been described, but all known mammalian synapses are chemical in nature. When an adequate stimulus is applied to the presynaptic neuron, it releases a chemical substance which diffuses across the synaptic cleft. The chemical substances are called neurohumoral transmitters or neurotransmitters. They may increase or decrease the likelihood with which the postsynaptic neuron fires, so they are classified as being excitatory or inhibitory at particular synapses.

Ideally, psychoactive drugs would be classified according to their effects on the process of neurohumoral transmission within specific parts of the CNS. Unfortunately, even though many sub-

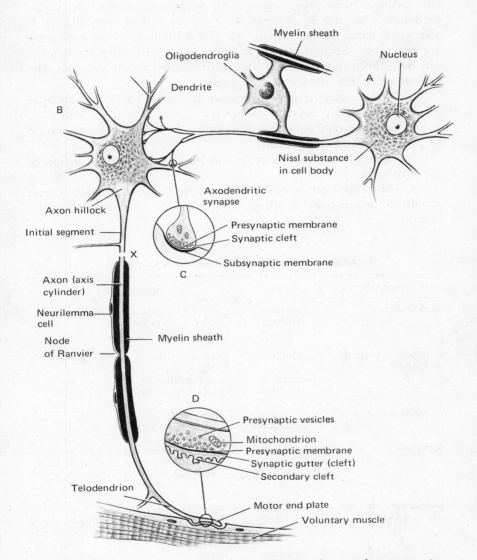

Figure 1-3 Diagram of (A) a neuron located within the central nervous system and (B) a lower motor neuron located in both the central and peripheral nervous systems. The latter synapses with a voluntary muscle cell to form a motor end-plate. Note the similarities, as reconstructed from electron micrographs, between (C) a synapse between two neurons and (D) a motor end-plate. The hiatus in the nerve at X represents the border between the central nervous system (above the X) and the peripheral nervous system (below the X). (From C. Noback and R. Demarest, *The Nervous System: Introduction and Review*, New York, McGraw-Hill, 1972, p. 15.)

stances have been proposed as CNS neurotransmitters, conclusive evidence is lacking in all cases, save for the role of acetylcholine at a single synapse in the spinal cord. The difficulties of the enterprise are enormous. Several criteria must be satisfied before a substance can be established as a neurotransmitter at a specific synapse. McLennan's criteria (10) are widely quoted:

1. The presumptive neurotransmitter at a particular synapse must occur in the presynaptic neuron.

2. The enzymes necessary for synthesis of the substance should be present within the neuron.

3. There should be a mechanism for terminating the action of the substance.

4. Direct application of the substance to the postsynaptic neuron should be equivalent in effect to stimulation of the presynaptic neuron.

TABLE 1.3   **Some Probable Neurotransmitters***

NEUROTRANSMITTER	ACTION	SITE OF ACTION
acetylcholine	excitatory	reticular formation
	inhibitory	reticular formation
	excitatory	visual system
5-hydroxytryptamine (serotonin)	inhibitory	medial geniculate bodies (pathway in the auditory system)
	excitatory	some cortical cells
	inhibitory	some cortical cells
norepinephrine	excitatory	some cortical cells
	inhibitory	some cortical cells
dopamine	inhibitory	caudate nucleus (area which underlies the cerebral cortex, and which probably has extensive connections with the motor cortex)
gamma-aminobutyric acid (GABA)	inhibitory	cerebral cortex
	inhibitory	Purkinje cells of cerebellum (concerned with movement, balance, and muscle tonus)
	inhibitory	retina
	inhibitory	spinal cord
glycine	inhibitory	spinal cord
glutamate	excitatory	spinal cord
glutamic acid	excitatory	spinal cord
aspartic acid	excitatory	spinal cord

*Adapted from Hebb, C. CNS at the cellular level: identity of transmitter agents. Ann. Rev. Physiol., 1970, 32:165–192.

5. When the synapse is activated, the substance should be detectable within the area of the synapse.

6. Drugs which interfere with the synthesis of the substance, or its reaction with the postsynaptic membrane, should block the effects of neuronal stimulation.

7. Drugs which block the enzyme which normally inactivates the substance should lead to a prolongation of its effects and of the effects of neuronal stimulation.

Hebb (7) suggested that the criteria such as given by McLennan are too stringent, and that satisfaction of criteria 4, 6, and 7, and perhaps 2, is sufficient. Hebb reviewed evidence on the prime candidates for neurotransmitters. Her conclusions are summarized in Table 1.3. Note that a given neurotransmitter may be excitatory at one site and inhibitory at another.

AUTONOMIC NERVOUS SYSTEM DRUGS

The autonomic nervous system (ANS) regulates activities of smooth muscle, cardiac muscle, and glands. Among the structures innervated are digestive, sweat, and lacrimal glands; urinary bladder; gastrointestinal tract; heart; blood vessels; iris of the eye; and glands such as the adrenals, pancreatic islets, and gonads. Fibers of the ANS arise from neurons within the spinal cord and brain stem. The fibers send axons to masses of nerve cell bodies, called ganglia, which are outside the CNS. These axons synapse with cells within the ganglia, which send their axons to the effector organs. The first neuron is called preganglionic, and the second, postganglionic. The two transmitters within the ANS have been identified and form a basis for classifying many drugs.

The autonomic nervous system is divided into two parts, sympathetic and parasympathetic, which are different both anatomically and functionally. They act in opposite directions on most, but not all, of the organs which they innervate. (See Table 1.4.) The neurotransmitter acetylcholine (ACh) is released by all preganglionic autonomic fibers, by postganglionic parasympathetic fibers, and by some postganglionic sympathetic fibers. ACh is also released at neuromuscular junctions, thus innervating skeletal muscles. Norepinephrine, also called noradrenaline, is released by the remaining sympathetic fibers. Drugs can mimic, promote the release of, or retard the destruction of ACh or norepinephrine, thereby producing effects similar to those seen upon parasympathetic or sympathetic stimulation. They may also interfere with stimulation of either system. Table 1.5 lists the various classes of autonomic drugs, their mechanisms of action, and representative drugs in each class. The characteristic effects of each class of drugs can be determined by

TABLE 1.4   Responses of Effector Organs to Autonomic Nerve Impulses*

| Effector Organs | Adrenergic Impulses | | Cholinergic Impulses |
	Receptor Type†	Responses ▲	Responses ▲
Eye			
Radial muscle iris	α	Contraction (mydriasis) (++)	———
Sphincter muscle iris		———	Contraction (miosis) (+++)
Ciliary muscle	β	Relaxation for far vision (slight effect)	Contraction for near vision (+++)
Heart			
S-A node	β	Increase in heart rate (++)	Decrease in heart rate; vagal arrest (+++)
Atria	β	Increase in contractility and conduction velocity (++)	Decrease in contractility and (usually) increase in conduction velocity (++)
A-V node and conduction system		Increase in conduction velocity (++)	Decrease in conduction velocity; A-V block (+++)
Ventricles	β	Increase in contractility, conduction velocity, automaticity, and rate of idiopathic pacemakers (+++)	Slight decrease in contractility claimed by some
Blood Vessels			
Coronary	α,β	Constriction (+); Dilatation ‡ (+++)	Dilatation (±)
Skin and mucosa	α	Constriction (+++)	Dilatation§
Skeletal muscle	α,β	Constriction (++); dilatation‖ (++)	Dilatation# (+)
Cerebral	α	Constriction (slight)	Dilatation§
Pulmonary	α,β	Constriction (+); dilatation (+)	Dilatation§
Abdominal viscera	α,β	Constriction (+++); dilatation‖ (+)	———
Salivary glands	α	Constriction (+++)	Dilatation (++)
Lung			
Bronchial muscle	β	Relaxation (+)	Contraction (++)
Bronchial glands		Inhibition (?)	Stimulation (+++)
Stomach			
Motility and tone	β	Decrease (usually)§§ (+)	Increase (+++)
Sphincters	α	Contraction (usually) (+)	Relaxation (usually) (+)
Secretion		Inhibition (?)	Stimulation (+++)
Intestine			
Motility and tone	α,β	Decrease§§ (+)	Increase (+++)
Sphincters	α	Contraction (usually) (+)	Relaxation (usually) (+)
Secretion		Inhibition (?)	Stimulation (++)

TABLE 1.4 *Continued*

Effector Organs	Adrenergic Impulses		Cholinergic Impulses
	Receptor Type†	Responses ▲	Responses ▲
Gallbladder and Ducts		Relaxation (+)	Contraction (+++)
Urinary Bladder			
Detrusor	β	Relaxation (usually) (+)	Contraction (+++)
Trigone and sphincter	α	Contraction (++)	Relaxation (++)
Ureter			
Motility and tone		Increase (usually)	Increase(?)
Uterus	α,β	Variable**	Variable**
Sex Organs		Ejaculation (+++)	Erection (+++)
Skin			
Pilomotor muscles	α	Contraction (++)	———
Sweat glands	α	Slight, localized secretion†† (+)	Generalized secretion (+++)
Spleen Capsule	α	Contraction (+++)	———
Adrenal Medulla		———	Secretion of epinephrine and norepinephrine
Liver		Glycogenolysis	———
Pancreatic Acini		———	Secretion (++)
Salivary Glands	α	Thick, viscous secretion‡‡ (+)	Profuse, watery secretion (+++)
Lacrimal Glands		———	Secretion (+++)
Nasopharyngeal Glands		———	Secretion (+++)

*From "Neurohumoral Transmission and the Autonomic Nervous System" by George B. Koelle, pp. 406–407, *The Pharmacological Basis of Therapeutics,* Fourth Edition, L. S. Goodman and A. Gilman, (eds.). Macmillan Publishing Co., Inc., New York 1970.

†Where adrenergic receptor type has been established.

▲Responses are designated 1+ to 3+ to provide an approximate indication of the importance of adrenergic and cholinergic nerve activity in the control of the various organs and functions listed.

‡Dilatation predominates *in situ* due to indirect effects.

§Cholinergic vasodilatation at these sites is of questionable physiological significance.

‖Over the usual concentration range of physiologically released, circulating epinephrine, β-receptor response (vasodilatation) predominates in blood vessels of skeletal muscle and liver; α-receptor response (vasoconstriction), in blood vessels of other abdominal viscera.

#Sympathetic cholinergic system causes vasodilatation in skeletal muscle.

**Depends on stage of menstrual cycle, amount of circulating estrogen and progesterone, and other factors; responses of pregnant uterus differ from those of nonpregnant uterus.

††Palms of hands and some other sites ("adrenergic sweating").

‡‡Parotid glands lack adrenergic innervation.

§§May result predominantly from inhibition of parasympathetic ganglionic transmission by postganglionic adrenergic fibers terminating on ganglion cells of Auerbach's plexus (Norberg, 1964; Jacobowitz, 1965; Paton and Vizi, 1969).

14   **Classification of Drugs**

studying Table 1.4 in conjunction with Table 1.5. The physiological actions of the two divisions of the ANS can be recalled merely by remembering that the sympathetic system is activated when the organism is aroused. What happens when an individual prepares for fight or flight? The heart begins pumping rapidly, the pupils of the eyes dilate, body sugar is mobilized for energy, and defecation is common. Differences in chemical structure of drugs within each class account for differences in rates of absorption, ease of penetration into the brain, resistance to degradation by metabolic enzymes, and, ultimately, relative potency and specificity of action on the

TABLE 1.5   ANS Drugs

Drug Class	Mechanism of Action	Representative Drugs
anticholinesterases	inhibit AChE, the enzyme which inactivates ACh, hence produce effects like those produced by continuous stimulation of cholinergic sites	*physostigmine:* readily enters the brain, so is a popular research tool for studying cholinergic synapses within the brain *neostigmine:* used in treatment of myasthenia gravis, a disease characterized by rapid fatigability of skeletal muscle *tabun, sarin,* and *soman:* they inactivate AChE irreversibly, so are lethal; they are nerve gases *parathion* and *malathion:* insecticides
parasympathomimetics	direct stimulation of cholinergic fibers	*carbachol:* is frequently applied directly to the brains of laboratory animals, where its resistance to degradation by AChE makes it very valuable for studying cholinergic synapses *muscarine:* occurs naturally in many mushrooms, and bestows hallucinogenic properties upon them *arecoline:* used as a euphoric in the East Indies *pilocarpine:* has many stimulant and depressant effects on the brain
antimuscarinics	inhibit action of ACh at post-ganglionic cholinergic sites	*scopolamine:* used in many preparations for inducing sleep; impairs memory; has played an important role in research on the role of ACh in memory formation; after large doses, disorientation, hallucinations, and euphoria are common *atropine:* similar peripheral effects but less powerful CNS effects than scopolamine *methyl scopolamine* and *methyl atropine:* unlike scopolamine and atropine, do not penetrate brain, so are used in research in conjunction with the latter to determine whether effects are due to central or peripheral actions
antinicotinics	inhibit action of ACh at neuromuscular junctions	*curare:* used by South American Indians to kill game, with death resulting from respiratory paralysis; useful laboratory tool for pharmacological studies, but should not be used in place of an anesthetic, because it does not reduce pain *succinylcholine:* very brief duration of action
ganglionic stimulants	mimic action of ACh at autonomic ganglia; stimulators and blockers affect all transmission at ganglia; thus, the final effect depends on initial predominance of sympathetic or parasympathetic tone	*nicotine:* its many CNS effects are discussed elsewhere; nicotine mimics the stimulant effects of ACh on skeletal muscles, and drugs which act similarly are said to have nicotinic actions.

(Table 1.5 continued on opposite page.)

effector organs. Many drugs have autonomic side effects. Tables 1.6 to 1.10, taken from Sigg (11), list many of them.

ACh and norepinephrine are almost surely neurotransmitters in widespread areas throughout the brain (see previous discussion). Therefore, it is not surprising that drugs which act upon the autonomic nervous system, and which penetrate the brain, are behaviorally active. Anticholinergics induce hallucinations, disordered thought, and impaired memory. Sympathomimetics are stimulants and mood-elevators. Adrenergic blockers are commonly used in treatment of the psychoses.

(Text continued on page 21.)

TABLE 1.5 *Continued*

Drug Class	Mechanism of Action	Representative Drugs
ganglionic blockers	a. In order for a neuron to discharge, there must first be an electrical gradient between the inside and outside of its cell membrane. The gradient is temporarily eliminated when the cell fires, and must be restored before the cell can fire again. One class of ganglionic blockers continuously stimulate neurons, thus producing a phenomenon called depolarization blockade, in which the gradient is not restored and the cell cannot fire	*nicotine*
	b. compete with ACh at receptor sites	*hexamethonium, mecamylamine,* and *tetraethylammonium:* of little importance in psychopharmacology
sympathomimetics	act by any or all of four different mechanisms: a. direct stimulation of postganglionic adrenergic sites b. release of the adrenergic transmitter, norepinephrine c. inhibition of monoamine oxidase, an enzyme which is important in the metabolism of norepinephrine d. prevent reuptake of released neurotransmitter by the nerve terminals, thus prolonging its action	*norepinephrine* and *epinephrine:* both are probably neurotransmitters, but have no powerful CNS action when administered outside the brain; epinephrine is often given along with local anesthetics, because its powerful vasoconstrictor action helps retard the systemic absorption of the anesthetic *amphetamine, methamphetamine,* and *cocaine:* these and many other stimulant drugs are sympathomimetics; they cross the blood-brain barrier, and are effective orally; the sympathomimetics relax bronchial muscles, so are used in the treatment of asthma and certain allergic reactions
alpha adrenergic blockers	inhibit certain responses to adrenergic sympathetic nerve activity (those listed as receptor type α in Table 1.4)	*phenoxybenzamine* and *dibenamine:* long acting *tolazoline* and *phentolamine:* short acting alpha adrenergic blockers have been used with some success in the treatment of hypertension
beta adrenergic blockers	inhibit some responses to adrenergic sympathetic nerve activity (listed as β in Table 1.4)	*dichloroisoproterenol* and *pronethalol:* little therapeutic importance
antiadrenergics	inhibit virtually all responses to adrenergic sympathetic nerve activity	*reserpine:* depletes stores of norepinephrine, epinephrine, and other catecholamines; is effective antipsychotic agent, but is no longer used much because it frequently produces severe depression *guanethidene:* used to treat hypertension

TABLE 1.6 Autonomic Side-effects of Psychostimulants*

Compound	Dry Mouth	Blurred Vision	Consti-pation	Increased Perspiration	Nausea and/or Vomiting	Dizziness	Micturition Difficulty
Iproniazid	22 (253)	11 (253)	23 (253)	4.7(253)	18 (253)		5.5(253)
Isocarboxazid	1.7(4660)	0.8(4660)	1.4(4660)	0.7(4660)	0.5(4660)	2.8(4660)	0.24(4660)
Phenelzine	8.2(257)	1.5(257)	7 (257)	5 (257)	4.6 (257)		1.2(257)
Nialamid	2.4(163)	1.8(163)	2.4(163)	2.4(163)	1.8 (163)		6.7(163)
Pargyline	10 (85)	10 (60)	3.3(60)	0 (60)	20 (60)		5.9(85)
Tranylcypromine	18.7(331)	9.1(110)	6.8(146)	13.6(22)	—	9.1(506)	5 (201)
d-Amphetamine	8.7(903)	6.9(29)	3.3(980)	1.3(555)	—	2.7(1226)	0.8(595)
Phenmetrazine	18 (122)	—	4.9(122)	—	14 (122)		—
Chlorphentermine	29 (24)	4.1(24)	4.1(24)	—	—	4.1(24)	—

*The numbers in italics represent the percentage of incidence of side effects.
The numbers in parentheses represent the total number of patients.

TABLE 1.7 Autonomic Side-effects of Tricyclic Antidepressants*

Compound	Dry Mouth	Blurred Vision	Consti-pation	Increased Perspiration	Nausea and/or Vomiting	Dizziness	Micturition Difficulty
Amitriptyline	23 (583)	7.5(546)	15 (546)	4.7(546)		9.3(546)	0 (546)
Desmethyl-amitriptyline	26 (1888)	6 (1888)	8 (1888)	<1 (1888)	1 (1888)	7 (1888)	<1 (1888)
Imipramine	18 (1998)	1.2(1998)	3 (1998)	15 (1998)	12 (1998)		0.2(1998)
Desmethyl-imipramine	10 (252)	2 (192)	8.7(192)	4.6(192)		9.8(192)	0 (192)
Dibenzepin	19 (355)	1.7(355)	1.4(355)	5.6(355)	21 (355)		2.5(355)
Protriptyline	31 (170)	8 (150)	2.7(150)	5.8(120)	1 (100)	11 (120)	4 (150)

*The numbers in italics represent the percentage of incidence of side effects.
The numbers in parentheses represent the total number of patients.

TABLE 1.8 Autonomic Side-effects of Phenothiazines*

Compound	Dry Mouth	Blurred Vision	Constipation	Nausea and/or Vomiting	Dizziness	Nasal Stuffiness	Micturition Difficulty
Chlorpromazine	*37.3*(4338)	*23.1*(251)	*12.6*(4785)	*4.1*(6430)	—	*22.9*(3764)	—
Promazine	*76* (1400)	—	*33.3*(1400)	—	*50* (1400)	*48* (1400)	—
Triflupromazine	*18.5*(23)	*8.3*(96)	*6.0*(182)	*10* (96)	—	*0* (20)	—
Trimeprazine	*11* (96) / *10.5*(243)	None	*15* (96) / None	*2.1*(333)	*2.6*(422)	—	None
Prochlorperazine	*12.6*(1292)	*2.9*(443)	*0.3*(2169)	*1.6*(2701)	*6.8*(1222)	*6.4*(1884)	—
Perphenazine	*9.5*(566)	*7.4*(203)	*8.0*(691)	*9* (128)	—	—	—
Trifluoperazine	*3.4*(1144)	*10.3*(838)	*3.6*(191)	*6* (853)	*4.2*(1495)	—	—
Fluphenazine	*12.0*(160)	*1.2*(160)	*12* (50)	—	*10* (50)	*0.9*(110)	—
Thipropazate	*0.96*(104)	*1.2*(104)	*7.5*(52)	*10* (52)	—	*23* (92)	—
Mepazine	*20.5*(432)	*38.5*(622)	*23.8*(551)	*4.8*(103)	—	—	—
Thioridazine	*6.7*(1445)	*0.6*(1445)	*1.6*(1445)	*4.4*(1445)	*3.3*(1445)	*1.5*(1445)	*0.8*(1445)
Chlorprothixene	*4.0*(3575)	*0.4*(3575)	*0.2*(3575)	*0.6*(3575)	*1.7*(3575)	*0.4*(3575)	*0.2*(3575)

*The numbers in italics represent the percentage of incidence of side effects.
The numbers in parentheses represent the total number of patients.

TABLE 1.9 Autonomic Side-effects of Reserpine-like Agents, Butyrophenones and Minor Tranquilizers*

Compound	Dry Mouth	Blurred Vision	Consti-pation	Nausea and/or Vomiting	Dizziness	Nasal Stuffiness	Micturition Difficulty
Reserpine	3.5ᵃ(28)	2.5ᵇ(28)	2.1(237)	9.0(112)	6.8(308)	39.0(501)	0 (62)
Tetrabenazine	Occasionally	—	0	Occasionally	.34(862)	0	0
Chloridiazepoxide	0 (17702)	0.1(17702)	0.4(17702)	0.34(17702)	0.64(17702)	—	0.08(17702)
Diazepam	0.2(14975)	0.14(14975)	0.4(14975)	0.7(14975)	0.1	—	0.4(14975)
Phenobarbital	11.6(129)	8.5(129)	8.5(129)	5.4(129)		—	—
Meprobamate	0.3(340)	1.1(340)	0 (340)	3.5(312)	8.8(312)	—	—
Haloperidol	20.5(63)	16.0(313)	12.6(63)	7.8(63)		—	—

*The numbers in italics represent the percentage of incidence of side effects.
The numbers in parentheses represent the total number of patients.
ᵃDryness of mucosa
ᵇMiosis

TABLE 1.10   Autonomic Side-effects of Placebo and Miscellaneous Drugs*

Compound	Dry Mouth	Blurred Vision	Consti-pation	Nausea and/or Vomiting	Dizziness	Micturition Difficulty
Pretreatment Controls	9.5(211)	0.3(211)	9.0(211)	27.0(211)		1.9(211)
Placebo (Tranquilizer studies)	6.2(286)	0.7(286)	2.1(286)	5.3(286)		0 (286)
Placebo (Antidepressant and stimulant drug studies)	20.0(105)	0 (105)	8.0(105)	11.0(105)		0 (105)
Miscellaneous Drugs^c	1.4(11115)	0.1(11115)	0.5(11115)	0.7(11115)		—

^c 71 different drugs
*The numbers in italics represent the percentage of incidence of side effects.
The numbers in parentheses represent the total number of patients.

Tables 1.6–1.10 are taken from Sigg, E. Autonomic side effects induced by psychotherapeutic agents. *In* Efron, D. *Psychopharmacology,* U.S. PHS Pub. No. 1836, 1968, pp. 582–583.

The preceding survey of classificatory schemata is by no means exhaustive. Several overlap considerably, and will eventually be discarded. Yet, each is of some current value, because each helps to organize the vast amount of data on drug actions.

REFERENCES

1. Balter, M., and Levine, J. The nature and extent of psychotropic drug usage in the United States. Psychopharm. Bull., 1969, 5:3–13.
2. Cerletti, A., and Rothlin, E. Role of 5-hydroxytryptamine in mental diseases and its antagonism to lysergic acid derivatives. Nature, 1955, 176:785–786.
3. Fink, M. EEG classification of psychoactive compounds in man: a review and theory of behavioral associations. In Efron, D. (Ed.) Psychopharmacology, U.S. PHS Pub. No. 1836, 1968.
4. Fink, M. EEG and human psychopharmacology: clinical antidepressants. In Efron, D. (Ed.) Psychopharmacology, U.S. PHS Pub. No. 1836, 1968.
5. Fink, M., and Itil, T. Neurophysiology of phantastica: EEG and behavioral relations in man. In Efron, D. (Ed.) Psychopharmacology, U.S. PHS Pub. No. 1836, 1968.
6. Goldstein, L., and Beck, R. Amplitude analysis of the electro-encephalogram (review of the information obtained with the integrative method). Int. Rev. Neurobiol., 1965, 8:265–312.
7. Hebb, C. CNS at the cellular level: identity of transmitter agents. Ann. Rev. Physiol., 1970, 32:165–192.
8. Jarvik, M. The psychopharmacological revolution. Psychology Today, May, 1967, 51–59.
9. Leslie, A. Ethics and practice of placebo therapy. Am. J. Med., 1954, 16:854–862.
10. McLennan, H. Synaptic Transmission. Philadelphia: W. B. Saunders Company, 1963.
11. Sigg, E. Autonomic side-effects induced by psychotherapeutic agents. In Efron, D. (Ed.) Psychopharmacology, U.S. PHS Pub. No. 1836, 1968.
12. Usdin, E. Classification of psychopharmaca. In Clark, W., and del Guidice, J. (Eds.) Principles of Psychopharmacology. New York: Academic Press, 1970.

CHAPTER 2

PRINCIPLES OF
DRUG ACTION

Drugs differ in their sites of action. Caffeine acts primarily on the brain, digitalis on the heart, and penicillin on infectious bacteria throughout the body. Some drugs act directly, others indirectly. For example, norepinephrine raises blood pressure by a direct action on many arterioles. Ephedrine also raises blood pressure, but it does so by promoting the release of stored norepinephrine. Blood pressure may also be secondarily increased by the administration of drugs which cause pain.

The brain has both inhibitory and excitatory areas. The mechanism of action of amphetamine has not been conclusively determined, but it may activate behavior by lowering the discharge thresholds of cells within excitatory areas. Low doses of alcohol activate behavior by suppressing inhibitory areas. Conversely, behavioral depression may result from suppression of an excitatory area or release of an inhibitory one.

For a drug to produce an effect, it must achieve an adequate concentration at its site of action. An obviously relevant factor is the amount administered. Others include the extent and rate of absorption from the area of administration into the bloodstream, distribution to various parts of the body from the blood, binding or localization in tissues, and mechanisms of inactivation.

DETERMINANTS OF DRUG EFFECT

Absorption

Drugs may be prepared either in solid form such as capsules, or in solution. The rapidity of absorption of a drug in solution varies

22

with the concentration of the drug. When a drug is administered in solid form, it must go into solution before it can be absorbed; therefore, its solubility is very important in determining the latency of onset of effects, i.e., how quickly the drug acts. Another important factor, the surface from which absorption occurs, is dependent upon method of administration. The lungs, stomach, and intestines all offer large surface areas, and so promote rapid absorption. When a drug is injected intravenously, it reaches maximal blood level concentration immediately. Table 2.1 lists various common routes of administration, and advantages and disadvantages of each. Figure 2–1 shows how the blood concentration of penicillin is affected by route of administration (13).

Absorption rate is affected by blood flow, which can be increased by massage, heat, or vasodilation. Some drugs, such as methacholine, dilate blood vessels and thus increase their own absorption rate. As a result they have a rapid onset of action. Conversely, a decrease in blood flow retards the rate of absorption. For example, cocaine constricts blood vessels, thereby slowing its own diffusion throughout the body. Consequently, it has negligible systemic effects and a long duration of action; its value as a local anesthetic is greatly enhanced.

Absorption rate is also affected by the pH gradient between the drug and absorbing surface. Weak acids such as salicylic acid are absorbed readily from the highly acidic stomach. Weak bases such as quinine tend to accumulate within the stomach. The intestine is very slightly acidic, and here the bases are absorbed better and the acids more poorly.

The passage of orally administered drugs from stomach to intestine is influenced by the temperature of the solution. Cold solutions pass more quickly than warm ones. This can be a very important consideration; for example, a cold solution of aqueous neostigmine hydrobromide is much more toxic than the same dose of a warm solution (53).

Distribution

After a drug reaches the bloodstream, via absorption or injection, it must cross various barriers to reach its final site of action. The pattern of distribution is different for each drug. For example, the distribution of some drugs is slowed because they combine readily with proteins within the blood plasma. While a drug is bound to a plasma protein, it cannot diffuse out of the blood stream. Eventually, an equilibrium is reached between the unbound drug, and the complex of plasma protein and drug. As the unbound drug is metabolized or excreted, the equilibrium changes, and the bound drug is released. When a drug becomes bound to plasma proteins, its

TABLE 2.1   Routes of Administration

Route	Advantages	Disadvantages
Oral	convenience	may cause emesis; some drugs are destroyed by digestive enzymes; food in stomach retards absorption, but some drugs are irritating when taken on empty stomach; some drugs are metabolized by the liver before they pass into the systemic circulation; patient must be awake and cooperative
Injection	often the only route which provides complete absorption, it is generally more rapid and predictable, thus dose can be selected with greater accuracy	pain; difficulty of self-administration; need for aseptic technique to minimize danger of infection; greater likelihood of systemic reaction
a. intravenous	greatest precision in obtaining particular blood concentration; effects are immediate; only route for certain irritating substances; dose does not have to be given all at once, but can be adjusted to response of patient	unfavorable reactions are more likely to occur than with other routes; more skill is required; once a drug is injected, there is no retreat (with other routes, absorption can be slowed or stopped); if injection is too rapid, patient may suffer "speed shock"
b. intramuscular	some irritating substances can be given by this route; muscle forms a depot for some drugs such as penicillin, so permits	

(Table 2.1 continued on opposite page.)

latency and duration of action are greatly modified. This can be utilized to clinical advantage; for example, sulfamethoxypyridazine is a sulfonamide drug which has a long-lasting anti-infective action because of protein binding.

Entry into the Brain

Drugs which are soluble in lipids enter the brain more easily than water soluble drugs. They also dissolve readily in neutral fat deposits, where they are often stored. Lipid solubility is greatest in drugs which have chemical structures least like the water molecule (HOH); lipid solubility can be measured by a method described by Dewhurst (6): the drug is added to a mixture of equal parts of

TABLE 2.1 *Continued*

Route	Advantages	Disadvantages
	continuous action over many days	
c. subcutaneous (under the skin)	absorption rate is slow and even, so sustained effects can be achieved; some hormones can be implanted under the skin, and will slowly be absorbed over months	drugs must be nonirritating to tissues
d. intraperitoneal (into the peritoneal cavity)	very convenient for small laboratory animals	very painful to humans
e. intrathecal (into the spinal subarachnoid space)	rapid local effects on central nervous system; bypasses blood-brain barrier	possibility of damage to spinal nerves
Inhalation	inhaled gases and volatile drugs gain rapid access to the circulation; used when there is lung disease and drug is meant to act on lungs	difficult to regulate dose; may produce irritation of pulmonary endothelium
Implanted Cannulae	important in behavioral research; hollow needles are permanently implanted in specific parts of the brain; drugs are administered in liquid or crystalline form, producing very localized effects. See Grossman (17) for description.	

olive oil and water, and shaken well; then the two phases are separated, and the amount of drug in the oil is divided by the amount in water.

The barbiturate thiopental is extremely soluble in lipids, and so enters the brain very rapidly to provide an anesthetic reaction. Then, as blood flows from the brain, the thiopental is carried out to neutral fat in tissues where it is stored. Thus, the duration of anesthesia is extremely long. The fat acts as a storage depot, and slowly releases the thiopental; this may cause a small depressant effect for a long time after recovery from anesthesia.

Lipid solubility, and thus ability to penetrate the brain, is reduced by addition of an OH group to a molecule. When an OH group is added to tryptamine, a drug with powerful effects upon the brain,

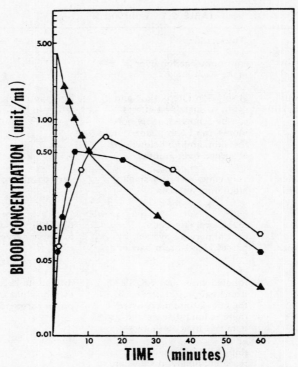

Figure 2–1 The effect of the route of administration on blood concentration of penicillin as a function of time following the injection of 15,000 units. The shaded triangle represents intravenous administration; the shaded hexagon indicates intramuscular administration; the unshaded hexagon stands for subcutaneous administration. (From D. Francke and H. Whitney, Jr., *Perspectives in Clinical Pharmacy*, Hamilton, Illinois, Hamilton Press, Inc., 1972, p. 392, based on material in Lancet, 1944, 2: pp. 621–624.)

the new compound is 5-hydroxytryptamine, which is not active unless injected directly into the brain.

Two other characteristics which affect the entry of a molecule into the brain are size and degree of ionization. Small, un-ionized molecules penetrate best. Un-ionized molecules are also absorbed much better from the alimentary tract than are highly ionized molecules. Therefore, Paton (41) made the interesting generalization that if a drug acts on the central nervous system, then it can be taken orally. Amphetamines, barbiturates, alcohol, LSD, marijuana, and narcotics are all active when taken orally, although injection may yield much more intense effects.

The entry of drugs into the brain is affected both by the presence of other drugs (30, 31) and by conditions within the central nervous system such as cerebral blood flow (12). Lorenzo et al. (32) used the easily detectable drug sodium sulfate to show that external stimuli are also important. Lorenzo and his co-workers injected the drug into cats, and then exposed the animals either to rapid flashes of light or to tones of various loudnesses and frequencies. The animals were then killed, and their brains assayed for sulfate. In those animals which had received visual stimulation, sulfate penetration was found to be increased over that in controls in both the visual cortex and lateral geniculate nuclei, two important stations in the visual pathway. There were no differences in penetration in other areas of the brain between the cats that received visual stimulation and the control group. Similarly, penetration was greater in the auditory pathway, but nowhere else, for cats which had been exposed to tones. These findings are of special interest because music festivals, with light shows as accompaniment, are very common settings for illicit use of drugs.

Many drugs which are injected outside the central nervous system are unable to enter the brain. This phenomenon can be clearly demonstrated with acidic dyes. It is attributed to a blood-brain barrier which, however, has no well-defined anatomical basis. The blood-brain barrier is present in adult chickens, but undeveloped in baby chicks until they are about 30 days of age. Research workers have used this knowledge to advantage is studying sites of action of drugs. For example, although norepinephrine produces an arousal response in adult chickens, it probably does not do so by any direct action on the central nervous system. This is presumed because in immature chicks, norepinephrine induces responses resembling those of sleep (26).

Removal of Drug from Body

Metabolism

Metabolic reactions involve several different enzyme systems, most of which are located in the liver. However, some metabolic reactions take place in plasma, kidneys, and other tissues. Drugs are usually, but not always, metabolized into inactive substances. One notable exception is codeine; about 10 per cent of administered codeine is metabolized to the much more powerful morphine. Another is the hypnotic (sleep-inducing) drug chloral hydrate, which owes its action primarily to trichloroethanol, to which it is rapidly reduced.

Metabolic enzymes are deficient in certain pathological conditions, in which case drug effects are amplified. For example, succinylcholine paralyzes skeletal muscles, including the muscles of respiration. It is used in small doses during surgery to obtain skeletal muscle relaxation. Some otherwise normal people have an enzyme deficiency which prevents them from properly metabolizing succinylcholine; thus the paralysis is dangerously prolonged.

Molecules such as water, which are positively charged at one end and negatively charged at the other, are called polar compounds. Most centrally active drugs are relatively nonpolar, and most drugs are metabolized to compounds which are more polar than the form in which administered. Polar compounds are excreted more efficiently than nonpolar ones.

Some drugs influence the metabolism of other drugs, even though they themselves may have few independent effects. Perhaps the best known enzyme inhibitor is SKF 525-A. (The name derives from the initials of Smith, Kline, and French, the pharmaceutical house in which it was developed.) When it is administered with hexobarbital, the sedative effect of the latter drug is greatly prolonged (5). Another drug, phenobarbital, produces effects in the opposite direction. It promotes the action of drug-metabolizing enzymes, and consequently shortens the effects of many drugs.

It is essential that physicians understand these types of drug interactions. For example, diphenylhydantoin, which is used for the symptomatic treatment of epilepsy, is normally free of serious toxic effects. Yet, it may be very dangerous when administered with dicoumarol (19), because dicoumarol greatly prolongs the effects of diphenylhydantoin. Other examples are given below.

Excretion

Drugs can be excreted in the urine, feces, expired air, sweat, and the milk of the nursing mother. The primary excretory pathway is via the kidneys. The rate at which a substance is excreted is pH-dependent. Overall, those drugs which are basic are excreted most rapidly when the urine is acidic, while acidic drugs are excreted fastest when the urine is alkaline. Knowledge of these factors may assume critical importance in the event of poisoning. Thus, if a person has taken an overdose of phenobarbital, a weak acid, excretion rate can be increased by administering the weak base sodium bicarbonate.

Some drugs are excreted unchanged. The mushroom *Amanita muscaria* was used as a hallucinogen by Siberian tribesmen; it was common custom among some of the tribes to collect for subsequent reuse the urine excreted after drinking *Amanita muscaria*.

Rebound Effects

The withdrawal of drugs which modify physiological or behavioral systems is often accompanied by changes in the opposite direction, called rebound effects. For example, the stimulant effects of amphetamine are generally followed by depression. Withdrawal from chronic use of high doses of barbiturates can precipitate severe seizures. Many drugs suppress dreaming, and dream time is increased upon discontinuance of these drugs.

REASONS FOR ADJUSTMENT OF DOSAGE

Barnes and Eltherington (1) have compiled a useful manual for drug researchers; it provides information on the appropriate dosage for producing various behavioral effects in several popular laboratory species. Quantitative and qualitative differences among species are common. For example, low doses of morphine sedate animals of most species, including man; however, morphine acts as a stimulant in cats, pigs, cows, and sheep. Clearly, one determinant of drug dosage is the species used.

The *Physicians' Desk Reference* is an indispensable handbook for dosage information in man. It lists drugs by class, and indicates dosages and contraindications. Physicians should, however, use the listed dosage ranges only as starting points from which to make adjustments in accordance with factors specific to the individual patients. Drugs are too often prescribed in routine fashion, without regard for differences among patients. Furthermore, in many cases the physician-patient relationship ends with diagnosis and the prescription of a drug, unless the patient fails to improve. As a result, dosages are rarely titrated to adjust for less than optimal responsiveness, and suffering may be prolonged even though cures are eventually effected.

RESPONSIVENESS TO DRUGS:
FOUR IMPORTANT INFLUENCES

The factors which influence responsiveness to drugs may be grouped under four broad headings: (1) organismic variables; (2) drug variables; (3) environmental variables; and (4) task variables.

Organismic Variables

AGE.   Children are often hyperreactive to drugs because of incomplete development of their enzyme systems. Older people may also be hyperreactive because of impaired metabolic or excretory mechanisms.

HEIGHT AND WEIGHT.   Dose must be adjusted to the weight of the drug recipient. In animal work, dosages are calculated on the basis of number of milligrams of drug per kilogram of body weight (mg/kg). Greater precision is often desirable in clinical practice, so the proportion of body fat is taken into account. The reader may be interested in how dosages are calculated.

Let W = weight of the recipient in kg
$\quad D$ = suggested dosage, in mg/kg
$\quad M$ = total number of mg administered
$\quad C$ = concentration of solution, if drug is in solution, in mg/cc
$\quad Q$ = quantity of drug injected in cc

Then, $DW = M$ if the drug is administered in pill form, so simply give the appropriate number of milligrams. $DW/C = Q$ if the drug is in solution, so give Q. To administer 0.05 mg/kg of a drug which is supplied in 1 cc vials containing 20 mg, to a man weighing 70 kilograms:

$\quad D = 0.05$
$\quad W = 70$
$\quad C = 20$

Then $DW/C = 0.05 \times 70/20 = 0.175$ cc. Give 0.175 cc of solution.

Height may also be a relevant consideration. Porter (42) found that women who reported side effects to imipramine were significantly taller than those who did not. He suggested that genes which influence height also influence the metabolism of imipramine.

SEX. Quinn et al. (45) reported that the sleeping time of female rats exceeds that of males after a similar dose of hexobarbital. The reason is that the metabolic enzyme activity in males is greater. Enzymatic activity is partially under hormonal control and can be modified by administering testosterone to females or estradiol to males; then sleeping time changes accordingly. Goldberg et al. (16) found that male schizophrenics were more responsive to placebos than females, whereas women showed the greater improvement after treatment with phenothiazine drugs.

BIOLOGICAL RHYTHMS.   Physiological systems undergo rhythmic variations in activity. Rhythmicity has been observed in organisms as simple as single cells and in more complex animals, including man (36). Responsiveness to many drugs is rhythmic in nature. Thus, 80 per cent of mice which were injected with the toxic substance *Escherichia coli endotoxin* during early evening died, whereas only 15 percent of those injected 8 hours later died (36). Short term cycles of susceptibility to toxins have also been described (29). In another study (48), rats injected at 6:00 P.M. with pentobarbital slept an average of 91 minutes, whereas those injected at 9:00 A.M. slept 53 minutes. In man, insulin has a more powerful effect when it is given very early in the morning. Mollerstrom (37) utilized this knowledge, and probably saved many lives, by giving the morning insulin very early to diabetic patients. Reinberg et al. (46) made the interesting observation that, in man, allergic responses to house dust, penicillin, and histamine were greatest during the period between 17.5 and 19.5 hours following the midpoint of the daily sleep span. Thus, a person who sleeps from midnight to 8 A.M. is maximally susceptible between the hours of 9:30 and 11:30 P.M.

GENETICS. Several recent articles and books (15, 25, 35) have emphasized genetic influences on drug response. An important early study in pharmacogenetics was by Thompson and Olian (54). They injected pregnant mice of three different strains with epinephrine, and then compared the activity of the offspring of each strain with that of offspring (from the same strain) that had untreated mothers. Activity was elevated above control levels in one strain, depressed in another, and not significantly changed in the third. Their results would seem to have important implications for anyone interested in deriving general laws about behavior.

Kalow (24) described a case in which a physician's failure to recognize that an untoward reaction to a drug may have a genetic basis had tragic consequences. A young boy died after receiving a general anesthetic and, when his sister subsequently required an operation, the troubled parents consulted with their anesthesiologist. He assured them that the boy's death had been an extremely rare occurrence and that no special precautions were needed. The girl died under the same circumstances. One of the goals of pharmacogeneticists is to develop techniques for anticipating such idiosyncratic responses.

PERSONALITY. Physicians used to be puzzled by the differential responsiveness of patients to therapeutic drugs; some patients responded excellently, while others were extremely refractory. The lack of homogeneous response inspired research on personality variables which influence drug effects. A representative experiment from the animal literature is that of Souskova and Bohdanecky (51). They showed that the depressant effects of physostigmine are determined in part by the initial level of excitability. Highly excitable rats were depressed to a greater extent than less excitable ones.

Frostad et al. (14) used human subjects. They took male volunteers and divided them into two groups on the basis of scores on the 16 PF_1 test, which distinguishes between action-oriented and non-action-oriented people. Subjects were also categorized on the basis of the Taylor Manifest Anxiety Scale, which measures anxiety. They were then given diazepam, which is an antianxiety agent. It provided the greatest therapeutic benefits, but also the most side effects, in the nonaction-oriented, low anxiety group. The action-oriented, low anxiety group responded least to diazepam.

The response to morphine is also personality-dependent. Euphoria is commonly observed when small doses are given to people suffering from pain, anxiety, or tension. On the other hand, when a similar dose is given to a happy, pain-free individual, mild anxiety and fear often follow (23).

Perhaps the best known work on personality variables and drug response is that of Eysenck (11). He made a simple dichotomy: people who seek stimulation were labeled extroverts and those who avoid stimulation, introverts. He predicted that stimulant drugs such as caffeine, amphetamine, and pipradrol, and depressants like alcohol, barbiturates, and meprobamate, would have differential effects in a wide variety of experimental situations. Many of his predictions have been borne out, but there have been many counterexamples as well (2, 34).

Kornetsky and his co-workers (summarized in 27) have shown that people who respond strongly to one drug tend also to respond strongly to others. Shagass and his colleagues (summarized in 49) have argued that thresholds of response to drugs are useful diagnostic tools. They showed that there was a high degree of reliability in individual patients, in their sedation and sleep thresholds to amobarbital and thiopental. In addition, patients who were resistant to the effects of the barbiturates were also resistant to the excitatory effects of methamphetamine. Responsiveness to amobarbital was different in different types of clinical populations and was sensitive to changes in clinical status. Further, responsiveness to amobarbital was predictive of the outcome of convulsive therapy and was influenced by changes in affective state, such as anger.

ETHNIC AND RACIAL VARIATIONS. Ethnic groups differ from each other both in gene frequencies and in personality variables. Therefore, it is not surprising that they respond differentially to drugs. Murphy (38) wrote to psychiatrists in several countries, asking them if they had noticed differential responsiveness in various ethnic groups. Three main findings emerged:

1. American schizophrenics required greater doses of chlorpromazine than did Europeans, for equivalent results.

2. European and American schizophrenics required greater doses of chlorpromazine than did Malayan schizophrenics, for equivalent results.

3. Anglo-Protestant geriatric patients responded in the expected ways to the tranquilizer thioridazine and the stimulant dextroamphetamine; Irish-Catholics, however, frequently responded paradoxically to both drugs.

Interpretation of Murphy's study is made difficult by the unavoidable confounding of experimental variables. Thus, it may have been the case that psychiatrists in one country more readily diagnosed patients as schizophrenic than did psychiatrists in another country; that the psychiatrists, or the patients, differentially interpreted responsiveness to drugs, irrespective of any actual changes which the drugs produced; that the treatment procedures, aside from the drugs, were different; or that the patient populations differed greatly in some critical variable such as age, sex, or socioeconomic status. In a more carefully designed study, native Americans, Japanese, Taiwanese, and Koreans, both adults and infants, were tested for responsiveness to alcohol. The three Mongoloid groups were much more sensitive, as evidenced by facial flushing and other symptoms of intoxication (57).

PHYSIOLOGICAL STATE. Many pathological physiological conditions modify drug actions, most frequently because mechanisms for metabolism or excretion become impaired. Anyone suffering from liver or kidney ailments must be suspect in this regard. Even normal alterations of physiological function may influence drug reactivity, as was noted in the previous discussion of biological rhythms. The pressor response to epinephrine varies with the initial arterial pressure, being greatest when initial arterial pressure is low (28). A second example is that the sleeping time of female mice following injection of hexobarbital is shortest during that phase of the estrus cycle when estrogen levels are highest (3). A third example is that pain reduces the respiratory depression produced by morphine. In fact, pain is a useful antidote for morphine-induced respiratory depression (23).

Drug Variables

THE DOSE-RESPONSE CURVE. Small doses of barbiturates often induce excitement and increase sensitivity to pain. Large doses produce sleep and are analgesic. Thus, the pharmacology of barbiturates is dependent upon dosage considerations. Similarly, while very small doses of strychnine may facilitate learning, larger doses cause convulsions and death. More generally, the characterization of any drug requires a description of the relationship between dosage and magnitude of effect. The plot of effects as a function of dosage is called the dose-effect or dose-response curve. It is usually, but not always, sigmoid in shape. Figure 2–2 is an example of a dose-effect curve showing a change from baseline heart rate in experienced and inexperienced marijuana smokers. The curves are approximately sigmoid.

DRUG INTERACTIONS. Two or more drugs should not be administered concurrently unless their mechanisms of action are thoroughly understood or unless their interactions have been fully studied. Drugs which are capable of combining with the same receptors to initiate a response are called agonists. Their actions are qualitatively similar. A drug which combines with receptors, thus

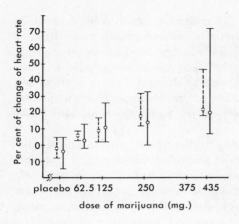

Figure 2-2 Heart rate response to placebo and marijuana, expressed as percent of change from the baseline heart rate. The solid line and circle are the mean and range, respectively, of heart rate changes of experienced subjects. The broken line and circle are the mean and range of heart rate changes of inexperienced subjects. (From Renault, P., Schuster, C., Heinrich, R., and Freeman, D. Marijuana: standardized smoke administration and dose effect curves on heart rate in humans. Science, 1971, *174*: pp. 589–591.)

preventing them from reacting maximally with an agonist, but which fails to initiate a response, is called a competitive antagonist. A noncompetitive antagonist is a drug which may permit an agonist to combine with its receptors, but which nevertheless blocks the initiation of a response. The choice of the terms agonist and antagonist to indicate opposite actions is unfortunate, since they have similar dictionary (nonpharmacological) meanings. When the effects of two drugs given in combination are greater than the sum of their individual effects, the drugs are called synergists.

Many interactions between drugs are extremely dangerous. For example, the monoamine oxidase inhibitors (MAOI's) are useful for treating certain types of depression. Patients who use MAOI's are warned against eating several foods, such as certain cheeses, bananas, and schmalz pickled herring; and against drinking Chianti wine and caffeine-containing beverages. Both caffeine and tyramine, which is found in the wine and the foods listed, may interact with MAOI's to produce hypertensive crises in which blood pressure becomes dangerously high. McIver (33) has summarized many other interactions.

In light of the foregoing it is frightening that, as late as 1964, hospital patients were receiving an average of seven different drugs, with some receiving as many as 35 distinct medications (39).

REPEATED ADMINISTRATIONS OF THE SAME DRUG. Chronic usage of a drug may lead to cumulation, so that a given dose will produce effects which are greater than normal in both intensity and duration. Cumulative effects can be avoided by limiting the dosage so that the amount administered does not exceed the amount removed from the body. The danger of cumulation is especially great with drugs which are excreted very slowly, such as bromides.

Tolerance develops to many drugs. Tolerance is said to occur when a given dose produces a smaller effect than it did initially. The development of tolerance to many drugs is striking; the usual therapeutic dose of amphetamine is 10 mg, but addicts have taken doses as high as 1700 mg without ill effect (21). Cross tolerance often develops among related drugs. An example of cross tolerance is that between mescaline and LSD. Reverse tolerance, in which responsiveness to a drug increases with repeated administrations, has been postulated for marijuana (see p. 73).

Tolerance does not develop equally to all aspects of drug action. In the case of morphine, rapid tolerance develops to its euphoric action, but the constipating effect remains largely unchanged over time. The nonuniform development of tolerance changes the therapeutic effectiveness of many drugs during the course of repeated administrations.

Environmental Variables

PHYSICAL ENVIRONMENT. Ambient temperature affects responsiveness. When the external temperature was low, chlorpromazine produced neurological depression in rats and mice; at higher external temperatures, administration of chlorpromazine produced hyperexcitability (44). To further illustrate the importance of environmental factors, amphetamine in high doses was toxic to mice, but to a much greater extent when they were grouped together rather than isolated (4). Similarly, the effects of pentobarbital were dependent upon whether mice were tested singly or in groups, as well as on the novelty and level of illumination of the environment (55).

EXPECTATIONS. Several years ago, an enterprising friend of the author wanted to market a new substance, which he would have called PLEEZBO. He intended to claim that it offered significant relief from cough, headache, postoperative pain, mood change, seasickness, anxiety, tension, pain from angina pectoris, cold, and virtually every other ailment known to man. Amazingly, he would have been telling the truth. Nevertheless, he was deprived of an opportunity to make a fortune when the Food and Drug Administration passed a law requiring that active ingredients of drugs be listed. The drug he planned to market, the placebo, has no active ingredients. Yet, Dubois claimed in 1946 that placebos were more widely used than any other class of drugs (10). Interestingly, 75 percent of physicians responded to a questionnaire on placebo use by saying that they use less than their colleagues (20). The defensiveness of their responses is not warranted. As long as it is the case that belief in the efficacy of a treatment is itself curative, the placebo will serve a useful function.

The effectiveness of active drugs may also be modified by expectations. Wolf (56) reported that atropine, which normally inhibits gastric secretion, produced hypersecretion in a patient who believed that he was receiving a drug which had previously caused him to hypersecrete. In one dramatic study, Wolf administered ipecac, which normally *causes* nausea and vomiting, to a pregnant woman who was suffering intensely from those very symptoms. She was told that the drug would cure her, and it did within 20 minutes.

Nisbett and Schachter (40) modified expectations in an ingenious way. They gave placebos to two groups of people, and provided them with false descriptions of probable symptomatology. Group 1 was given a descriptive list which included the symptoms normally associated with fearful situations: hand tremor, breathing rate changes, and a sinking feeling in the pit of the stomach. Group 2 received descriptions which were unrelated to fear: itching and numb feet. Both groups were then placed in a situation designed to generate fear: they were asked to self-administer shocks from a machine which had an adjustable dial. They were to increase the intensity until the pain was intolerable. Subjects in the first group withstood considerably greater intensities than those in the second. The authors' explanation is that the unpleasantness of the shock is greatly augmented by symptoms of fear, and that subjects who were told to expect such symptoms attributed them to the drug rather than the shock.

Task Variables

SCHEDULE OF REINFORCEMENT.   For almost 20 years, Dews (7–9) has been stressing that the action of a drug is influenced to a great extent by the ongoing behavior of the recipient. His work does not seem to have received the attention it deserves, except among scientists of the operant persuasion, i.e., those who study behavior with the techniques devised by B. F. Skinner and his colleagues. Therefore, the work of Dews is described in some detail below. In all cases, pigeons were the experimental subjects.

The first relevant study involved the drug pentobarbital, which is normally classified as a central nervous system depressant. Hungry pigeons pecked at a recessed disc of light translucent plastic, called a key, for food reward. They were tested under two different schedules of reinforcement. In one, the bird was required to peck at the key 50 times in order to gain brief access to food. This type of schedule is called a fixed ratio (FR); since every fiftieth response was rewarded, the abbreviation FR[50] is used. In the second schedule, called a fixed interval (FI), a specified period of time must elapse before a response is rewarded. Dews chose an FI[15'], which means that the first response after an interval of 15 minutes had elapsed, was rewarded. Responses emitted prior to the end of the interval went unrewarded. Following low doses of pentobarbital, pigeons working on FI$^{15'}$ made fewer responses than they did after being injected with saline. The results are consonant with the classification of pentobarbital as a general depressant. However, the same doses increased response rates when the birds were working on FR^{50}.

Dews next showed that his finding on the importance of schedules of reinforcement had considerable generality. Pigeons working on FR^{900} or FI$^{15'}$ greatly increased their response output over a wide range of doses of methamphetamine. However, when the behavior was maintained by FR^{50} or VI$^{1'}$, the birds were much less stimulated by methamphetamine, regardless of dose. (VI is a variable interval schedule—a schedule in which the subject is rewarded for the first response it makes after some specified time interval has elapsed, the length of the interval varying from trial to trial. In this case, the time interval varied around a mean of one minute.) Dews noted that the FR^{900} and FI$^{15'}$ schedules gave rise to intermittent responding, with periods in which the pigeons did not peck. By contrast, pecking under the other two schedules was steady and sustained. He concluded that amphetamines only affect responses which are being emitted intermittently, and he gave additional examples:

1. When reward is delayed following a response, very low response rates are generated, and methamphetamine increases rate.

2. Intermittent responding is generated when an animal is required to make a response which postpones punishment. In such situations, for example when each bar press by a rat delays electric shock for some predetermined time interval, amphetamine augments responding.

3. DRL schedules, in which reward is given after the first response following a predetermined period of no responding, also give rise to low response rates. These, too, are increased by amphetamines, with the result that the animals are rewarded less frequently. (DRL designates differential reinforcement of low rates.)

Dews also tested drug effects on two separate discrimination tasks. Both required pigeons to distinguish between lights of different colors, but the combinations of lights associated with reward and nonreward were different in the two cases. The drugs used were methamphetamine, pentobarbital, and scopolamine. The latter had no effect in either situation. However, the effects of the other two drugs were situation-specific; they impaired discriminations in one task, but not the other.

Terrace (52), in a related experiment, showed that the schedule of reinforcement prior to drug administration greatly influenced the effects on discrimination performance. Two pigeons were trained to discriminate between vertical and horizontal lines in the traditional fashion, i.e., by appropriately rewarding or not rewarding their responses. Two others were trained with a procedure which abolishes errors: the correct and incorrect stimuli are alternated, but the incorrect one is initially presented for such short intervals that there is no time to respond to it; then the interval is gradually lengthened until it is equal in intensity and duration to the other. Yet the organism rarely responds to it. The two training procedures give rise to several differences in performance, the relevant one here being responsiveness to drugs. Chlorpromazine and imipramine did not affect the behavior of the two pigeons which had been trained without errors, but both drugs greatly impaired discrimination performance of the other two birds. The implications of Terrace's work for studies on drug-induced sensory changes are clear; performance decrements are not necessarily the result of sensory deficits. For another example of a very dramatic drug-environment interaction, see the description of the effects of sensory deprivation on reaction to LSD, page 231.

SOME DRUG TERMINOLOGY

The *intensity* of a drug refers to its peak effect. A more useful characteristic is *maximum efficacy,* which is the strongest effect not accompanied by undesirable side effects.

LSD is often described as an extremely potent drug. It is, but potency is unimportant except in rare instances when a very potent drug is difficult to handle because it is also volatile, or when it can be readily absorbed through the skin. *Potency* refers to the amount of drug needed to reach peak effect. One drug may be more potent than another, yet have a much smaller maximum efficacy. Television pitchmen who exhort viewers to buy their brand of aspirin often try to exploit differences in potency, i.e., they say that one tablet of their brand is as powerful as two of brand X. That would be an irrelevant consideration if two brand X tablets were cheaper, safer, and more effective.

Consider the following problem:

> Drugs X and Y are equally capable of relieving headache pain. However, 50 per cent of people given 5 mg/kg of drug X complain of nausea. Drug Y does not produce undesirable side effects in 50 per cent of users until doses of 1000 mg/kg are given. Which drug is safer for headache sufferers?

Insufficient information has been provided. Before a decision can be reached, it is necessary to determine the dose of each drug which relieves headache. Suppose that the dose of X which relieves pain in 50 per cent of the cases is 0.005 mg/kg, and the corresponding Y dose is 500 mg/kg. Drug X would be vastly preferable because it has a much greater margin of safety between therapeutic and toxic doses. In general, the steeper the slope of a dose-effect curve, the greater the likelihood that an effective dose will produce annoying or dangerous side effects.

In the preceding example, doses were calculated with reference to their effects on 50 per cent of the people. This emphasizes what has already been indicated—that a given dose of drug has different effects on different people. The dose required to produce a specified intensity of effect in 50 per cent of the subjects is called the *median effective dose* (ED_{50}). The LD_{50} refers to the dose which is lethal to 50 per cent of the subjects. One of the most useful ways of characterizing a drug is by stating its *therapeutic index,* which is the ratio between the median dose at which any type of toxic effect becomes manifest (the TD_{50}) and the median effective dose, i.e., TD_{50}/ED_{50}. Sometimes the therapeutic index is defined by LD_{50}/ED_{50}; other proportions may also be used. Thus, the ratio TD_{25}/ED_{90} would refer to the dose which produces toxic effects in 25 per cent of recipients, and which is effective in 90 per cent. In general, the larger the therapeutic index the safer the drug. However, no hard and fast rule can be given about the size of the therapeutic index, because other factors are relevant as well. A very low therapeutic index would be acceptable for use with terminal cancer patients, but not with headache sufferers.

Irwin (22) advocates determination of the minimal dose of drug which produces clinically important effects. These may be therapeutic or toxic. He feels that a term should be invented to describe the minimum dose which produces side effects sufficiently toxic to make the drug therapeutically unacceptable.

SELECTIVITY. Drugs are usually described in terms of their most prominent effects, but it is important to realize that all drugs have many effects. LSD is classified as a hallucinogen or psychotomimetic, but it also may induce salivation, dilatation of the pupils of the eyes, rapid heart beat, elevated body temperature, increased adrenal cortical function, decreased thyroid function, nausea, muscular weakness, intensification of color perception, and euphoria. Drugs can be used safely, and their actions interpreted intelligently, only if an attempt is made to understand the full spectrum of their effects.

One of the goals of chemists who synthesize new drugs is to increase selectivity. For example, although chlorpromazine is effective in the treatment of psychotic behavior, it sometimes produces unpleasant side effects such as faintness, tremor, palpitations, nasal stuffiness, and postural hypotension. Many congeners (members of the same family of drugs) of chlorpromazine have been developed in the hopes of maintaining antipsychotic action while reducing side effects. To date, no compound has supplanted chlorpromazine, but the search continues.

Analysis of the relationship between the structure of a drug and its pharmacological effects often yields valuable clues toward the development of new compounds. For example, when the length of the side chain on one particular carbon atom of sodium barbital is increased, the latency of onset and the duration of hypnotic activity are reduced. Both latency and duration of action, and hypnotic potency, may also be modified by other specific types of substitutions. Still others confer convulsant or anticonvulsant activity on the barbiturates (50).

NEW DRUGS

The United States government does not permit new drugs to be marketed for general use until they have been subjected to rigorous tests of efficacy and safety. First they must be tested on several species of animals, for both acute and chronic effects. It should be noted that the requirement of the Food and Drug Administration (FDA) for toxicity studies of a year or more is not without its critics. Both Gross and Paget (58) claimed that the requirement often results in unnecessary delays in releasing useful medicines, and that little additional information about long-term toxicity can be gained by prolonging test periods beyond three months. Gross noted that long-term testing is especially foolish in cases where the drug is meant to be administered only once, e.g., as an antidote for acute poisoning.

Should the results of the animal screening be promising, the drug is then released for tests with select groups of humans, both patients and volunteers. The purpose is to establish that the drug is safe; if it passes this hurdle, it is subjected to carefully controlled clinical trials. Even when a drug is approved, the FDA retains the right to order its removal from the market if new evidence suggests that it is dangerous.

When a drug is approved for manufacture, it is given an official name. When it is marketed, the manufacturer gives it a proprietary name or trademark. If many companies market the same drug, it will have many proprietary names but only one official name. Although manufacturers may differ somewhat in the quality of their preparations, FDA regulations assure that all meet a certain level of acceptability. Therefore, there is no great advantage in using one proprietary name rather than another, unless one brand is marketed in a special dose form. When physicians prescribe by official name rather than proprietary name, the patient is often able to purchase his medicine at considerable savings. One additional useful term is the generic name, which designates a class of drugs with similar structure and properties, e.g., the amphetamines or the barbiturates.

REFERENCES

1. Barnes, C., and Eltherington, L. *Drug Dosage in Laboratory Animals: A Handbook.* Berkeley: University of California Press, 1965.

2. Callaway, E., III. The influence of amobarbital (amylobarbitone) and methamphetamine on the focus of attention. J. Ment. Sci., 1959, 105:382–392.

3. Catz, C., and Yaffe, S. Strain and age variations in hexobarbital response. Sleeping time in female mice varies with menstrual cycle, being shortest when estrogen levels are highest. J. Pharm. Exp. Ther., 1967, 155:152–156.

4. Chance, M. Aggregation as a factor influencing the toxicity of sympathomimetic amines in mice. J. Pharmacol. Exp. Therap., 1946, 87:214–219.

5. Cook, L., Toner, J., and Fellows, E. Effect of diethylaminoethyl 2,2-diphenylvalevate -HCl (SKF 525-A) on hexobarbital. J. Pharmacol. Exp. Ther., 1954, 111:131–141.

6. Dewhurst, W. The blood-brain barrier and other membrane phenomena in psychopharmacology. In Clark, W., and del Guidice, J. (Eds.), Principles of Psychopharmacology. New York: Academic Press, 1970.

7. Dews, P. Analysis of effects of psychopharmacological agents in behavioral terms. Fed. Proc., 1958, 17:1024–1030.

8. Dews, P. The effects of pentobarbital, methamphetamine, and scopolamine on performances in pigeons involving discriminations. J. Pharmacol. Exp. Therap., 1955, 115:380–389.

9. Dews, P. Studies on behavior. I. Differential sensitivity to pentobarbital of pecking performance in pigeons depending on the schedule of reward. J. Pharmacol. Exp. Therap., 1955, 113:393–401.

10. Dubois, E. Cornell Conference on Therapy, N.Y. State J. Med., 1946, 46:2, 1718.

11. Eysenck, H. Experiments With Drugs. New York: The MacMillan Co., 1963.

12. Firemark, H., Barlow, C., and Roth, L. The entry, accumulation, and binding of diphenylhydantoin-2-C^{14} in brain. Internat. J. Neuropharm., 1963, 2:25–38.

13. Fleming, A., Young, M., Suchet, J., and Rowe, A. Penicillin content of blood serum after various doses of penicillin by various routes. Lancet, 1944, 247:621–624.

14. Frostad, A., Forrest, G., and Bakker, C. Influence of personality type on drug response. Am. J. Psychiat., 1966, 122:1153–1158.

15. Fuller, J. Pharmacogenetics. In Clark, W., and del Guidice, J. (Eds.), Principles of Psychopharmacology. New York: Academic Press, 1970.

16. Goldberg, S., Schooler, N., Davidson, E., and Kayce, M. Sex and race differences in response to drug treatment among schizophrenics. Psychopharm., 1966, 9:31–47.

17. Grossman, S. Eating and drinking elicited by direct adrenergic or cholinergic stimulation of hypothalamus. Science, 1960, 132:301–302.

18. Halberg, F. Temporal coordination of physiologic function. Cold Spring Harbor Symp. Quant. Biol., 1960, 25:289–308.

19. Hansen, J., Kristensen, M., Skovsted, L., and Christensen, L. Dicoumarol-induced diphenylhydantoin intoxication. Lancet, 1966, 2:265–266.

20. Hofling, C. The place of placebos in medical practice. Gen. Pract., 1955, 11:103.

21. Innes, I., and Nickerson, M. Drugs acting on postganglionic adrenergic nerve endings and structures innervated by them (sympathomimetic drugs). In Goodman, L., and Gilman, A. (Eds.), The Pharmacological Basis of Therapeutics. New York: The MacMillan Co., 1965.

22. Irwin, S. Considerations for the pre-clinical evaluation of new psychiatric drugs: a case study with phenothiazine-like tranquilizers. Psychopharm., 1966, 9:259–287.

23. Jaffe, J. Narcotic analgesics. In Goodman, L. and Gilman, A. (Eds.), The Pharmacological Basis of Therapeutics. New York: The MacMillan Co., 1965.

24. Kalow, W. Pharmacogenetics and the predictability of drug responses. In Wolstenholme, G., and Porter, R. (Eds.), Drug Response in Man. Boston: Little, Brown & Co., 1967.

25. Kalow, W. Pharmacogenetics: Heredity and the Response to Drugs. Philadelphia: W. B. Saunders Company, 1962.

26. Key, B., and Marley, E. The effect of the sympathomimetic amines on behavior and electrocortical activity of the chicken. EEG, 1962, 14:90–105.

27. Kornetsky, C. Alterations in psychomotor functions and individual differences in responses produced by psychoactive drugs. In Uhr, L., and Miller, J. (Eds.), Drugs and Behavior. New York: John Wiley & Sons, 1960.

28. Korol, B., and Brown, M. Influence of existing arterial pressure on autonomic drug responses. Am. J. Physiol., 1967, 213:112–114.

29. Lindsay, J., and Kullman, V. Pentobarbital sodium: variation in toxicity. Science, 1966, 151:576–577.

30. Lorenzo, A., Barlow, C., and Roth, L. Effect of metrazol convulsions on S^{35} entry into cat central nervous system. Am. J. Physiol., 1967, 212:1277–1287.

31. Lorenzo, A., and Barlow, C. Effect of strychnine convulsions upon the entry of S^{35} sulfate into the cat central nervous system. J. Pharmacol. Exp. Ther., 1967, 157: 555–564.

32. Lorenzo, A., Fernandez, C., and Roth, L. Physiologically induced alteration of sulfate penetration into brain. Arch. Neurol., 1965, 12:128–132.

33. McIver, A. Drug interactions. Pharmaceut. J., 1967, 199:205–210.

34. Marley, E. Response to drugs and psychiatry. J. Ment. Sci., 1959, 15:19–43.

35. Meier, H. *Experimental Pharmacogenetics*. New York: Academic Press, 1963.

36. Menaker, M. Biological clocks. BioScience, 1969, 19:681–689.

37. Mollerstrom, J. Om diabetes och diabetes behandling. Nord. Med. Tidskr., 1937, 14:1693.

38. Murphy, H. Ethnic variations in drug response. Transcult. Psychiat. Res. Rev., 1969, 6:5–23.

39. Nat. Health Fed. Bull., 1964, 10:29.

40. Nisbett, R., and Schachter, S. The cognitive manipulation of pain. J. Exp. Soc. Psychol., 1966, 2:227–236.

41. Paton, W. The principles of drug action. Proc. R. Soc. Med., 1960, 53:815–820.

42. Porter, A. Body height and imipramine side-effects. Brit. Med. J., 1968, 2:406–407.

43. Porter, I. The genetics of drug susceptibility. Dis. Nerv. Syst., 1966, 27:25–36.

44. Quadbeck, G. Effects of phenothiazine derivatives on blood brain barrier system. Psychopharm. Serv. Cent. Bull., 1962, 2:83.

45. Quinn, G., Axelrod, J., and Brodie, B. Species, strain, and sex differences in metabolism of hexobarbitone, amidopyrine, antipyrine, and aniline. Biochem. Pharmacol., 1958, 1:152–159.

46. Reinberg, A., Zagula-Mally, Z., Ghata, J., and Halberg, F. Circadian reactivity rhythm of human skin to house dust, penicillin, and histamine. J. Allergy, 1969, 44:292–306.

47. Renault, P., Schuster, C., Heinrich, R., and Freeman, D. Marijuana: standardized smoke administration and dose effect curves on heart rate in humans. Science, 1971, 174:589–591.

48. Scheving, L., Vedral, D., and Pauly, J. A circadian susceptibility rhythm in rats to pentobarbital sodium. Anat. Rec., 1968, 160:741–750.

49. Shagass, C. Drug thresholds as indicators of personality and affect. *In* Uhr, L., and Miller, J. (Eds.), *Drugs and Behavior*. New York: John Wiley & Sons, 1960.

50. Sharpless, S. Hypnotics and sedatives I. The barbiturates. *In* Goodman, L., and Gilman, A. (Eds.), *The Pharmacological Basis of Therapeutics*. New York: The MacMillan Co., 1965.

51. Souskova, H., and Bohdanecky, Z. Differences in the effect of atropine, physostigmine and certain combinations of drugs on the higher nervous activity of rats with different excitability levels. Physiol. Bohemoslov., 1965, 14:191–200.

52. Terrace, H. Errorless discrimination learning in the pigeon: Effects of chlorpromazine and imipramine. Science, 1963, 140:318–319.

53. Ther, L., and Winne, D. Drug absorption. In *Annual Review of Pharmacology*, 1971, Palo Alto: Annual Reviews, Inc., 1971, p. 67.

54. Thompson, W., and Olian, S. Some effects on offspring behavior of maternal adrenalin injection during pregnancy in three inbred mouse strains. Psychol. Rep., 1961, 8:87–90.

55. Watzman, N., Barry, H., III, Kinnard, W., Jr., and Buckley, J. Some conditions under which pentobarbital stimulates spontaneous motor activity of mice. J. Pharm. Sci., 1968, 57:1572–1576.

56. Wolf, S. Effects of suggestion and conditioning on the action of chemical agents in human subjects – the pharmacology of placebos. J. Clin. Invest., 1950, 29:100–109.

57. Wolff, P. Ethnic differences in alcohol sensitivity. Science, 1972, 175:449–450.

58. Wolstenholme, G., and Porter, R. (Eds.), *Drug Responses in Man*. Boston: Little Brown & Co., 1967, pp. 14–15.

CHAPTER 3

EFFECTS OF DRUGS

Western man uses an awesome variety of substances to manipulate his mood, affect, energy level, and sense of well-being. Even so, many powerful drugs which are widely used in other cultures are unknown to most westerners. In a fascinating book edited by Daniel Efron (6), a group of internationally known scientists provided descriptions of current and historic worldwide drug practices. The effects of the drugs range from sedation to stimulation, from muscular lassitude and incoordination to increased strength, and from enhanced ability to attend to external stimuli to inattentiveness to, or distortion of, the external world. It is not obvious what they have in common. However, laboratory animals, even the lowly rat, press levers or make other kinds of responses in order to gain exposure to novel stimuli (17); perhaps the attractiveness of drugs lies not so much in their specific effects, as in their novelty and their ability to transform the reality of the user in some (any?) direction.

Schultes (33) noted that in the Western hemisphere there are more than 40 species of plants which are used for hallucinogenic purposes. Although the structures of hallucinogenic substances vary enormously (15), most plants owe their hallucinogenic properties to alkaloids, which are cyclic structures containing nitrogen. At least 5000 higher plants contain alkaloids, and the recent interest in pharmacognosy may well augur the uncovering of a great many more plants with psychoactive substances.

The most prominent effects of a few psychoactive drugs which are used throughout the world, whether they are licit or illicit, are outlined below. Several are described in greater detail elsewhere

43

in the book. A great many of the descriptions are of necessity anecdotal. Although there are individual differences in response to all drugs, some, such as alcohol, seem to produce much more variable effects than others. The role of extradrug factors must be emphasized. Alcohol, because of its cultural acceptance and legal status, is used by a broader range of individuals, and in more diverse settings, than other drugs. That alone may account for the greater variability of effect. Perhaps Efron's book will spur other scientists to begin conducting well-controlled research on exotic drugs. Another area which, hopefully, will begin to attract increasing numbers of research-oriented scientists is that of dietary influences on behavior. Some recent provocative findings on diet and behavior are described after the following survey of various drugs.

For those who are tempted to try some of the drugs mentioned on the next few pages, a warning is in order. Information on acute and chronic toxicity is lacking, but it is reasonable to assume that drugs which produce powerful psychoactive effects have enormous potential for danger if misused. *Please do not experiment.*

Since data on many of the substances listed below are very scanty, it did not seem appropriate to use an elaborate classification system. The drugs are listed merely as stimulants, depressants, euphorics, hallucinogens, opiates, or miscellaneous. As previously mentioned, all such categories are overlapping and largely arbitrary.

STIMULANTS

Cocaine

Cocaine is derived from the plant *Erythroxylon coca* and is widely used in the highlands of Columbia, Peru, Bolivia, and northwestern Argentina. It is one of the most powerful antifatigue agents known, and produces feelings of great muscular strength and increased mental capacities. The most prominent psychic changes in man include euphoria, decreased hunger, and indifference to pain. Euphoric excitement and hallucinatory episodes are common.

Cocaine potentiates the effects of sympathetic nerve stimulation and of injected epinephrine and norepinephrine. It produces a notable rise in body temperature, partly because it increases muscular activity and partly because it constricts blood vessels. The duration of action of cocaine is brief, and it is not physically addictive.

Amphetamines

The amphetamines are in many respects qualitatively similar to cocaine. The amphetamines alleviate fatigue, increase mental

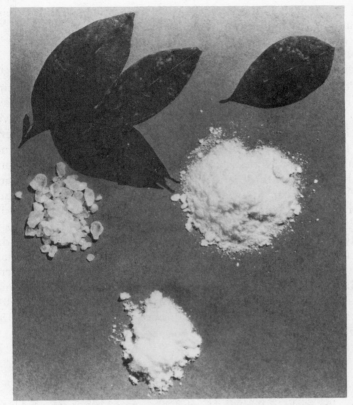

Figure 3–1   Cocaine, in processed and unprocessed forms. The *erythroxylon coca* leaves are shown above cocaine crystals and powders. (AFIP Neg. 71-3778-4.)

alertness, and promote a sense of well-being, with methamphetamine producing the most powerful central effects of the group. They also enhance physical capacities (47). Large doses, especially when administered intravenously, produce hallucinations and paranoid delusions. Tremor, restlessness, and increased motor activity are common effects. Amphetamine is a strong appetite suppressant.

Amphetamine increases sympathetic functioning, possibly by a direct action on sympathetic neurons, and probably by releasing norepinephrine. Normal doses have effects for about four hours.

Caffeine

Caffeine is a CNS stimulant and antifatigue agent. It increases endurance and motor activity, and makes thought processes clearer. The caffeine in a cup of coffee is effective for about two to three hours. In 1965, a billion kilograms of coffee were being consumed annually in the United States alone (30, p. 354).

Nicotine

People smoke for a variety of reasons, including taste, stimulation, relaxation, and, to a great extent, as a result of social pressures. Many smokers begin when they are adolescents, eager to prove that they have become adults. People also smoke because advertisers have been effective in suggesting a link between smoking and sex appeal and fun. In past years, there was even an implication that smoking was healthful, and there were slogans such as "Reach for a Lucky instead of a sweet." Athletes endorsed popular brands, as did singers. The extent to which advertising influences smoking of cigarettes is difficult to determine, but in any case tobacco is more widely used than any other psychoactive substance in the world.

The nicotine from tobacco has several physiological effects. It increases metabolic rate, heart rate, and blood pressure. The secretion of epinephrine, which mediates both stress and arousal responses, is increased. Moreover, smoking increases hand steadiness (10) and lowers skin temperature. The duration of action of the nicotine in one cigarette is about an hour.

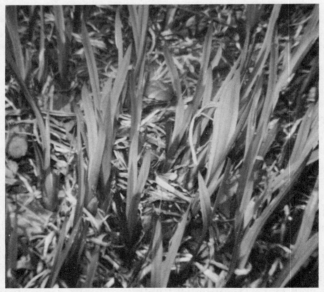

Figure 3–2 The *acorus calamus* plant. The elongated, leafy plants can produce stimulant or hallucinogenic effects, depending on the dosage. (Courtesy of Robert Gustafson.)

Asarone

Asarone is the active principle of *Acorus calamus,* a plant of widespread distribution throughout Asia, Europe, and North America. It helps to banish fatigue, and in high doses produces effects similar to the LSD experience. It is regularly used by adult Indians of Northern Canada (15, p. 55).

Khat

Khat is derived from the plant *Celastrus edulis.* It is used in Ethiopia and many parts of Africa, and in Yemen, about 80 percent of the adult population uses khat. An amphetamine-like substance, khat produces stimulation, loquacity, clarity of thought, and euphoria. Fatigue is removed, hunger is suppressed, and sometimes libido is also suppressed. Tolerance does not develop, and there is no physical dependence (15, p. 47).

DEPRESSANT DRUGS

Alcohol

In 1962, in the United States, 12 billion dollars were spent for the purchase of alcoholic beverages, excluding wines and beers (9, p. 3). Alcohol has variable effects, but generally produces relaxation, drowsiness, a sense of well being, and euphoria. Alcohol is an emetic, and users vomit once the blood level reaches about 120 mg percent (120 mg alcohol per 100 ml blood, or .12 percent). Vomiting is a safety device, which does not always function if the critical level is approached slowly (indeed, fatal amounts may then be ingested). The approximate blood level of alcohol can be calculated by assuming .05 per cent in blood for every 2½ ounces of 86 proof liquor ingested by a 75 kg person (subtract .05 percent for each hour since drinking began). The approximate behavioral effects of various blood levels of alcohol are:

.09–.21	stimulation
.15	legally drunk
.20–.30	confusion, slurred speech, ataxia
.30	severe intoxication
.50–.80	death occurs

Alcohol promotes gastric secretions and urine flow. It dilates peripheral blood vessels, so that increased amounts of blood circulate through the skin. (One consequence of the increase is that alcoholics often have red noses.) The increased blood flow brings a feeling of warmth, but also leads to a loss of body heat (on cold days, peripheral blood vessels normally constrict so that flow to the skin and hence heat loss is reduced). Therefore, although the popular custom of drinking alcohol at outdoor events like football games may serve some function, staving off the cold is not it.

Barbiturates

Barbiturate intoxication closely resembles alcohol intoxication, and withdrawal symptoms are also similar. Alcohol suppresses many of the barbiturate withdrawal symptoms, and vice versa (see p. 80 for a description of alcohol withdrawal syndrome).

Barbiturates sedate, and produce relief from anxiety and stress. The user often becomes more sociable, garrulous, and good-humored. Incoordination, ataxia, and slurred speech are observed, as with alcohol. There are more than 2500 barbiturates, and they have varying durations of action. An intoxicating dose of those which are most frequently abused generally lasts about four hours. The barbiturate-like drug methaqualone has been increasing in popularity during the past few years. Users prefer it to barbiturates because less drowsiness is produced, and because withdrawal symptoms are less severe.

EUPHORICS

Marijuana

Marijuana is used primarily because it is a euphoriant. It also produces increased sociability and a host of other effects, including hilarity, occasional anxiety and restlessness, confusion, difficulty in concentration, flights of ideas, and distortions of space and time. The effects appear very rapidly when the drug is smoked — often within seconds — but when marijuana is eaten or drunk as a tea, the effects take considerably longer to appear. Eating also prolongs the duration of action. When taken in large enough doses, the effects of marijuana are very similar to those of LSD (37).

Tart (40) questioned experienced users about the frequency of occurrence of various effects. Among those occuring most often were absorption in what one is doing, seemingly meaningful insights, religious or spirtual experiences, and enjoyment of eating. Tart's subjects were also asked to compare marijuana with alcohol. With respect to somatic processes, such as unpleasant body sensations or changes in perception, there was a distinct preference for marijuana. Similarly, cognitive processes were believed by users to be improved by marijuana and worsened by alcohol. They also felt that they did not lose control with marijuana, and that, if the

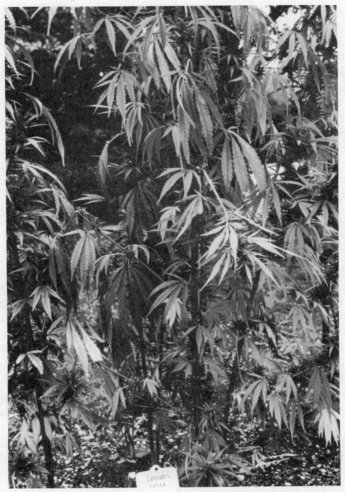

Figure 3-3 The marijuana plant, *Cannabis sativa L.*, grows throughout the world and reaches seven to eight feet in height. (Department of Justice Photo.)

situation demanded it, they could cope with an emergency. Overall, marijuana was the drug of choice, but alcohol, which was claimed to lower inhibitions more reliably, was preferred for large social settings. The responses may not reflect real differences between the drugs, since Tart's sample consisted of people who had used marijuana at least 12 times, and most had used it much more than that. As a result, the sample was biased toward those who had enjoyed their experiences; it is possible that many people who tried marijuana once or twice decided that they preferred alcohol, and stopped using marijuana. If these users had been questioned, perhaps the overall preference would have shifted toward alcohol.

Hollister (16) summarized the effects of marijuana on man. It does not produce changes in pupil size (in spite of what law enforcement officials may think), respiratory rate, or deep tendon reflexes; it *does* produce increased pulse and heart rate, reddening of the conjunctiva of the eye, muscular weakness, and sleepiness. Drooping of the eyelids is often observed (5). These findings confirmed much of the work done earlier by Weil et al. (47). Weil and his co-workers also tested intellectual and psychomotor performance and found that first-time users showed substantial decrements, but chronic users were indistinguishable from controls.

Nutmeg

In *The Autobiography of Malcolm X,* the author described the regular use of nutmeg as an intoxicant. Prison inmates, cut off from their supply of marijuana, stirred nutmeg in water and drank it. The result, according to Malcolm X, was a marijuana-like experience.

Nutmeg and mace, two related household spices, both come from the nutmeg tree, *Myristica fragrans.* The approximate dose is 10 to 30 grams (a whole spice tin) dissolved in juice or water. Reactions to the drugs vary considerably, perhaps because there is no quality control over the hallucinogenic potency of spice tins. Some people feel no effects, while others equate the experience with that of marijuana or even LSD. The latency of onset is two to five hours, and the effects last up to two days. There are several reports on nutmeg poisoning (12, 29), which should serve as a warning to self-experimenters. A fuller description of the pharmacology of nutmeg can be found in Reference 6.

Kava

The freshly harvested roots of the kava plant, *Piper methysticum,* provide the basis for a drink which is enjoyed on many of the Pacific islands. In 1966, the late United States President Lyndon Johnson visited American Samoa and partook of a kava ceremony (6, p. 117). The main effect of drinking kava is a sleep-like state which is very pleasant and relaxed. Abnormal sensations are common. In laboratory animals of several different species, kava depresses reflexes which involve more than one synapse, while leaving monosynaptic reflexes unaffected (24); in this respect kava resembles mephenesin, which was once commonly prescribed for relief of anxiety.

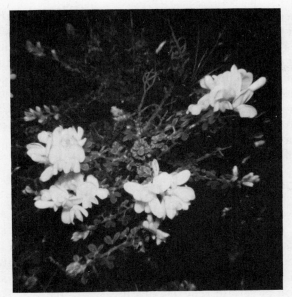

Figure 3–4 Canary Island Broom, or *Cytisus canariensis*. Smoking the blossoms produces mild euphoric effects. (Courtesy of Robert Gustafson.)

Canary Island Broom

Fadiman (7) investigated the psychic effects of Canary Island Broom (*Cytisus canariensis,* formerly called *Genista canariensis*), a plant which grows wild in northern California. When the dried blossoms were smoked in hand-rolled cigarettes, subjects reported feelings of relaxation and friendliness. When several cigarettes were smoked, intellectual clarity and flexibility were increased and colors appeared more intense. Headache was frequently reported as a side effect. The closely related plant Scotch Broom (*Cytisus scoparius*) is also used to get high, but it is a fairly powerful cardiac stimulant and as such, can be quite dangerous.

Inhalants

Several of the anesthetic gases have been employed for their psychic effects. Perhaps the best known is "laughing gas," nitrous oxide, which is still used by physicians and dentists to relax their patients and relieve their anxieties. The famous psychologist William James was a great believer in the use of nitrous oxide to reveal significant truths. For an example of one of his revelations, see page 294.

In recent years, gasoline, model airplane glues, paint thinner, and lighter fluid have been used as inhalants, primarily by teenagers. Authorities disagree about the likelihood that the practice leads to permanent organic brain damage. However, there is no dispute over the fact that several deaths have occurred because of suffocation from the plastic bags in which the material is placed, and which are held over the head to prevent the volatile substance from escaping. Still other deaths have been attributed to the actions of aerosol propellants on the heart and lungs.

HALLUCINOGENS

LSD

LSD is a sympathomimetic drug. Thus, it produces several somatic effects, such as dilated pupils, increased mobilization of free fatty acids (which are also mobilized during stressful situations), exaggeration of certain reflexes, dizziness, and nausea. The primary subjective alteration is a facilitation of focusing on subjective experience. After ingestion of LSD, colors appear to be more saturated, stationary objects may appear to move, everyday objects become endowed with beauty and meaning, there is a feeling of omnipotence, time is slowed, the body concept may alter, and thought becomes disordered and often dreamlike. Users frequently report profound religious and esthetic experiences and self-insights (although attempts at in-depth self-analysis often become quite aversive). Euphoria is regularly reported. The effects take about an hour to occur, and last for about 12 hours.

Osmond (28) summarized his experiences with LSD and other hallucinogens as follows: ". . .most subjects find the experience valuable, some find it frightening, and many say that it is uniquely lovely. . . .For myself, my experiences with these substances have been the most strange, most awesome, and among the most beautiful things in a varied and fortunate life. These are not escapes from but enlargements, burgeonings of reality."

Unger (41) illustrated beautifully the importance of extradrug variables in determining the outcome of LSD experiences by placing in apposition quotes from several psychiatrists who had used hallucinogenic drugs to treat their patients. Consider these negative views:

Hoch: Actually, in my experience, no patient asks for it (LSD) again.
Katzenelbogen: I can say the same.
Denber: I have used mescaline in the office. . . and the experience was such that the patients said 'Once is enough.' The same thing happened

in the hospital. I asked the patients there if, voluntarily, they would like to take this again. Over 200 times the answer has been 'No.' [p. 208]

Unger contrasted the above exchange with the following comment by Abramson:

During the past four years we have administered the drug (LSD) hundreds of times to nonpsychotics in doses up to 225 micrograms. . . . Those who have participated in these groups are nearly always definitely benefited by their experiences. Almost invariably they wish to return and to participate in new experiments. [p. 208]

Peyote and Mescaline

Several authors (19, 49) have reported that subjects were unable to distinguish between the effects of LSD, peyote, and mescaline. The latencies of onset and durations of action are similar. Yet, Schultes (34) emphatically stated that the intoxications of peyote and mescaline are very different. Peyote, *Lophophora williamsi*, is a hallucinogenic cactus which contains at least 15 active alkaloids, mescaline being the most important among them. Mescaline has a close structural resemblance to epinephrine. Its primary effects are on vision. It induces vivid hallucinations consisting of brightly colored lights and geometric designs, and brilliantly colored objects which are treated as sources of wonder. Euphoria and feelings of mental and physical energy are the rule. Kluver (20) and Huxley (18) have provided rich descriptions of the mescaline experience.

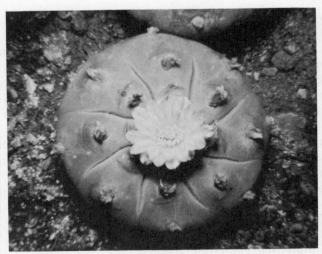

Figure 3-5 The peyote cactus, *Lophophora williamsi*. Along with its powerful hallucinogenic effects, peyote produces nausea and vomiting. (Courtesy of Robert Gustafson.)

Mescaline (and peyote to an even greater extent) causes nausea and vomiting. Mitchell (cited in 15, p. 4) wrote that "these shows are expensive.... The experience, however, was worth one such headache and indigestion, but was not worth a second." The alkaloids other than mescaline contribute to peyote intoxication, which often includes auditory and tactile hallucinations, and synesthesia.

Other Cacti

Many cactaceous plants are rich in alkaloids, and are employed as hallucinogens. McLaughlin and his colleagues (2, 23, 27) have identified several possible hallucinogenic alkaloids in the genera *Coryphantha* and *Ariocarpus*. Several species of *Mammilaria* and *Echinocactus*, which are sold in plant nurseries in the United States, are used under certain circumstances by the Tarahumare Indians of Mexico for hallucinogenic effects (34).

Mescal Beans

The seeds of the shrub *Sophora secundiflora* are called mescal beans, and are commercially available. They were commonly used by Indian tribes of Texas and northern Mexico, both as a stimulant and a hallucinogen. However, mescal beans are extremely dangerous, producing respiratory failure often leading to death. Peyote has a much greater margin of safety, and has replaced mescal beans in popularity (32).

STP and MDA

The compound 2,5-dimethoxy-4-methylamphetamine achieved great popularity for a while in the hippie culture, and was known as STP (36). It is similar to LSD in its effect on mood, although with much more variable results. Users experienced either euphoria or dysphoria. STP has mild hallucinogenic and psychotomimetic effects, and is believed by users to enhance self-awareness. A related sympathomimetic drug is MDA (3,4-methylenedioxyamphetamine). MDA, in doses of about 125 mg, increases the sense of physical well-being, and enhances the enjoyment of esthetic experiences. Hallucinations are rare. The duration of action of MDA is about eight hours.

DMT and DET

N,N-dimethyltryptamine (DMT) and N,N-diethyltryptamine (DET) are two other drugs which enjoyed a brief vogue in the hippie culture and whose names were, mercifully, shortened to their initials. Both produce LSD-like symptoms, but for much briefer durations (39). In fact, the brevity of the DMT trip earned it the nickname "businessman's LSD," because it can be squeezed into the schedule during a normal workday.

Morning Glory Seeds

Morning glory seeds (*Ipomoea violacea,* although usually decribed as *I. purpurea*) are sold in plant nurseries throughout the country. They contain D-lysergic acid amide, which is closely related to LSD. Low doses (20 to 50 seeds) are claimed to produce enhanced rapport with others, heightened awareness of objects and of nature, and a feeling of tranquility. Medium doses (100 to 150 seeds) produce effects which parallel those for medium dose LSD experiences; and high dose (200 to 500 seeds) effects resemble those of high doses of LSD. Nausea and drowsiness are common side effects. The best varieties of seeds are Heavenly Blue and Pearly Gates. Measures were taken to combat the increase in popularity of morning glory seeds, and most nurseries now sell only seeds which have been chemically treated to produce severe discomfort if ingested.

Harmaline

Harmaline is an alkaloid which is found in many plants and is very similar in structure to a substance manufactured in our bodies by the pineal gland (25). It gives rise to several unpleasant physical sensations, such as nausea, vomiting, dizziness, and numbness. Noises cannot be ignored, and become bothersome. Harmaline-induced imagery is very vivid and realistic. In contradistinction to LSD or mescaline, the perception of objects is largely undistorted; however, images or imaginary scenes are superimposed on surrounding objects. Changes in the affective sphere are small.

Fly Agaric

Fly agaric is the English name for the mushroom *Amanita muscaria* (see Fig. 3–6). The mushroom is poisonous when taken in large doses, and several deaths are caused each year by people who mistake *Amanita* for an edible mushroom. It grows wild in many parts of the United States and is used in several parts of the world. When taken in doses of approximately one mushroom, it is a strong intoxicant. The powerful mind-altering effects of certain mushrooms have been recognized for centuries. In addition, the mushroom has been used throughout history by widely disparate cultures, as Figures 3–7 and 3–8 indicate. The properties of the fly agaric have been summed up by Wasson (42):

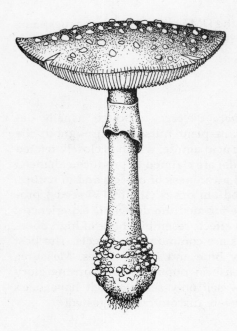

Figure 3–6 The *Amanita muscaria* mushroom, or fly agaric. In addition to producing powerful hallucinogenic effects, *Amanita muscaria* is somewhat toxic, and ingestion of the mushroom entails considerable risk. (From *Color Treasury of Mushrooms and Toadstools,* Crescent Books, p. 20.)

a. It begins to act in 15 or 20 minutes and the effects last for hours.

b. First it is a soporific. One goes to sleep for about 2 hours, and the sleep is not normal. One cannot be roused from it, but is sometimes aware of the sounds round about. In this half-sleep sometimes one has coloured visions that respond, at least to some extent, to one's desires.

c. Some subjects enjoy a feeling of elation that lasts for 3 or 4 hours after waking from the sleep. In this stage it is interesting to note that the superiority of this drug over alcohol is particularly emphasized: the fly agaric is not merely better, it belongs to a different and superior order of inebriant, according to those who enjoyed the experience. During this state the subject is often capable of extraordinary feats of physical effort, and enjoys performing them.

d. A peculiar feature of the fly agaric is that its hallucinogenic properties pass into the urine, and another may drink this urine to enjoy the same effect. Indeed it is said that the urine of 3 or 4 successive drinkers may be thus consumed without noticeable loss of inebriating effect. This surprising trait of fly agaric inebriation is unique in the hallucinogenic world, so far as our present knowledge goes.

Wasson added that the *Amanita* is very different in effects from the genus *Psilocybe*.

Figure 3–7 Seventeenth-century Chinese representation of a philosopher contemplating the Divine Mushroom. (Drawing of Chen Hung-Shon courtesy of Wan-Go H. C. Weng Collection, New York.)

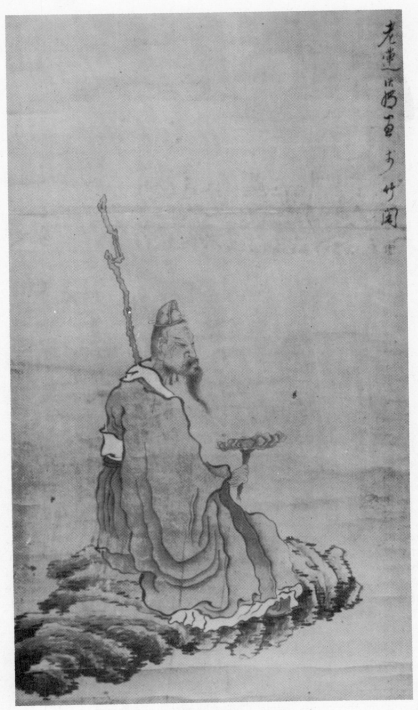

Figure 3–7 See opposite page for legend.

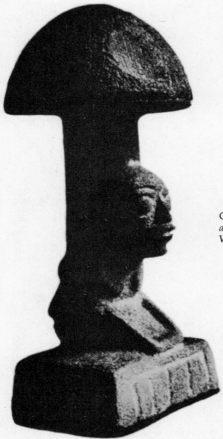

Figure 3–8 A mushroom stone from Guatemala. (From *Mushrooms, Russia, and History,* © by R. G. Wasson and V. Wasson, 1957, Pantheon Books, Inc.)

Dream Fish

Bufotenine, which is a major constituent of fly agaric mushrooms, is also manufactured by a fish, *Kyphosus fuscus,* which inhabits the area around Norfolk Island. Natives call it the dream fish, because eating it induces vivid dreams. Roughly (31) ate some of the fish, and verified the claims, reporting that his dreams were indeed vivid and weird. A relative of *Kyphosus fuscus* called the rudder fish is found in the United States.

Salvia divinorum, _Coleus pumila_ and _blumei_, and _Brunfelsia hopeana_

These are all close relatives of common house plants. The herb sage is in the genus *Salvia, Coleus blumei* is the common coleus, and the handsome shrubs "Brazil raintree" and "Yesterday-today-and-tomorrow" are in the genus *Brunfelsia*. All are employed as hallucinogens by various South American tribes (34). Scientific studies of their efficacy and toxicity are lacking.

Datura and Other Anticholinergics

Datura is a genus of plants, several of which grow wild in the United States or are sold in nurseries. Jimson weed is a member of the genus. Species of *Datura* are used in South America as hallucinogenic substances. The initial effect is one of extreme violence which is followed by a deep, disturbed sleep during which hallucinations are experienced. Members of the genus *Datura* are extremely toxic. Anticholinergic alkaloids — atropine, scopolamine, and hyoscyamine — are the active principles. Others plants with similar active principles include *Atropa belladona* (Deadly Nightshade) and *Hyoscyamus niger* (Henbane). Longo and de Carolis (22) reviewed the behavioral pharmacology of the anticholinergic drugs. The characteristic syndrome includes impaired memory, slurred speech, drowsiness, impaired motor ability, a state of confusion and disorientation, feelings of unpleasantness, and both visual and auditory hallucinations.

OPIATES

Opium is derived from the poppy plant *Papaver somniferum*. Its most important constituent (about 10 percent by weight) is the alkaloid morphine. Other alkaloids of opium include codeine, a common ingredient of cough suppressants, thebaine, papaverine, noscapine, and narcine. Heroin, which is synthetic, is very similar in structure to morphine (see Fig. 3–11), and is made from it.

Morphine is one of the most powerful analgesics known (see p. 234). It is selective in its actions. Compared to equianalgesic doses of nitrous oxide, ether, or barbiturates, morphine causes less drowsiness, fewer affective changes, and less impairment of the sensory modalities (except that of pain). The abuse of opiate drugs is due in large part to their analgesic effects. People suffering from physical or mental pain often become euphoric when the pain is relieved. Not only pain, but also hunger, sex, and aggressive drives are reduced by morphine. Heroin has similar effects, and when it is given subcutaneously the results cannot be distinguished from those of morphine, even by experienced users (11). Heroin is more potent, and of smaller bulk.

Among the many side effects of morphine are nausea, consti-

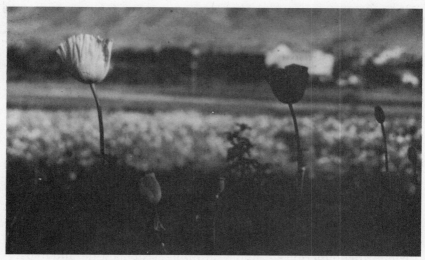

Figure 3–9 The poppy plant (*Papaver somniferum*) in a field in the Middle East. (AFIP Neg. 71-3778-1.)

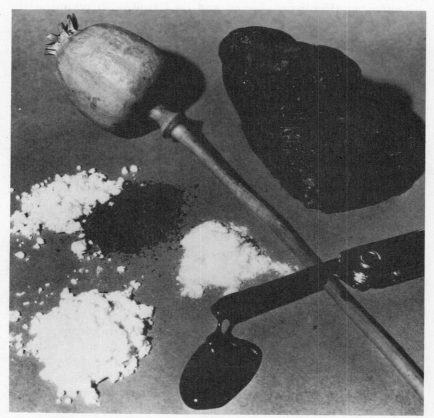

Figure 3–10 The opium poppy and its derivatives. The white powders are heroin, codeine, and morphine. The black substances are crude and smoking opium. (AFIP Neg. 71-3778-1.)

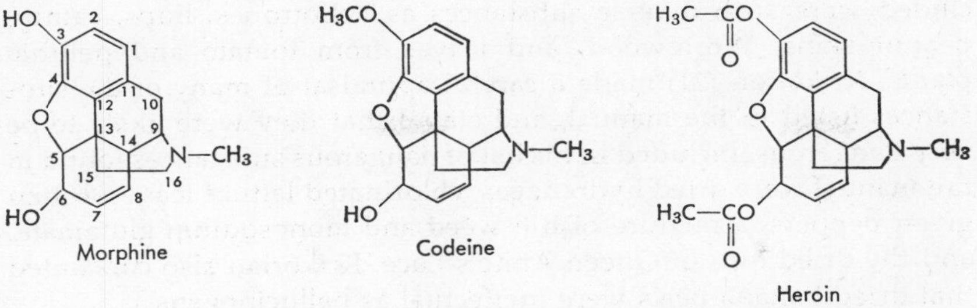

Morphine   Codeine   Heroin

Figure 3–11   Chemical structures of morphine, codeine, and heroin.

pation, miosis (pinpoint pupils), and respiratory depression, which is the principal cause of death. Meperidine, which is marketed under several trade names (including Demerol) is similar to morphine in most respects, but without the pupillary effects. It is commonly used as an analgesic in obstetrics. Methadone, like meperidine, is a synthetic narcotic. The effects of methadone are described in Chapter 6.

MISCELLANEOUS

In a little manual written in 1970 (38), several readily available substances which might alter consciousness were described. The purpose was to provide readers with ways to get legally high. In-

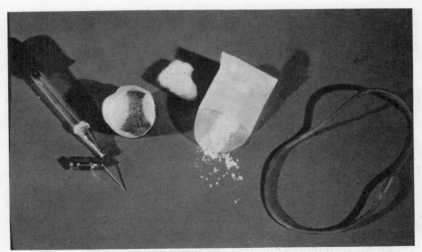

Figure 3–12   The paraphernalia of the narcotic addict. Shown are a medicine dropper with attached flange, hypodermic needle, bottle cap (which can be replaced by any similar small container) used as a "cooker," cotton, drug packet, and an elastic band (which serves as a tourniquet). (Courtesy, Office of Chief Medical Examiner, Baltimore, Maryland.)

cluded were such diverse substances as heliotropes, hops, catnip, peanut skins, Wormwood, and leaves from tomato and petunia plants. Krikorian (21) made a careful appraisal of many of the substances listed in the manual, and stated that they were likely to be very dangerous. Included in his list of dangerous substances found in the manual were dried hydrangeas, chlorinated lettuce leaves, rotten green peppers, a mixture of dill weed and monosodium glutamate, and the dried tops of Queen Anne's Lace. Krikorian also concluded that dried banana peels were ineffectual as hallucinogens.

Ginseng

Ginseng, which is listed in many herbals, has been used as a medicine by the Chinese for at least 4000 years. It is very expensive, and the extraordinary claims which have been made for it have been met with skepticism by Western scientists. Baranov (1) described the prominent physiological effects of each of the active principles of ginseng: panagulon stimulates endocrine secretions, ginsenin is antidiabetic; panaxic acid acts as an aid to the heart and blood vessels; and panacen is an analgesic and tranquilizer.

Ginseng is employed by the Chinese to treat anemia, diabetes, insomnia, neuroses, gastritis, various types of sexual problems, and some debilitative diseases. Baranov mentioned the possibility that *Eleutherococcus senticosus,* a very common Far Eastern shrub, may have the same properties as ginseng. Is ginsent a panacea or a quack medicine? Careful experimentation will perhaps determine the final verdict.

DIET

It is well known that mental performance is impaired by malnutrition. (A review of some of the evidence relevant to this fact can be found in Cravioto [4].) Moreover, it is becoming apparent that wide variations in even so-called normal diets may profoundly influence behavior. Concentrations of neurotransmitters within the CNS, upon which behavior ultimately depends, are affected by dietary factors (8), and patterns of sleep in man have been modified by manipulation of protein intake (49). The possible increase in learning and memory capacity following ingestion of glutamic acid or vitamin B_{12} is reviewed elsewhere (see Chap. 11). There is evidence that breast-fed children are smarter than bottle-reared babies (14), although the differences might be the result of psychological factors associated with breast feeding rather than some special nutrient in human milk. Recently Cheraskin et al. (3) reviewed studies which indicate that dietary supplements, especially of the B vitamins, may substantially improve mental performance even in the nondeprived.

Although Cheraskin and his colleagues carefully selected their cases, and did not discuss many relevant experiments in which the outcomes were negative, the many positive findings should serve as incentive to additional research.

Table 3.1, taken from Gregory and Paul (13), implicates dietary factors in the genesis of psychological disorders. It is clear from the table that substantial numbers of patients with such disorders suffer from dietary deficiencies. Of course, two additional bits of data must be obtained before the possibility of any causal link should seriously be entertained: first, it must be shown that psychologically normal individuals do not suffer to the same extent from dietary deficiencies (Gregory and Paul did have some control data which indicated this); and second, that the deficiencies predate the disease, rather than simply being a consequence of the fact that people who become mentally ill stop eating properly.

Another researcher who believes that improper attention to diet is the basis for many emotional disorders is Watson (44–46). He feels that mood, outlook, and energy level can be improved by first determining one's metabolic pattern, and then taking dietary supplements in accord with the findings. Watson's thesis, while intriguing, has not yet been subjected to careful experimental scrutiny, such as statistical analyses of double blind experiments. The work of Hoffer on the use of massive doses of vitamins to cure certain forms of mental illness is discussed in Chapter 7. He believes that nicotinic acid and vitamin C are powerful antidepressants. It may be worthwhile to study the effects of normal variations in the intake of vitamins on mental functioning.

ADDITIONAL RESEARCH

The reader who is interested in further exploration of the psychoactive properties of exotic substances can refer to several sources.

TABLE 3.1 Percentages of Selected Diagnostic Groups Showing Relative Nutritional Deficiencies*

	THIAMINE	RIBO-FLAVIN	NIACIN	ASCORBIC ACID	VITAMIN A	CARO-TENE	PRO-TEIN
Schizophrenia	15.5	25.8	10.5	27.9	15.5	7.2	18.6
Affective psychoses	7.7	13.5	11.5	17.3	19.3	9.6	17.3
Organic psychoses or senility	16.7	16.7	14.3	16.7	11.9	19.1	28.6
Psychoneuroses and pathologic personality	15.7	37.4	13.7	27.5	7.8	3.9	7.8
Alcoholism and alcoholic psychoses	9.1	31.8	9.1	22.7	18.2	9.1	9.1
Other diagnoses	12.5	25.0	20.9	33.4	10.4	4.2	16.7

*From Gregory, I., and Paul, R. Nutritional deficiencies in patients admitted to mental hospitals. Canad. M.A.J., 1959, *80*: p. 187.

TABLE 3.2   Comparative Pharmacological Effects of Δ⁹-THC* with Various Psychoactive Drugs†

PHARMACOLOGICAL PARAMETERS	Δ⁹THC	E+OH	Morphine	LSD-25	N₂O	Scopolamine	Phencyclidine
Euphoria	yes	yes	yes	yes	yes	no	yes
Panic reaction	yes	no	no	yes	yes	yes	yes
Stupor with large doses	yes	yes	yes	no	yes	yes	yes
Analgesia	yes (animals)	no	yes	yes	yes	no	yes
Hallucinations (acute dose)	yes	no	no,→	yes	yes,→	yes,→	yes
Auditory and visual sensations	←	→	—,→	←	←,→	—,→	→,?
Tolerance	yes (animals)	yes	yes	yes	no	yes (animals)	?
Cross-tolerance to narcotic analgesics	no	no	yes	no	no	no	no
to sedatives	?	yes	no	no	yes	no	no
Physical dependence	no	yes	yes	no	no	no	?
Psychic dependence	yes	yes	yes	yes	yes	no	yes
Short-term memory loss	yes	no	no	no	yes	yes	yes
Antagonists Specific Pharmacologic	none amphetamines (poor)	none amphetamines (poor)	Naloxone —	none CPZ Diazepam	none	none physostigmine	none
Selective blockade conditioned avoidance	yes	no	yes	no	?	no	no
Brain ACh Content	←→	←→	←→	—	?	→←	—,→
Release				—	?	←	—,→
EEG Activity	slow	slow	slow	fast	slow	slow	slow-fast

*Δ⁹THC is one of the active principles in marijuana.

†From Domino, E. Neuropsycho-pharmacologic studies of marijuana—some synthetic and natural THC derivatives in animals and man. Ann. N.Y. Acad. Sci., 1971, 191: p. 187.

The journal *Economic Botany* periodically publishes descriptions of plants which are used for their abilities to alter consciousness. The book edited by Efron (6) offers a wealth of information on psychoactive substances. Schultes and Holmstedt (35) have discussed South American snuffs, and Wasson and Wasson (43) hallucinogenic mushrooms. For those interested in synthesis and structure-activity relationships, Nieforth (26) has written an important paper, but one which requires substantial background in organic chemistry and biochemistry. Finally, Table 3.2, taken from Domino (5), is a comparison of the effects of various psychoactive drugs.

REFERENCES

1. Baranov, A. Recent advances in our knowledge of the morphology, cultivation and uses of ginseng (*Panax ginseng* C. A. Meyer). Econ. Botany, 1966, *20*:403–406.
2. Braga, D., and McLaughlin, J. Cactus alkaloids V. Isolation of hordenine and N-methyltyramine from *Ariocarpus retusus*. Planta Medica, 1969, *17*:87–94.
3. Cheraskin, E., Ringsdorf, W., and Clark, J. *Diet and Disease*. Emmaus, Penna.: Rodale, 1968.
4. Cravioto, J. Nutritional deficiencies and mental performance in childhood. *In* Glass, D. (Ed.) *Environmental Influences*. New York: Rockefeller Univ., 1968.
5. Domino, E. Neuropsychopharmacologic studies of marijuana: some synthetic and natural THC derivatives in animals and man. Ann. N.Y. Acad. Sci., 1971, *191*:166–191.
6. Efron, D. (Ed.) *Ethnopharmacologic Search for Psychoactive Drugs*. U.S. PHS Pub. No. 1645, 1967.
7. Fadiman, J. Psychedelic properties of *Genista canariensis*. Econ. Bot., 1965, *19*:383.
8. Fernstrom, J., and Wurtman, R. Brain serotonin content: increase following ingestion of carbohydrate diet. Science, 1971, *174*:1023–1025.
9. Forney, R., and Hughes, F. *Combined Effects of Alcohol and Other Drugs*. Springfield, Ill.: Chas. Thomas, 1968.
10. Frankenhauser, M., Myrsten, A., Waszak, M., Neri, A., and Post, B. Dosage and time effects of cigarette smoking. Psychopharmacologia, 1968, *13*:311–319.
11. Fraser, H., Van Horn, G., Martin, W., Wolbach, A., and Isbell, H. Methods for evaluating addiction liability. (A) "Attitude" of opiate addicts toward opiate-like drugs. (B) A short-term "direct" addiction test. J. Pharmacol. Exp. Ther., 1961, *133*:371–387.
12. Green, R., Jr. Nutmeg poisoning. J.A.M.A., 1959, *171*:1342–1344.
13. Gregory, I., and Paul, R. Nutritional deficiencies in patients admitted to mental hospitals. Canad. M.A.J., 1959, *80*:186–189.
14. Hoefer, C., and Hardy, M. Later development of breast-fed and artificially-fed infants. J.A.M.A., 1929, *92*:615–619.
15. Hoffer, A., and Osmond, H. *The Hallucinogens*. New York: Academic Press, 1967.
16. Hollister, L. Marijuana in man: three years later. Science, 1971, *172*:21–29.
17. Hughes, R. Behavior of male and female rats with free choice of two environments differing in novelty. Anim. Behav., 1968, *16*:92–96.
18. Huxley, A. *The Doors of Perception*. New York: Harper, 1954.
19. Isbell, H. Comparison of the reactions induced by psilocybin and LSD-25 in man. Psychopharmacologia, 1959, *1*:29–38.
20. Kluver, H. *Mescal and Mechanisms of Hallucinations*. Chicago: Univ. Chicago, 1966.
21. Krikorian, A. The psychedelic properties of banana peel: an appraisal. Econ. Botany, 1968, *22*:385–389.

22. Longo, V., and de Carolis, A. Anticholinergic hallucinogenics: laboratory results versus clinical trials. *In* Bradley, P., and Fink, M. (Eds.) *Anticholinergic Drugs and Brain Functions in Animals and Man.* Amsterdam: Elsevier, 1968.
23. McLaughlin, J., and Paul, A. The cactus alkaloids. I. Identification of N-methylated tyramine derivatives in *Lophophora williamsii.* Lloydia, 1966, *29*:315–327.
24. Meyer, H. Pharmacology of kava. *In* Efron, D. (Ed.) *Ethnopharmacologic Search for Psychoactive Drugs.* U.S. PHS Pub. No. 1645, 1967.
25. Naranjo, C. Psychotropic properties of the harmala alkaloids. *In* Efron, D. (Ed.) *Ethnopharmacologic Search for Psychoactive Drugs.* U.S. PHS Pub. No. 1645, 1967.
26. Nieforth, K. Psychotomimetic phenethylamines. J. Pharmaceut. Sci., 1971, *60*: 655–665.
27. Norquist, D., and McLaughlin, J. Cactus alkaloids VIII: Isolation of N-methyl-3,4-dimethoxy-beta-phenethylamine from Ariocarpus fissuratus var. fissuratus. J. Pharmaceut. Sci., 1970, *59*:1840–1841.
28. Osmond, H. A review of the clinical effects of psychotomimetic agents. Ann. N.Y. Acad. Sci., 1957, *66*:418–434.
29. Payne, R. Nutmeg intoxication. New Eng. J. Med., 1963, *269*:36–38.
30. Ritchie, J. Central nervous system stimulants. II. The xanthines. *In* Goodman, L., and Gilman, A. *The Pharmacological Basis of Therapeutics.* New York: Macmillan, 1965.
31. Roughly, T. Bounty descendants live on remote Norfolk island. Nat. Geograph. Mag., 1960, *118*:559–584.
32. Schultes, R. Pharmacognosy. The Pharmaceut. Sci., 1960, Third Lect. Series, 138–185.
33. Schultes, R. The search for new natural hallucinogens. Lloydia, 1966, *29*:293–307.
34. Schultes, R. Hallucinogens of plant origin. Science, 1969, *163*:245–254.
35. Schultes, R., and Holmstedt, B. De plantis toxicariis e mundo novo tropicale commentationes II. The vegetal ingredients of the Myristicaceous snuffs of the Northwest Amazon. Rhodora, 1968, *70*:113–160.
36. Snyder, S., Weingartner, H., and Faillace, L. DOET (2,5-dimethoxy-4-ethylamphetamine) and DOM (STP) (2,5-dimethoxy-4-methylamphetamine), new psychotropic agents; their effects in man. *In* Efron, D. (Ed.) *Psychotomimetic Drugs.* New York: Raven, 1970.
37. Soveif, M. Hashish consumption in Egypt, with special reference to psychosocial aspects. Bull. Narc. Drugs, 1967, *19*:1–12.
38. Superweed, M. *Herbal Highs.* San Francisco: Stone Kingdom, 1970.
39. Szara, S. DMT (N,N-dimethyltryptamine) and homologues: clinical and pharmacological considerations. *In*: Efron, D. (Ed.) *Psychotomimetic Drugs.* New York: Raven, 1970.
40. Tart, C. *On Being Stoned.* Palo Alto: Sci. and Behav., 1971.
41. Unger, S. Mescaline, LSD, psilocybin and personality change. *In* Solomon, D. (Ed.) *LSD: The Consciousness-Expanding Drug.* New York: Putnam, 1966.
42. Wasson, R. Fly agaric and man. *In* Efron, D. (Ed.) *Ethnopharmacologic Search for Psychoactive Drugs,* U.S. PHS Pub. No. 1645, 1967.
43. Wasson, V., and Wasson, R. *Mushrooms, Russia, and History.* New York: Pantheon, 1957.
44. Watson, G. Differences in intermediary metabolism in mental illness. Psychol. Rep., 1965, *17*:563–582.
45. Watson, G. *Nutrition and Your Mind.* New York: Harper and Row, 1972.
46. Watson, G., and Currier, W. Intensive vitamin therapy in mental illness. J. Psychol., 1960, *49*:67–81.
47. Weil, A., Zinberg, N., and Nelsen, J. Clinical and psychological effects of marijuana in man. Science, 1968, *162*:1234–1242.
48. Weiss, B., and Laties, V. Enhancement of human performance by caffeine and the amphetamines. Pharmacol. Rev., 1962, *14*:1–36.
49. Williams, H., Lester, B., and Coulter, J. Monoamines and the EEG stages of sleep. Activities Nervosa Sup., 1969, *11*:188–192.
50. Wolbach, A., Miner, E., and Isbell, H. Comparison of psilocin with psilocybin, mescaline and LSD-25. Psychopharmacologia, 1962, *3*:219–223.

CHAPTER 4

DANGERS OF DRUGS

Controversy about dangers of drug use have generally been intertwined with arguments about legalization, although there is no logical linkage between the two. Certain religions, such as the Mormon and Christian Science faiths, forbid their members to use many substances for reasons that are quite independent of considerations of safety. On the other side, the philosophy enunciated by John Stuart Mill appeals to many; he argued that dangerous behavioral practices should not be legally proscribed so long as the risks are confined to the behaving person. The present-day "do your own thing" philosophy derives from Mill. Adherents of views at either polar extreme, upon being presented with favorable or unfavorable evidence concerning toxicity, would remain unchanged on questions of legalization.

NEED FOR ADEQUATE CONTROLS

More than 50 percent of people who are treated with the drug methotrexate die within a year. However, it would be a terrible error to withdraw the drug on the grounds that it causes the deaths, for methotrexate is most commonly administered to children suffering from acute leukemia, and before its discovery the average survival of such children was only about four months. In order to avoid similar errors of interpretation, scientists should make statements about causality only when they are based on evidence derived from carefully controlled experiments. Statements like "one percent of LSD users have bad trips" are not indictments of LSD un-

67

less it is established that the incidence of unpleasant reactions in nonusers of similar emotional health, during the same time span, is smaller. It is conceivable that people take LSD primarily when they are depressed, and that if it were unavailable many more than one percent would be unhappy. Despite the inadequacy of such data for determining the hazards of drug use, they are common, and furnish fuel for controversy: opponents interpret the data as proof that LSD users run considerable risk of having bad trips; advocates counter that the drug may actually be prophylactic.

The importance of adequate control is illustrated nicely by a report of Reidenberg and Lowenthal (56). Of 414 normal people they surveyed who had had no illnesses and had taken no medications during the previous three days, only 19 percent were free from all the 25 symptoms commonly listed as side effects of drugs. The percentage of subjects who experienced each symptom is given in Table 4.1.

Unfortunately it is exceedingly difficult for both practical and

TABLE 4.1   Percentage of Normal Nondrugged Subjects Reporting Each Symptom*

Symptom	Medical Group	Nonmedical Group
Skin rash	8	3
Urticaria	5	1
Bad dreams	8	3
Excessive sleepiness	23	23
Fatigue	41	37
Inability to concentrate	25	27
Irritability	20	17
Insomnia	7	10
Loss of appetite	3	6
Dry mouth	5	3
Nausea	3	2
Vomiting	0	0
Diarrhea	5	2
Constipation	4	3
Palpitations	3	3
Giddiness or weakness	2	3
Faintness or dizziness on first standing up	5	5
Headaches	15	13
Fever	3	1
Pain in joints	9	5
Pain in muscles	10	11
Nasal congestion	31	13
Bleeding or bruising	3	3
Bleeding from gums after brushing teeth	21	20
Excessive bleeding from gums after brushing teeth	1	1

*Reprinted, by permission, from the New England Journal of Medicine, 1968, 279: p. 679, of "Adverse nondrug reactions," by M. Reidenberg and D. Lowenthal.

ethical reasons to employ adequate controls in human drug research. Even prior to their first drug experience, drug users differ from non-users (see Chapter 5). Consequently, the difficulty of forming adequate control groups cannot be surmounted by equating users and nonusers on relevant variables such as age, sex, intelligence, income, or political views. Some unknown variable (or variables), perhaps with far-reaching consequences, must be differentially operative or else there would be homogeneity of usage. That unknown variable, whether genetic or experiential, may also account for other, observed differences, like susceptibility to various pathological conditions. For example, smokers are more prone to heart disease than are nonsmokers—the evidence is incontrovertible (33). But smokers may differ genetically from nonsmokers (61), and the genetic factor may be the crucial one in predisposing certain individuals to heart disease (but, see p. 78). The point bears repetition: if two groups of people differ in their use of a drug, then they *must differ* in at least one other respect as well—specifically, in some factor which predisposes to drug use or to abstinence. This predisposing factor, rather than the drug, may account for other differences between the groups.

How then can we ever disentangle real effects of drugs from factors which predispose to use? The answer is conceptually simple. In properly designed experiments, subjects are assigned to groups by purely random means, such as by flipping coins. If the groups are made large enough, then prior to the administration of a drug they are considered to be essentially equal in all important respects. Then, if they are exposed to different experimental conditions, it is safe to conclude that differences between them are the result solely of their differential treatment. Unfortunately, however, such experiments are easier to design than to conduct. For instance, in order to get at the relationship between smoking and heart disease, some people would have to be selected at random and directed to smoke a specified number of cigarettes per day, while others would be directed to refrain from smoking. Volunteers would be hard to find.

An alternative to the use of human volunteers is research with animals, which has many practical advantages. Rats, for example, are inexpensive to buy and maintain. Their past histories and current experiences can be fully controlled by the experimenter, and ethical standards are less stringent than they are with human subjects. Animal research constitutes the bulk of experimentation reported in this book, and the findings are often relevant for man. But until animal experiments are formally replicated with human subjects, any findings can be regarded only as suggestive. In Chapter 9, several examples are given of substantial differences between animals and man in responsiveness to drugs.

To summarize, evidence of drug toxicity is obtained from three sources. First, information is gathered from properly controlled experiments in man; these are relatively rare, for both practical and ethical considerations. Even when experiments are properly conducted, certain types of individuals — physically unhealthy, mentally unstable, very old or young — are generally excluded from the subject sample. Yet these same individuals may be the ones for whom the drugs are intended, or who tend to abuse them. A second source

TABLE 4.2   Potential Toxicity of Common Substances

Substance	Where Found or How Obtained	Effects of Overdose
vitamin A	mammalian and fish liver, egg yolk, butter, cream, cod liver oil, many vegetables	hemorrhage, thickening of cortex of bone, loss of appetite, muscular weakness, fragility of bones, death
thiamin	liver, kidney, lean pork, brewer's yeast, wheat germ, oatmeal, rice, peanuts, peas, beans, egg yolk, milk, potatoes	nervousness, tremor, sweating, tachycardia, asthmatic attack, urticaria, nausea, death
vitamin D	milk, cod liver oil, sunlight	kidney stones, peptic ulcer, skeletal deformities
thyroid hormone	iodized salt, sea foods	restlessness, irritability, anxiety, exophthalmos, diarrhea, hypertension, tachycardia, hyperphagia, weakness
aspirin		confusion, dizziness, tinnitus, high-tone deafness, delirium, psychosis, stupor, coma, genetic damage
caffeine	coffee, tea, cocoa, cola drinks	insomnia, restlessness, excitement, mild delirium, ringing in the ears, tachycardia
antihistamines	used to treat hayfever, allergy, asthma, itch, motion sickness .	hallucinations, excitement, ataxia, incoordination, fever, convulsions, death
milk of magnesia	gastric antacid, cathartic	neurological, neuromuscular, cardiovascular impairment
calcium carbonate	antacid	constipation, nausea, hypercalcemia
tragacanth	bulk-forming cathartic	urticaria, rhinitis, dermatitis, asthma, gastrointestinal disturbances
potassium chlorate	mouthwash	abdominal pain, nausea, vomiting, kidney damage, death

of information on drug toxicity is uncontrolled experimentation, of which physicians' reports on idiosyncratic reactions of patients may be regarded as special examples. Such reports lack crucial information—the frequency of similar or worse reactions in people who have not used the drug, for instance. Finally, there is experimentation with animals, which may not always be relevant for man. Therefore, the need for extreme caution in evaluating claims about the safety or hazardousness of drugs can scarcely be overemphasized.

Some people may conclude that the limitations upon our knowledge constitute sufficient reason for abstinence from drugs. The argument has some appeal, but it ignores the positive aspects of drug use. *All substances, in some doses and in some individuals, are dangerous.* Table 4.2 lists some potential dangers of overindulgence in items found in most households. It should be recognized that the appropriate question is not whether a particular drug is dangerous, because indiscriminate use of any chemical substance is dangerous, but rather whether the potential benefits outweigh the risks. As the benefits are increased, greater risks can be incurred. The therapeutic index provides an estimate of the relationship between benefits and risks.

THE THERAPEUTIC INDEX

In animal research the therapeutic index* is often defined as the ratio ED_{50}/LD_{50}. The ratio of the TD_{25} or TD_{50} (dose at which the first signs of toxicity appear in 25 percent or 50 percent of the subjects) to the ED_{50} is more common in therapeutic practice. Even a very high therapeutic index does not insure that a drug will be safe. There are idiosyncratic reactors to virtually all drugs. In addition, many people have the notion that "you can't get too much of a good thing." Figure 4–1 illustrates how they can be fatally wrong. It presents data for a hypothetical drug. The LD_{50}/ED_{50} is $900/30 = 30$, which is high. Despite the wide margin of safety, a 1 mg dose, which is a very small absolute quantity, would be extremely hazardous.

The therapeutic index is rarely calculated directly for most drugs used in clinical practice, but it can be reliably estimated from the incidence of side effects from therapeutic doses. Estimates are much more difficult for illicit drugs. Figures on usage and adverse side effects are, at best, gross approximations. The reasons for usage are diverse, hence there is considerable variability in the endpoint required before a dose is considered effective. For example, a user who experiences euphoria from some drug may regard the experience as a failure if his goal had been to improve creativity, while another user may take the same drug solely for its euphoric effects.

---

*The therapeutic index is discussed on p. 39.

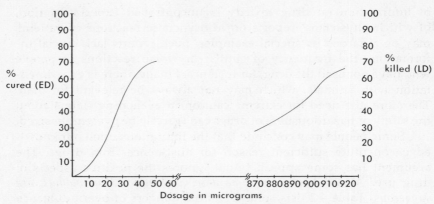

Figure 4–1 Dose-response curves for a hypothetical drug.

Many abstainers do not regard the pharmacological search for euphoria, relief from stress, or esthetic or religious experiences as appropriate goals. For them, there can never be an effective dose. An additional problem is that drug effects, such as disorders of memory or hallucinations, which under other circumstances would be regarded as toxic, are often ignored, tolerated, or actually desired by users. Finally, the therapeutic index refers to the effects of acute administration of drug; the primary danger of some drugs, such as the nicotine in tobacco, comes from chronic usage. Grinspoon (32, p. 227) modified a table of Mikuriya to give approximate therapeutic indexes of secobarbital, alcohol, and tetrahydrocannabinol, which is the active principle in marijuana (listed in Table 4.3).

Despite the many areas of imprecision, certain comments can be made about the dangers associated with certain drugs. The following drugs are considered: marijuana, LSD, nicotine in tobacco, caffeine, alcohol, opiates, and amphetamines. The dangers

TABLE 4.3 Margins of Safety of Secobarbital, Alcohol, and Tetrahydrocannabinol*

	Effective Dose	Lethal Dose	Safety Factor (Lethal Dose/ Effective Dose)
Secobarbital	100–300 mg	1,000–5,000 mg	3–50
Alcohol	0.05–0.1%	0.4–0.5%	4–10
Tetrahydro-cannabinol	50 mcg/kg	2,160,000 mcg/kg†	40,000†

*From Grinspoon, L. *Marihuana Reconsidered* (Cambridge: Harvard University Press, 1971), p. 227.

†Because no human fatalities have been documented, the figures given are for the human effective dose and the lethal dose for mice.

of barbiturates are considered in Chapter 15. First, the physical dangers of each drug are discussed, then the psychological dangers. Afterward, there is a section on dangers caused by the attitudes of our society toward the drugs.

DANGERS INHERENT IN THE DRUGS THEMSELVES

Physical Dangers

Marijuana

TOLERANCE AND WITHDRAWAL.   The development of tolerance to a drug creates dangers because of the possibility of overdose due to changes in effective and toxic doses. Addicts may, upon resuming usage after a temporary hiatus, take their customary large doses. The effects are often disastrous. Overdose is very rarely a problem when, as is usually the case with marijuana, smoking is the route of administration. The reason is that absorption from the lungs is very rapid, so that onset of action is almost immediate. As soon as the user feels high, he stops smoking. A second problem with tolerance is that it does not develop equally to all drug actions. Should there be rapid development of tolerance to the euphoric effects of a drug but none to the effects on respiratory depression, then addicts might begin taking doses dangerously close to the lethal one. Finally, tolerance is usually associated with physical dependence and withdrawal symptoms, which make it difficult to discontinue the drug.

The AMA Committee on Alcoholism and Drug Dependence (17) recently endorsed the position that tolerance does not develop to marijuana. In fact, it is widely believed that chronic users require less of the drug than do novices. Less is required because many aspects of the high state are learned and are detected more readily by experienced users. Snyder (65) has suggested a physiological mechanism for the reverse tolerance: the active component of marijuana is one of the drug's metabolites, and with repeated use the efficiency of the liver in forming the psychoactive metabolic product is increased. On the other hand, Domino (21, p. 169 to 173) has summarized evidence, both from his own laboratory and others, showing that tolerance does occur. However, withdrawal symptoms, if they occur, are very mild. Williams et al. (76) reported that abrupt discontinuation of synhexyl, a synthetic marijuana-like drug, resulted in mild stress reactions. In the same study he found no evidence of an abstinence syndrome with marijuana itself.

ADVERSE SIDE EFFECTS.   Bronchitis and bronchial asthma, fairly common complaints (12), are more prominent in smokers than in oral users. Since marijuana is often mixed with tobacco, the latter may be the sole causative agent. According to one study, a related mild respiratory ailment known as "hash throat" is seen in substantial numbers of people who smoke three or four marijuana cigarettes a day (69). In the same study, although users of moderate amounts of marijuana showed no disturbances of personality, very heavy users (17 to 200 cigarettes per day) were characterized as suffering from apathy, dullness, and lethargy, with impairment of judgment also evident. However, even 17 cigarettes per day is an incredibly large number, and there is good reason to wonder about the pre-drug judgmental abilities of such heavy users.

There was a report in 1969 (40) that marijuana might impair liver function, but subsequent research on 31 very heavy users (61) showed no impairment at all. Another adverse effect was publicized by Wesley Hall (70), a former president of the American Medical Association. In an amazing display of irresponsibility, Hall asserted that marijuana "makes a man of 35 sexually like a man of 70." Hall added that chronic use causes birth defects. He later retracted his statement (60), admitting that it was not based on any evidence. His purpose had been to reduce marijuana use, irrespective of facts. In light of such attitudes on the part of some members of the medical profession, and the fact that there have been a huge number of recent studies on marijuana, the absence of reports on toxicity is testimony to the relative safety of the drug.

Common physical symptoms include rapidly beating heart, hypotension, dry mouth, and ptosis. They are not perceived as being unpleasant during the drug high, and do not persist beyond it. The most reliable physical symptom is reddening of the conjunctiva (the membrane in the front part of the eye). Chopra and Chopra (12) reported that 72 percent of marijuana users whom they examined had conjunctival inflammation.

CHROMOSOMAL DAMAGE AND TERATOGENICITY.   I know of no reports of chromosome damage or teratogenicity in humans. There may be teratogenic effects in hamsters, rabbits, and rats after very high doses (24, 49). However, virtually any drug, if administered in high enough doses during the early stages of pregnancy, can produce teratogenic effects (23).

INTERACTIONS.   Concurrent administration of two or more drugs can be hazardous. For example, therapeutic doses of MAOIs and amphetamine form a lethal combination. Marijuana is synergistic with at least two drugs: it prolongs barbiturate sedation and augments amphetamine stimulation (25). Any unsupervised use of another drug with marijuana is inadvisable.

BENEFICIAL EFFECTS.   Snyder (65) has suggested that marijuana might have a place in medical practice. He listed the following as conditions which might respond favorably to marijuana: pain, anxiety, insomnia, cough, excessive menstrual bleeding, withdrawal from narcotics and alcohol, stimulation of appetite, and epilepsy. It might also be useful in the treatment of migraine headaches (10).

LSD

TOLERANCE AND WITHDRAWAL.   Tolerance develops rapidly to both LSD and mescaline, and there is cross tolerance between them (3). There are no withdrawal symptoms.

ADVERSE SIDE EFFECTS.   Adey (1) has reported that discharges within the hippocampal region of the brain persist for several weeks in cats given large doses of LSD and exposed to stress in the form of electric shock. The abnormal brain wave patterns were not permanent, and were of lesser extent than changes produced by reserpine (21, p. 11). Lucas and Jacques (46) reported that rats pretreated with anticoagulant drugs were prone to hemorrhage after being given 0.5 mg/kg LSD. The dose is enormous when compared with that used in humans, where 0.01 mg/kg is considered very large. Nevertheless, LSD is probably contraindicated in patients taking anticoagulant drugs.

Somatic symptoms which are frequently reported are dizziness, weakness, nausea, paresthesias (abnormal sensations), and tremors.

CHROMOSOME DAMAGE.   In 1967, Cohen et al. (14) published the first paper implicating LSD as an agent which damages chromosomes. Cells with damaged chromosomes represent a danger to the individual, because of the possibility that they will establish new, possibly cancerous, cell lines. There is also danger to unborn children because the genes, which carry the genetic message, are encoded in damaged chromosomes in the reproductive cells.

At the outset it should be noted that cells are often damaged and die during illness. Damaged organisms, whether human beings or single cells, have difficulty in duplicating themselves. If LSD-induced chromosome damage is to be regarded as dangerous, the damage must be shown to persist for relatively long periods of time. Dishotsky et al. (20) recently reviewed the results of 68 studies during the period 1967 to 1970 which dealt with the question of possible chromosome damage in LSD users. The highlights of this paper are summarized and discussed below. (Their references are omitted.)

The paper by Cohen et al. described chromosome damage to laboratory cultures of white blood cells, after high doses of LSD had been added to them for periods ranging from 4 to 48 hours. (The mean circulation time in humans is about four hours.) Although most subsequent investigations with in vitro preparations have corroborated the initial findings, the significance of these findings remains obscure. In the first place, the process of culturing cells stimulates them to enter a reproductive phase which is abnormal for them. Cells in test tubes are extremely susceptible to chromosome breakage; aspirin, caffeine, water, and changes in temperature or oxygen pressure are some of the many agents which induce breakage of the same order of magnitude as LSD. Moreover, the type of breakage produced by LSD is different from that caused by known mutagenic or carcinogenic agents. Secondly, animals in nature have evolved efficient metabolic and excretory systems to eliminate harmful substances, but these detoxification mechanisms are not available to cells in test tubes.

BREAKAGE RATES OF CELLS WITHIN HUMAN USERS. In only four studies were comparisons made of breakage rates before and after exposure to LSD. Only one of the studies was positive. In all other cases, breakage rates of users were compared with those of nonusers; again, the impropriety of such nonrandom assignment of subjects to groups, which has been discussed before, is important to consider. Some unknown factor may predispose individuals both to take LSD and to chromosome damage. For example, heavy drug users are more likely than nonusers to have suffered serious childhood illnesses (see p. 100).

Dishotsky et al. distinguished between studies in which known quantities of pure LSD were administered to human volunteers and those in which cells were collected from people who admitted to illicit use outside of the laboratory. In both paradigms the cells were studied for chromosome damage.

There had been (at the time of publication of Dishotsky's paper) a total of 126 subjects studied after administration of pure LSD, and a maximum of 18 were reported to have chromosome damage. The exact number is unknown because of incomplete data on nine of the subjects. Three of the eighteen positive cases received LSD intravenously, an unusual route, and one other had a viral infection. A follow-up of five of the subjects within eight months of the last dose indicated that the frequency of breakage had returned to the normal range. Eight of the eleven teams of investigators who employed pure LSD found no evidence of chromosome damage. However, because of the importance of the issue, additional data should be collected before the majority opinion is accepted. One disturbing fact is that the tables of Dishotsky and his colleagues indicate that in ten of the fifteen studies they listed, users of LSD had elevated breakage rates. In only five of the cases were the increases statistically significant. However, failure to find statistical significance may result from small sample size or insensitive testing procedures. Although the number of *cells* tested for damage was generally adequate (at least 200 cells in all cases but one), the number of LSD *users* ranged from one to 32. It is conceivable that LSD damages chromosomes in only some users, e.g., those with relatively inefficient metabolic or excretory systems. If so, even a sample size of 32 might be too small to detect chromosome damage, irrespective of the number of cells counted. Furthermore, Markowitz et al. (47) reanalyzed some of the negative data with a more powerful statistical test, and showed that significant damage was in fact indicated.

Three laboratories which investigated chromosome damage in users of illicit LSD reported positive results, while nine others found no difference between users and nonusers. The positive results are vitiated by two considerations. First, damage to chromosomes may be organized into two classes: breakage occurring in vivo, and damage occurring in the process of culturing cells. Only in vivo breakage is relevant to the question of the potential danger of LSD, yet in the positive studies, the examples of LSD-induced aberrations were primarily of the type produced by the culture process. The significance of the fact that LSD renders cells more susceptible to damage during culturing is unknown. Second, people who use LSD illicitly generally take other drugs as well. In addition, they are exposed to a variety of substances which are fraudulently sold as LSD. Marshman and Gibbins (43) found that 54 percent of 57 samples of allegedly pure LSD contained substantial quantities of adulterants. These adulterants, rather than the LSD, might account for increased breakage. Thus, although the data are insufficient to convict LSD unequivocally of damaging chromosomes, damage is nevertheless a likely consequence of illicit use of substances sold as LSD.

TERATOGENIC EFFECTS (ALSO FROM DISHOTSKY ET AL.). A total of 14 children whose mothers had ingested illicit LSD during pregnancy have been studied for numbers of chromosome breaks. All were healthy, but ten had elevated breakage rates. There have been six reports of congenital malformations in babies whose mothers had used illicit LSD prior to or during pregnancy, but it should be realized that birth defects occur in the offspring of nonusers as well. There are no known instances of malformations in babies born to users of pure LSD. McGlothlin et al. (51) found that users of illicit LSD run an increased risk of spontaneous abortion; perhaps they have a greater than normal percentage of malformed, unhealthy fetuses, which are unable to survive to term.

Tobacco

TOLERANCE AND WITHDRAWAL. Some tolerance develops to tobacco (31, p. 583) and there are mild but never life-threatening withdrawal symptoms. These take the form of drowsiness (in 59 percent of males and 61 percent of females), nervousness (65 and 77 percent), anxiety (53 and 58 percent), headaches (41 and 47 percent), energy loss (39 and 52 percent), and several other symptoms (cited in 10). Other evidence of dependence is the pattern of smoking; Russell (58) noted that most smokers inhale one or more cigarettes per hour, an amount which ensures that the brain level of nicotine remains high throughout most of their waking life.

ADVERSE SIDE EFFECTS.   Common symptoms are nausea, vomiting, and dizziness.

EFFECTS OF CHRONIC USAGE.   The Surgeon General's Advisory Committee on Smoking and Health published a 387 page report in 1964 which summarized the results of several different types of studies, on both animals and man, concerning the relationship between smoking and health (72). The conclusion, which has been widely disseminated, is that smoking is unquestionably hazardous to health. Table 4.4 presents data on 14 disease categories for which the mortality ratio of smokers to nonsmokers is at least 1.5. When all causes of death are considered, the mortality rate of smokers is nearly 70 percent higher than that of nonsmokers. Various aspects of the report have been criticized, but the consensus of medical opinion (41) is that the overall conclusions are correct.

A point worth noting is that nicotine, when administered chronically in small doses, has low toxicity (72, p. 32). Therefore, other components of cigarette smoke, perhaps including the generated heat, may be responsible for the increased mortality rate of smokers. Other substances which are smoked, such as marijuana, should therefore be suspect. The danger for most marijuana users,

TABLE 4.4   Expected and Observed Deaths for Smokers of Cigarettes Only and Mortality Ratios in Seven Prospective Studies

UNDERLYING CAUSE OF DEATH	Expected deaths	Observed deaths	Mortality ratio
Cancer of lung	170.3	1,833	10.8
Bronchitis and emphysema	89.5	546	6.1
Cancer of larynx	14.0	75	5.4
Oral cancer	37.0	152	4.1
Cancer of esophagus	33.7	113	3.4
Stomach and duodenal ulcers	105.1	294	2.8
Other circulatory diseases	254.0	649	2.6
Cirrhosis of liver	169.2	379	2.2
Cancer of bladder	111.6	216	1.9
Coronary artery disease	6,430.7	11,177	1.7
Other heart diseases	526.0	868	1.7
Hypertensive heart	409.2	631	1.5
General arteriosclerosis	210.7	310	1.5
Cancer of kidney	79.0	120	1.5
All causes†	15,653.9	23,223	1.68

*From *Smoking and Health*. Report of the Advisory Committee to the Surgeon General of the Public Health Service (Washington). U.S. PHS Pub. No. 1103, 1964, p. 29.
†Includes all other causes of death as well as those listed above.

whose total weekly consumption may be only one or two shared cigarettes, is probably small.

Caffeine

TOLERANCE AND WITHDRAWAL. Tolerance develops to some of the effects of caffeine, but not to the central stimulation. Withdrawal is often accompanied by headache. In a carefully controlled study, Goldstein and Kaizer (29) made identically tasting preparations of coffee, which contained either no caffeine, or 150 mg or 300 mg of caffeine. Eighteen non-coffee drinkers and 38 heavy drinkers were tested three times with each preparation under double blind conditions. On days when the heavy drinkers drank the caffeine-free preparation, they reported several mood changes, including nervousness, irritability, and lack of alertness. The nondrinkers reported many similar unpleasant effects when they were given caffeine.

ADVERSE SIDE EFFECTS. A variety of unpleasant side effects are often reported after ingestion of as little as 1 gram of caffeine (seven to ten cups of coffee). These include insomnia and restlessness, sensory disturbances such as ringing in the ears and flashes of light, muscle tenseness and tremor, cardiac irregularities, exacerbation of the symptoms of peptic ulcer, and diarrhea. In fact, Reimann (57) believes that many instances of unexplained illness are caused by excessive ingestion of caffeine or the other xanthines. Recently (9) coffee drinking was shown to have a strong correlation (although not necessarily a causal relationship) with incidence of acute myocardial infarction. A total of 276 patients who were admitted to hospitals all over the world, who were diagnosed as having acute myocardial infarction (the death of an area of the heart muscle as a result of occlusion of a coronary artery), were matched with 1104 control patients who had other diseases. The former group drank much more coffee. The authors of the study analyzing the groups concluded that people who drink five or more cups of coffee per day have about twice the risk of acute myocardial infarction as nondrinkers. Although coffee drinking and cigarette smoking are highly correlated, the difference between the groups was shown not to be attributable to smoking. The role of the caffeine in coffee must still be clarified, since tea drinkers were not more prone to myocardial infarction than were controls, even though a cup of tea contains approximately the same amount of caffeine as a cup of coffee. The authors noted prior research which indicates that there is a positive correlation between coffee intake, but not tea intake, and serum cholesterol level. They therefore suggested that the cardiac damage caused by coffee may be mediated by the effects of coffee on serum cholesterol levels.

Alcohol

TOLERANCE AND WITHDRAWAL.   Tolerance develops, and withdrawal effects are invariable, after chronic use. The well-known hangover may actually be a form of withdrawal symptom (31, p. 295). In more severe cases, following chronic intoxication, the withdrawal syndrome is marked by tremulousness, hallucinations, seizures, and delirium.

ADVERSE EFFECTS.   There are at least five million alcoholics in the United States, and estimates by experts go as high as nine million. Alcoholics are far more prone than teetotalers to a wide variety of physical ailments, such as pellagra, peripheral neuropathies, nutritional amblyopia, Korsakoff's psychosis, and cirrhosis of the liver. Most of these may be the result of the inadequate dietary regimens of most alcoholics. The calories obtained from alcohol often lead to reductions in intake of other, more nutritionally valuable foods. Still, alcohol does have some toxic effects. Three male volunteers who received nutritional supplements along with doses of alcohol comparable to those ingested by chronic alcoholics suffered muscle pain, intracellular edema in muscles, and ultrastructural changes in muscle (66). The heart is a muscle, although different in several respects from skeletal muscle, so the results may be relevant to cardiac damage from consumption of alcohol.

BENEFICIAL EFFECTS.   Although excessive drinking is harmful, alcohol taken in moderation offers many health-promoting qualities. In fact, Pearl (54) observed that moderate drinkers had longer life expectancies than abstainers, while heavy drinkers had the shortest life expectancies (recall once again that correlation does not prove causation). Leake and Silverman (42) noted that the various forms of alcoholic beverages differ pharmacologically, and offered detailed descriptions of the medicinal, and other, uses of specific alcoholic beverages.

Alcohol is an appetite stimulant, and is especially valuable when lack of appetite is attributable to emotional factors. Goetzl, for instance, found red table wines to be helpful adjuncts in the management of patients suffering from anorexia nervosa (28). By the same token, when excessive eating is a symptom of anxiety, wine may help to normalize intake (44).

Diabetics respond well to alcohol (38), and it may serve as a prophylactic to diseases of the coronary arteries (49). Alcohol may reduce the pain and the frequency of occurrence of attacks of angina pectoris (35). Hypertensive states respond favorably to alcohol (43). Leake and Silverman prefaced their remarks on the use of alcohol in geriatric medicine with the comment that Osler had called it "the milk of old age," and then they quoted from Brooks: "Either as a food, as a medicine, or for its comfort-giving qualities, alcohol properly administered is one of the greatest blessings of old age." Chien (reported in Ref. 71) has recently shown that beer can be useful in facilitating social interactions in the aged.

Opiates

TOLERANCE AND WITHDRAWAL. Intermittent use of narcotics such as morphine, opium, or heroin may be continued indefinitely in some individuals, who eventually quit without difficulty (11, p. 23). However, with continuous use, tolerance develops rapidly to many of the drug's actions, including euphoric effects. Therefore, addicts must keep increasing their dosages. Cross tolerance among narcotics, even those with dissimilar chemical structures, is observed. Withdrawal is a painful process and of long duration, the

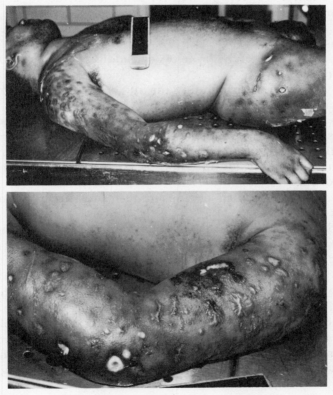

Figure 4–2 Subcutaneous or intramuscular self-administration of narcotics is called skin popping. It may be accomplished in any accessible location. Note the multiple ulcerating lesions and keloids of arms and right hip. (From Hirsch, Charles S. The dermatopathology of narcotic addiction. *In* Human Pathology, 3:1, March 1972, p. 45.)

Figure 4–3 Close-up of sites of skin popping on arm. (From Hirsch, p. 45.)

peak effects being reached about three days after the last dose. Some symptoms remain for seven to ten days.

ADVERSE SIDE EFFECTS.   Most addicts suffer nausea, vomiting, and constipation. Narcotic analgesics are very dangerous in individuals with reduced respiratory reserve, such as occurs in emphysema. The major therapeutic usefulness of narcotic analgesics, their ability to obtund pain, contributes to their dangerousness when taken illicitly, because addicts rendered insensitive to pain may remain unaware of symptoms of various diseases.

Baden (5) has debunked the myth that many — or possibly any — deaths are caused by heroin overdose. Still, in 1970, in New York City alone, there were 1046 deaths attributed to heroin overdose (63). Baden cited six lines of evidence to indicate the falsity of the attribution (note: although the deaths are not caused by overdose, they do result from heroin use):

1. Packets of heroin found near dead addicts do not differ from ordinary packets of heroin.

2. Syringes used by dead addicts do not contain more heroin than usual.

3. An analysis of the urine of dead addicts provides no evidence of overdose.

4. The tissues surrounding the site of the fatal injection show no signs of high heroin concentration.

5. Almost all deaths from heroin are in long-term users. But addicts develop extreme tolerance to the lethal effects of heroin and morphine, and evidence from several sources (cited in 5) indicates that the lethal dose for an addict is far in excess of even several street doses.

6. Groups of addicts often share the same supply, yet multiple deaths are rare.

What, then, causes death from heroin? Brecher (10) suggested two likely possibilities. The first is that some adulterant of heroin, perhaps quinine, causes the deaths. The second is that heroin interacts synergistically with other drugs, most notably with alcohol and barbiturates, so that an otherwise ordinary dose might prove fatal. The significance of these findings is that they place the responsibility for narcotics deaths on the drug laws. If heroin were obtainable through legal channels, there would be no improper adulteration of it; and if addicts could trust government officials, they would probably heed warnings to refrain from mixing heroin with other drugs.

CHRONIC EFFECTS.   Addicts who are able to obtain unadulterated supplies of morphine, and who maintain aseptic conditions for administration, do not evidence physiological damage (31, p. 292). Brecher devoted an entire chapter to "eminent narcotics addicts," people who were quite successful in their professions despite long-standing addiction. Brecher also quoted a 1956 unpublished study by Stevenson et al.:

> It was immediately apparent to us that the actual deleterious effects of addiction on the addict, and on society, should be clearly understood. . . . To our surprise we have not been able to locate even one scientific study on the proved harmful effects of addiction. Earlier investigators had apparently assumed that the ill effects were so obvious as not to need scientific verification.
>
> We have assembled over 500 documents on various phases of addiction . . ., but not one of them offers a clear-cut, scientifically valid statement on this problem.
>
> We finally wrote to some of the most eminent research workers in the field of drug addiction, explaining our problem and requesting scientific data on the deleterious effects of narcotic drugs. They indicated, in their reply, that there was no real evidence of brain damage or other serious organic disease resulting from the continued use of narcotics (morphine and related substances), but that there was undoubted psychological and social damage. However, they made no differentiation between such damage as might be caused by narcotics and that which might have been present before addiction, or might have been caused, at least in part, by other factors. Moreover, they were unable to direct us to any actual studies on the alleged harmful effects of narcotic drugs.
>
> At a later date we also consulted officials of the United Nations Commission on Narcotic Drugs, and they, too, were unable to direct us to any scientific studies on the actual damaging effects of morphine or heroin addiction. . . .
>
> The Narcotic Control Division of the Canadian Government's Department of Health and Welfare was likewise unable to direct us to scientific studies on this subject.

Brecher quoted several other authorities on the harmlessness of heroin and morphine. Two brief samples:

Dr. Nathan Eddy: "Given an addict who is receiving (adequate) morphine . . . the deviations from normal physiological behavior are minor (and) for the most part within the range of normal variations."

Dr. Vincent Dole: "Cigarette smoking is unquestionably more damaging to the human body than heroin."

Amphetamines

TOLERANCE AND WITHDRAWAL. Although tolerance is not usually observed with CNS stimulants, it does develop rapidly to the amphetamines. There are no serious withdrawal symptoms, though disturbances of sleep during withdrawal have been reported (53).

ADVERSE SIDE EFFECTS. The distinction between moderate and high dose amphetamine use must be emphasized. When taken orally, in moderate quantities, amphetamines cause few or no adverse effects. People who use large doses often grind their teeth, which causes ulcers of the lip and tongue (4). Brain damage is a possibility, although the evidence on which the suggestion is based is highly inferential (16). During high-dose usage there is generally insufficient sleep and inadequate attention to diet, which may contribute to circulatory collapse.

BENEFICIAL EFFECTS.   See Chapter 14.

Psychological Dangers of Drugs

The dangers to physical health of certain drugs like marijuana are minimal, but opponents of legalization often point to severe dangers to the psyche. One special hazard, which does not conveniently fit under the rubric of physical or psychological danger, is that of driving skills. DiMascio and Shader (19) noted that there is little statistical evidence for the assertion that psychotropic drugs enhance the likelihood of automobile accidents, despite the well-documented impairment of psychomotor performance attributed to the drugs. Data do exist on alcohol: the average driver with a blood alcohol concentration of 15 percent, which is associated with mild intoxication, is 33 times more likely to have an accident than the alcohol-free driver (31, p. 150).

There is some evidence that marijuana users, primarily inexperienced ones, have impaired performance of complex tasks (13, 50, 74). Since driving is a complex task, there is a good a priori reason for appraising the relationship between marijuana and driving. Crancer et al. (18) estimated driving ability by means of a simulator consisting of standard driving equipment. The subjects faced a screen which projected films of normal and emergency driving situations. They were exposed to a greater variety of hazardous situations than exist in typical road tests. The subjects were all experienced marijuana users, and were tested in each of three conditions: marijuana intoxication, alcohol intoxication, and control.

Total errors increased 15 percent under alcohol, but were unchanged with marijuana. The authors concluded that marijuana does not impair driving skill. However, since the subjects were experienced marijuana users, they were probably not unbiased about the outcome of the experiment, and may have tried harder in the marijuana condition. Duker (22) has shown the importance of motivational factors in psychopharmacological research. When his subjects received small doses of sedative and were motivated to sleep, sleep was rapidly induced. The same subjects, when given the same dose but required to concentrate on a continuous mental task, did not fall asleep but instead showed an improvement in their performance.

One way in which depressant drugs might increase the risk of accident is by reducing vigilance. That is, an intoxicated person might be quite capable of responding to emergencies, but not of maintaining full attention on the road during long, dull stretches of driving. The mere fact that experimental subjects were required to perform under observation undoubtedly increased their attentiveness, and the greater than normal number of simulated hazards minimized their likelihood of having lapses in vigilance. Therefore, although the Crancer et al. study is useful in demonstrating that experienced marijuana users do not suffer from gross impairment of driving skills, it is still possible that driving while under the influence of marijuana increases the risk of accident.

Kalant (30) criticized the comparison of marijuana with alcohol on the grounds that the doses were not comparable. When subjects were in the marijuana condition, they were asked to smoke until they experienced effects comparable to their previous experiences with marijuana. When they were in the alcohol condition, they drank an amount which Crancer et al. felt would result in a blood alcohol concentration of 0.10 percent; Kalant claimed, on the basis of independent data, that the actual concentration was probably about 0.15 percent. Kalant observed that the study would have been far more meaningful if dose-response curves had been obtained for both drugs.

Psychological Dependence on Drugs

Physical dependence is defined as a state characterized by the appearance of physical symptoms when administration of a drug is suspended. The concept of dependence has been broadened by substituting the word "psychological" for "physical." The World Health Organization (reported in 77, p. 21) defined drug dependence as ". . . a state of psychic or physical dependence, or both, on a drug, arising in a person following administration of that drug on a periodic or continuous basis." The wisdom of the expanded definition is disputable. Many drugs are used because of their ability to produce euphoria, a state of intense pleasure. People try to repeat pleasurable experiences, so it is not surprising that drug usage often becomes habitual. Psychological symptoms such as frustration and anxiety are to be expected when a potentially pleasurable experience is denied. The intensity of the symptoms may reflect the intensity of the experience. However, there is nothing about drugs which distinguishes them in this respect from other forms of pleasure.

Escape from Reality

It is often stated that drugs enable alienated, depressed people to escape from reality. The notion is a vague one. If escape from reality means nothing more than a drug-induced respite of several hours from the demands of everyday living, then it is not different in any important way from other forms of relaxation. Television, books, and football games fulfill the same needs. If, on the other hand, the phrase refers specifically to perceptual distortions, hallucinations, or disjointed thought, then not all psychoactive drugs produce escape from reality. Marijuana users commonly experience enhanced ability to attend to sensory stimuli; LSD, psilocybin, and amphetamine all improve certain aspects of sensory acuity; and the effects of heroin on sensory and perceptual processes and on thinking are minimal. Therefore, at least in some circumstances and with some doses, drugs may enhance reality rather than offer an escape from it. A special type of escape from reality is considered next.

Reliance on Drugs to Avoid Problems

In most societies (including our own), the period of adolescence is marked by an identity crisis. During this time, decisions which may be irreversible are made concerning ultimate lifelong goals. The process is often a painful one, and inability or unwillingness to cope with it has been suggested as one factor in the rapid spread of marijuana usage among young Americans. Unfortunately for individuals who use drugs as a way to avoid making difficult decisions, one's decisions cannot be postponed indefinitely. However, postponement may reduce alternatives—for example, someone who postpones choosing between entering college and taking a job may eventually opt for college, but be denied entry because of inability to compete on updated entrance examinations.

The incidence of drug use as a means of avoiding decisions may be substantial. It should not be confused with the deliberate usage of drugs for the purpose of dealing with problems which have been insoluble by traditional methods. In the latter instance, altered perspectives afforded by various drugs are viewed as enhancing chances of solution. Whether they actually do so is immaterial to the present discussion, because when taken for such purposes they do not constitute a danger.

Acute Adverse Reactions

Not all drug experiences turn out as anticipated. Acute panic reactions, depression, paranoia, and psychotic episodes occur with sufficient frequency to make the phrase "bad trip" an important part of the lexicon of the drug culture. Any potentially enjoyable event may prove to be a disappointment, as when rainy weather spoils a picnic, but the special quality of drug-induced bad trips is that they cannot be terminated easily.

Weil (73) estimated that about one percent of responses to marijuana, in supportive settings, are highly unpleasant. Cohen (15) determined that one of 2500 patients undergoing psychotherapy and taking LSD committed suicide, and 0.02 percent of normal subjects who took LSD experimentally experienced psychotic reactions of greater than 24 hours duration. To some extent, the first statistic persuaded Louria (45) to condemn the therapeutic use of LSD, a position which ignores the possibility that the suicide rate of patients in therapy and not given LSD may be higher than one in 2500. There have been several reports of severe acute reactions after ingestion of illicit LSD (71). Severe psychotic reactions are frequent concomitants of chronic high-dose amphetamine and phenmetrazine usage, and also occur frequently in cocaine addicts. The severity of the response is compounded by the stimulant nature of the drugs, and users may attack their alleged persecutors. Methamphetamine is occasionally used with LSD, and the combination appears to increase the likelihood of acute panic reactions (56).

Some data provided by Smith (62) emphasize the tenuousness of the link between marijuana and acute psychosis. He reported that none of 5000 acute drug intoxications which were treated at San Francisco General Hospital in 1967 could be labeled "marijuana psychosis." Furthermore, of almost 30,000 patients who visited the Haight-Ashbury Medical Clinic (of which Smith is Medical Director) none were diagnosed as having marijuana psychosis—this despite the fact that almost all of them were marijuana users, and that many of their problems were drug-related.

Instances of paranoia with any illicit drug are undoubtedly increased by the user's recognition of the very real dangers of arrest and imprisonment. The most effective treatment of adverse reactions to LSD and marijuana is reassurance by others. If users begin to feel distressed, they probably seek out friends and are unlikely to commit socially deviant acts.

People who use drugs probably have informal notions of a therapeutic index: if the ratio of untoward reactions to instances of euphoria is excessive, use declines. That appears to have been the fate of methamphetamine and STP. Marijuana use, by contrast, is steadily increasing.

Long-term Effects

Arguments have been advanced that both marijuana and LSD may precipitate long-lasting psychosis or depression, and that marijuana usage leads to a permanent reduction in motivation. The charges are too important to be casually dismissed; but they should be regarded with skepticism because of the rarity with which any event of relatively short duration, other than those which produce permanent brain damage, is capable of inducing permanent profound negative changes in adult personality. The argument that LSD may push borderline individuals over the brink into psychotic behavior (45) ignores the fact that there is no sharp line of demarcation between normal and psychotic personalities. A person who is adjudged to be "on the brink" is already exhibiting signs of psychopathology; if a drug then increases the severity of the symptoms even slightly, the individual may be reclassified as a psychotic. While such an outcome is, of course, undesirable, it should be viewed in proper perspective; statements by supposed authorities to the effect that LSD is extremely dangerous "because of its capability to induce attempted or completed homicide, attempted suicides, or even prolonged psychosis," (45, p. 254) are hardly informative.

Approximately two-thirds of individuals who suffer long-lasting psychoses after LSD ingestion present a history of psychopathology prior to drug use (8). LSD is frequently taken in a last ditch effort to solve an impending crisis which has proven refractory to other attempts at solution (27). When the hoped for beneficial effects are not forthcoming, a deterioration in symptomatology may be inevitable, but it would be erroneous to conclude that LSD is the causative agent. People who take drugs are likely to attribute to them *any* unusual emotional or physiological responses, even though such responses also occur in the absence of drugs. In addition, drug users are apt to be alerted to changes, and will therefore be more sensitive to them.

When considering the possibility that LSD or marijuana may precipitate psychotic behavior, the equally plausible argument that they protect against disruption of personality by reducing stress or providing self-insights should be appraised. Grinspoon (32, p. 267) has advanced such an argument. By way of proof, he cited figures for the incidence of psychiatric disturbance during recent wars involving American troops. In Vietnam the rate was 12 per 1000 men per year, which compares favorably with the Korean War (73 per 1000) and World War II (between 28 and 101 per 1000). Grinspoon acknowledged that there are undoubtedly many factors which contributed to the change, but suggested that one important reason may be the widespread use of marijuana in the Vietnam War. Up to 65% of soldiers in Vietnam have used marijuana at least once (68).

Several authors have described a marijuana-induced "amotivational syndrome," characterized by a rejection of the American work ethic (2, 75). Timothy Leary's well-known exhortation to college students to "turn on, tune in, and drop out," is taken as a model for the behavior of the "pothead." The proof offered in support of the proposition that marijuana reduces motivation is of two sorts:

comparisons of pre- and postdrug achievement motivation of pot-
heads, and observed personality differences between users and
nonusers. Neither of these "proofs" convincingly demonstrates a
causal relationship between marijuana use and motivation, the latter
because there are pre-existing personality differences in individuals
who do and do not begin using marijuana. One obvious difference
is that people who decide to try marijuana thereby show disrespect
for the belief that people should invariably obey all laws. With
respect to the first "proof," studies involving pre- and postdrug
comparisons generally neglect changes which occur just prior to
initiation of drug use. These changes have been described by West
and Allen (75), and typically include dissatisfaction with the world,
which leads to a search for value and meaning in life and to association with other searchers. Only then does drug use start.

In one important sense, discussion of the role of marijuana in
producing the amotivational syndrome is irrelevant. The position
that accumulation of material goods is unimportant, and should not
take precedence over a search for meaning in life, is surely defensi-
ble. Many respected historical personages, such as Thoreau, Emer-
son, Gauguin, and Gandhi held such views, views which did *not*
prevent them from enriching our culture.

Claims have been made that LSD users expose themselves to a
unique psychological hazard, the flashback. A flashback is a re-
experiencing of the drug trip several months or more after it has
ended. However, flashbacks have not been shown to be dangerous,
and there is no evidence that they occur with greater frequency than
the reliving of other types of experiences by nonusers. In any event,
since people frequently relive events which have had a strong emotional impact on them, it should not be surprising that the same
occasionally occurs with LSD users.

The Escalation Theory

One of the arguments advanced against the legalization of
marijuana is that it would lead to the abuse of other drugs, particularly narcotics. The evidence against such a position is overwhelming. Jaffe (31, p. 300) asserted that the medical community has
reached the consensus that marijuana usage does not cause heroin
addiction. In fact, Chopra and Chopra (12) showed that marijuana
may be used to wean people from alcohol or opium addiction. The
history of the myth that marijuana leads to heroin addiction has been
traced by Grinspoon (32), who emphasized that it is a myth. While it
is true that a person who uses marijuana is more likely than a non-
user to experiment with other drugs (7), and that because marijuana

is illicit, users are more likely than nonusers to gain access to other illicit drugs, it is also true that only a small proportion of marijuana users try heroin (30), and only a small proportion of these become addicted (36).

There have been several national committees formed to study the effects of marijuana. All of the following — British Report of the Indian Hemp Drug Commission (1894), Mayor's Committee on Marijuana (1944), President's Advisory Commission on Narcotic and Drug Abuse (1963), President's Commission of Law Enforcement and Administration of Justice (1967), Council on Mental Health and Committee on Alcoholism and Drug Dependence (1967), British Government Advisory Committee on Drugs (1969), and National Commission on Marijuana and Drug Abuse (1972) — concluded that the assertion that marijuana leads to escalation to opiates is untenable.

Although there is no normal progression from marijuana to heroin, frequent users may turn to other drugs if cut off from their regular supply. McGlothlin et al. (52) surveyed heavy users shortly after a period in which marijuana had been unavailable (because of the government's efforts in 1969 to block the smuggling of marijuana from Mexico). Seventy-six percent of UCLA students, and 84 percent of patients in attendance at the Los Angeles Free Clinic, reported that they had increased their consumption of other drugs, including opiates and cocaine, during the period of unavailability of marijuana.

DANGERS OF DRUGS WHICH RESULT FROM SOCIETY'S ATTITUDES TOWARD THEM

The illegality of most drugs which are abused should not be ignored in assessing their risk potentials. The penalties for possession of marijuana are severe — the federal penalty is a prison term of up to one year and/or a fine of as much as $5000, and some individual state penalties are even harsher. The mere threat of incarceration may increase both the likelihood of bad trips and the likelihood that minor, easily treated problems will be compounded because of reluctance to see a physician.

Four important consequences of illegality are that (1) prices are high; (2) the purchaser cannot be certain that the product is what it is claimed to be; (3) users remain ignorant about necessary precautions to prevent communicable diseases; and (4) patterns of use are determined largely by accessibility.

High Prices

The profits in heroin trafficking are enormous. A kilogram of heroin which costs about $2500 when bought in its land of origin has a retail value on the streets of New York of about $300,000. The cost to the addict has been estimated at $50 to 75 per day, an amount which far exceeds the earning powers of virtually all habitual users. As a result, addicts resort to crime. In New York City alone, the estimated daily cost of heroin is $10 million, most of which is obtained illegally (34). In addition, the overwhelming preoccupation of the addict with obtaining heroin leads to reduced concern for health. Certain physical problems are ignored, and diet is generally seriously inadequate.

Faith in Supplier

Truth in packaging does not apply to the illicit drug market. Dealers in drugs frequently adulterate their products, and often substitute entirely different substances for the one they claim to be selling. PharmChem Laboratories, based in Palo Alto, California, has some interesting data on misrepresentation. PharmChem charges a nominal fee for the confidential analysis of drugs, a service used by many people who buy illicit drugs and then want assurances about their purchases. In their January, 1972, newsletter, PharmChem reported that only 30 percent of the samples which they analyzed were, in fact, what the sellers had alleged them to be. The figures for other months are similar. One consequence of misrepresentation is that users are unable to determine dosage accurately, which may be one reason for adverse experiences with LSD, amphetamine, and barbiturates.

Failure to Protect Against Infectious Disease

Substantial numbers of heavy users of amphetamine and of heroin are carriers of infectious disease (37). The diseases are not inevitable consequences of drug use. They occur in part because needles and syringes are difficult to obtain, and because users are ignorant of the relationship between disease and the multiple use of syringes which are meant to be discarded after single use. It is probable that most addicts sterilize neither the needle nor the site of injection. These are not pharmacological but social problems. Still, the remedy is not obvious. In Great Britain, addicts are permitted to obtain heroin from licensed physicians, but the policy has not greatly influenced the incidence of infectious disease among addicts (6).

Accessibility Determines Use

The long history of human drug use makes it apparent that the demand for drugs is unlikely to be soon eliminated. However, patterns of use do change. The popularity of particular drugs, both licit and illicit, is determined by many factors: advertising and educational efforts, availability, price, legality, and legal sanctions. Then, even if there is a clear-cut drug of choice for a particular purpose, other, more readily obtainable drugs may be used in its stead. For example, the barbiturates are best for inducing sleep despite their many shortcomings (see Chapter 15), but since barbiturates can be purchased only by prescription, many nonprescription sleeping preparations command an imposing share of the market. A related phenomenon is that attempts to curtail marijuana use may precipitate abuse of more dangerous substances. It is to be hoped that drugs like mescal beans, which fell into disfavor because of their toxicity, do not become popular again because they are inexpensive and enjoy favorable legal status.

WHY ARE DRUGS ILLEGAL?

The case has been made that most commonly abused drugs, if used intelligently, are relatively free from serious side effects. At the least, they are considerably safer than certain cherished American institutions such as football, boxing, automobile and motorcycle racing, and skiing. It is interesting to speculate on the sociological reasons which have given rise to such widespread condemnation of drugs.

Biased Sample of Cases

People who are frequently called upon to deal with drug problems are generally exposed only to bad cases. Physicians and school administrators, for instance, are called upon for guidance during bad trips. The victims are likely to condemn the use of drugs which, after all, have brought them to their wretched states. Thus, the physicians and administrators—people in positions of influence—receive distorted pictures of drug effects, although the suffering which they see is very real. They never see favorable outcomes of drug use, although such are in the vast majority.

Police and narcotics agents constitute another group which helps determine public attitudes towards drugs, and which observes a very biased sample of cases. Law-enforcement officials tend to place too simple an interpretation on the fact that the capture of big-time sellers or smugglers of illicit drugs often uncovers large-scale criminal activity. Criminality devolves from drug-dealing, not from drugs themselves; the illegality of drugs assures that enormous profits can be realized from their sale, and makes an attractive enterprise for organized crime (63), thus involving big-volume dealers who often have criminal records and associate with other criminals. It does not follow that drugs increase the criminal activity of occasional users. Nor does it follow that drugs increase the tendency toward violence—rather, people who are faced with the prospect of a long prison term for the commission of an act which they regard as harmless may take extraordinary measures to escape, including violence.

Control of Groups with Unpopular Political Views or Life Styles

The life style espoused by many spokesmen for drugs is alien to the American ethic of hard work and accumulation of material goods. It is undoubtedly true that many Americans find the hippie philosophy repugnant. Perhaps one way of attacking this philosophy is by making drug use illegal and using these laws as a means to control certain groups. However, a convincing case must be made concerning the dangers of drugs if their illegality is to be justified. Currently, the legal status of drugs has nothing to do with their toxicity or lack thereof.

REFERENCES

1. Adey, W. Computer analysis of hippocampal EEG activity and impedance in approach learning: effects of psychotomimetic and hallucinogenic drugs. *In* Mikhelson, M., Longo, V., and Votava, Z. (Eds.) *Pharmacology of Conditioning.* New York: Pergamon, 1965.
2. Allen, J., and West, L. Flight from violence: hippies and the green rebellion. Am. J. Psychiat., 1968, 125:364–370.
3. Appel, J., and Freedman, D. The relative potencies of psychotomimetic drugs. Life Sci., 1965, 4:2181–2186.
4. Ashcroft, G., Eccleston, D., and Waddell, J. Recognition of amphetamine addicts. Brit. Med. J., 1965, 1:57.
5. Baden, M. Pathological aspects of drug addiction. *Proceedings of the Committee on Problems of Drug Dependence.* Wash., D.C.: Nat. Acad. Sci., 1969.
6. Bewley, T. Heroin addiction in the United Kingdom. Brit. Med. J., 1965, 2:1284–1286.
7. Blum, R. et al. *Students and Drugs II.* San Francisco: Jossey-Bass, 1969.
8. Blumenfield, M., and Glickman, L. Ten months experience with LSD users

admitted to county psychiatric receiving hospital. N.Y.S. J. Med., 1967, 67:1849–1853.

 9. Boston Collaborative Drug Surveillance Program. Coffee drinking and acute myocardial infarction. Lancet, 1972, 2:1278–1281.
10. Brecher, E. *Licit and Illicit Drugs.* Boston: Little, Brown & Co., 1972.
11. Chein, I., Gerard, D., Lee, R., and Rosenfeld, E. *Narcotics, Delinquency, and Social Policy.* London: Tavistock, 1964.
12. Chopra, R., and Chopra, G. The present position of hemp-drug addiction in India. Indian Med. Res. Memoirs, 1939, 31:1–119.
13. Clarke, L., and Nakashima, E. Experimental studies of marihuana. Am. J. Psychiat., 1968, 125:379–384.
14. Cohen, M., Marinello, M., and Back, N. Chromosomal damage in human leukocytes induced by lysergic acid diethylamide. Science, 1967, 155:1417–1419.
15. Cohen, S. Lysergic acid diethylamide: side effects and complications. J. Nerv. Ment. Dis., 1960, 130:30–40.
16. Connell, P. Clinical manifestations and treatment of amphetamine type of dependence. J.A.M.A., 1966, 196:718–723.
17. Council on Mental Health and Committee on Alcoholism and Drug Dependence. Dependence on cannabis (marijuana). J.A.M.A., 1967, 201:368–371.
18. Crancer, A., Dille, J., Delay, J., Wallace, J., and Haykin, M. Comparison of the effects of marihuana and alcohol on simulated driving performance. Science, 1969, 164:851–854.
19. DiMascio, A., and Shader, R. Behavioral toxicity. *In* Efron, D. (Ed.) *Psychopharmacology: A Review of Progress.* U.S. PHS Pub. No. 1836, 1968.
20. Dishotsky, N., Loughman, W., Mogar, R., and Lipscomb, W. LSD and genetic damage. Science, 1971, 172:431–440.
21. Domino, E. Neuropsychopharmacologic studies of marijuana: some synthetic and natural THC derivatives in animals and man. Ann. N.Y. Acad. Sci., 1971, 191:166–191.
22. Duker, H. Über Die Wirkung von Pharmaka auf die geistige Tätigkeit voll leistungsfähiger Personen. Arzneimittel-Forschung, 1964, 14:570–573.
23. Freedman, D. The psychopharmacology of hallucinogenic agents. Ann. Rev. Med., 1969, 20:409–418.
24. Freedman, D. The use and abuse of psychedelic drugs. Bull. Atom. Sci., April, 1968, 6–14.
25. Garriott, J., King, L., Forney, R., and Hughes, F. Effects of some tetrahydrocannabinols on hexobarbital sleeping time and amphetamine induced hyperactivity in mice. Life Sci., 1967, 6:2119–2128.
26. Geber, W., and Schramm, L. Effect of marihuana extract on fetal hamsters and rabbits. Toxicol. Applied Pharmacol., 1969, 14:276–282.
27. Glickman, L., and Blumenfield, M. Psychological determinants of "LSD reactions." J. Nerv. Ment. Dis., 1967, 145:79–83.
28. Goetzl, F. A note on the possible usefulness of wine in the management of anorexia. Oakland, Calif.: Permanente Foundation, 1953.
29. Goldstein, A., Kaizer, S., and Whitby, O. Psychotropic effects of caffeine in man. IV. Quantitative and qualitative differences associated with habituation to coffee. Clin. Pharmacol. Ther., 1969, 10:489–497.
30. Goode, E. Multiple drug use among marijuana smokers. Social Prob., 1969, 17:48–64.
31. Goodman, L., and Gilman, A. (Eds.) *The Pharmacological Basis of Therapeutics.* New York: Macmillan, 1965.
32. Grinspoon, L. *Marihuana Reconsidered.* Cambridge: Harvard, 1971.
33. *The Health Consequences of Smoking.* U.S. PHS Pub. No. 1696, 1967.
34. Hekimian, L., and Gershon, S. Characteristics of drug abusers admitted to a psychiatric hospital. J.A.M.A., 1968, 205:125–130.
35. Helwig, F. Beverage alcohol and heart disease. J. Missouri M.A., 1940, 37:204–206.
36. Hoch, P. Comments on narcotic addiction. Comp. Psychiat., 1963, 4:143.
37. Howard, J., and Borges, P. Needle sharing in the Haight: some social and psychological functions. *In* Smith, D. and Gay, G. (Eds.) *It's So Good Don't Even Try it Once.* Englewood Cliffs, N.J.: Prentice-Hall, 1972.

38. Joslin, E. *The Treatment of Diabetes Mellitus.* Phila.: Lea and Febiger, 1959.
39. Kalant, H. Marihuana and simulated driving. Science, 1969: 640.
40. Kew, M., Bersohn, I., and Siew, S. Possible hepatotoxicity of cannabis. Lancet, 1969, *1*:578–579.
41. Kotin, P. The cigarette-lung cancer imbroglio and public opinion. J.A.M.A., 1970, *211*:506.
42. Leake, C., and Silverman, M. *Alcoholic Beverages in Clinical Medicine.* Cleveland: World, 1966.
43. Lintz, W. Practical consideration of essential hypertension. Clin. Med., 1934, *41*:534–543.
44. Lolli, G. Role of wine in treatment of obesity. N.Y. J. Med., 1962, *62*:3438–3443.
45. Louria, D. Abuse of lysergic acid diethylamide—an increasing problem. *In* Wilson, C. (Ed.) *Adolescent Drug Dependence.* Oxford: Pergamon, 1968.
46. Lucas, O., and Jacques, L. Effects of E-A.C.A in spontaneous hemorrhage due to stress with anticoagulants in rats. Can. J. Physiol. Pharmacol., 1964, *42*: 803–808.
47. Markowitz, E., and Klotz, J. LSD and chromosomes. J.A.M.A., 1970, *211*:1699.
48. Marshman, J. and Gibbins, R. The credibility gap in the illicit drug market. Addictions, 1969, *16*:22–25.
49. Master, A., Dack, S., and Jaffe, H. Factors and events associated with onset of coronary artery thrombosis. J.A.M.A., 1937, *109*:546–549.
50. Mayor's Committee on Marihuana. *The Marihuana Problem in the City of New York.* Lancaster, Penna.: Cattell, 1944.
51. McGlothlin, W., Sparkes, R., and Arnold, D. Effect of LSD on human pregnancy. J.A.M.A., 1970, *212*:1483–1487.
52. McGlothlin, W., Jamison, K., and Rosenblatt, S. Marijuana and the use of other drugs. Nature, 1970, *228*:1227–1229.
53. Oswald, I., and Thacore, V. Amphetamine and phenmetrazine addiction: physiological abnormalities in the abstinence syndrome. Brit. Med. J., 1965, *1*:57.
54. Pearl, R. *Alcohol and Longevity.* New York: Knopf, 1926.
55. Persaud, T., and Ellington, A. The effects of Cannabis sativa L. (ganja) on developing rat embryos—preliminary observations. West Ind. Med. J., 1968, *17*: 232–234.
56. Reidenberg, M., and Lowenthal, D. Adverse nondrug reactions. New Eng. J. Med., 1968, *279*:678–679.
57. Reimann, H. Caffeinism. A cause of long-continued low-grade fever. J.A.M.A. 1967, *202*:1105–1106.
58. Russell, M. Cigarette smoking: natural history of a dependence disorder. Brit. J. Med. Psychol., 1971, *44*:1–16.
59. San Francisco Chronicle, March 2, 1971.
60. San Francisco Chronicle, April 3, 1971.
61. Seltzer, C. Constitution and heredity in relation to tobacco smoking. Ann. N.Y. Acad. Sci., 1967, *142*:322–330.
62. Smith, D. Acute and chronic toxicity of marijuana. J. Psychedelic Drugs, 1968, *2*:37–47.
63. Smith, D., and Gay, G. Introduction. *In* Smith, D. and Gay, G. (Eds.) *It's So Good Don't Even Try it Once.* Englewood Cliffs, N.J.: Prentice-Hall, 1972.
64. Smith, D., and Rose, A. The use and abuse of LSD in Haight-Ashbury. Clin. Pediat., 1968, *7*:317–322.
65. *Smoking and Health.* Report of the Advisory Committee to the Surgeon General of the Public Health Service (Washington). U.S. PHS Pub. No. 1103, 1964.
66. Snyder, S. *Uses of Marijuana.* New York: Oxford, 1971.
67. Song, S., and Rubin, E. Ethanol produces muscle damage in human volunteers. Science, 1972, *175*:327–328.
68. Talbott, J., and Teague, J. Marihuana psychosis: acute psychosis associated with the use of cannabis derivatives. J.A.M.A., 1969, *210*:299–302.
69. Tennant, F., and Groesbeck, C. Psychiatric effects of hashish. Arch. Gen. Psychiat., 1972, *27*:133–136.
70. Tennant, F., and Prendergast, T. Medical manifestations associated with hashish. J.A.M.A., 1971, *216*:1965–1969.

71. *Time* Magazine, June 29, 1970.
72. Ungerleider, J., Fisher, D., and Fuller, M. The dangers of LSD. J.A.M.A., 1966, *197*:389–392.
73. Weil, A. Adverse reactions to marihuana. New Eng. J. Med., 1970, *282*:997–1000.
74. Weil, A., Zinberg, N., and Nelsen, J. Clinical and psychological effects of marihuana in man. Science, 1968, *162*:1234–1242.
75. West, L. and Allen, J. Three rebellions: red, black, and green. *In* Masserman, J. (Ed.) *The Dynamics of Dissent: Scientific Proceedings of the American Academy of Psychoanalysis.* New York: Grune and Stratton, 1968.
76. Williams, E., Himmelsbach, C., Wikler, A., Ruble, D., and Lloyd, B. Studies on marijuana and pyrahexyl compound. Pub. Health Rep. No. 2732, 1946, *61*: 1059–1083.
77. Wilson, C. (Ed.) *Adolescent Drug Dependence.* Oxford: Pergamon, 1968.

CHAPTER 5

PROFILES OF
DRUG USERS

Any book which attempts to characterize people who use drugs is out of date even before it is published. The reason is that patterns of use have been changing with extreme rapidity, and many once taboo substances are now sanctioned by large segments of society, even though the legal status of the substances may remain unchanged. Therefore, while many of the studies cited in this chapter are useful because they indicate very general characteristics of users, others are of little more than historic interest.

Even works of recent vintage are often misleading because they set up a false dichotomy between users and nonusers, while they neglect distinctions between one-time experimenters, occasional indulgers, and heavy abusers. Such distinctions are vital. For example, occasional low dose use of amphetamine improves performance, and moderate indulgence in alcohol may increase longevity — but heavy use of either endangers both physical and emotional health.

Many studies yield differences between abstainers and users which, although statistically significant, are unimpressive. When many subjects are used, even very small differences between groups will show up as significant.* Bakan (4) illustrated the point by ob-

*Statistical significance refers to the probability that observed differences between two or more groups are due to chance factors. Significance in scientific research generally implies probability values of .05 or less, which means that the likelihood that differences between groups are due to chance is less than 1 in 20. However, although differences between two groups may be genuine, i.e., not due to chance, they may nevertheless be very small and of no practical consequence.

taining data on 60,000 subjects and then arbitrarily dividing them into such groups as east versus west of the Mississippi, and Maine versus the rest of the country. All of his results were statistically significant, although of no predictive value. Smith (76), who was interested in personality characteristics of smokers, elaborated upon the point. He said that if members of two groups, e.g., smokers and nonsmokers, meaningfully differ with respect to some trait, then measurement of the trait should enable accurate assignment of individuals to the groups. Smith found that the accuracy of classification in most studies of smokers ranges from 50 percent, which is chance, to 60 percent.

A final important introductory point, which has already been emphasized ad nauseum, is that interpretation of differences is difficult. If users of and abstainers from a drug differ with respect to some trait, it may be that drug use modifies expression of the trait, or that people with characteristic amounts of the trait tend toward use of the drug, or that some other factor influences both drug use and expression of the trait.

OVERVIEW

An important study by Davis and Miller (26) is one of the very few well-controlled demonstrations of the genesis of a drug habit. They used rats as subjects, and amobarbital as the drug. The rats were randomly assigned to one of four groups, two of which received brief electric shocks every 60 seconds for one hour per day. Rats in groups 3 and 4 did not receive shocks. Rats in group 1 (shocked) and group 3 (unshocked) had access to a lever which, when pressed, caused them to be injected with a small dose of amobarbital. Each rat in group 2 was paired with an animal in group 1, and each rat in group 3 was paired with one in group 4. Although the levers of the rats in groups 2 and 4 were nonfunctional, the animals received a dose of amobarbital every time the rat with which they were paired pressed the lever which prompted injection.

Rats in groups two to four were indistinguishable from each other in bar pressing, while rats in group 1 pressed significantly more often. The similarity of groups 2 and 4 showed that shock by itself does not increase lever pressing, and the similarity of groups 3 and 4 showed that amobarbital is not rewarding to rats under all circumstances. The increased responding of rats in the first group showed that animals which are subjected to a painful stimulus will, if given the opportunity, self-inject amobarbital. The authors suggested that the amobarbital might act by reducing either fear or pain. Their finding, that a painful, unpleasant life situation increases drug use, presages much of the work with humans.

The person who takes two aspirins whenever he has slight head pains, or who takes pills to help fall asleep, stay awake, lose weight, or have bowel movements with clocklike regularity, is akin to the marijuana smoker or heroin user—that is, whether the drug is licit or illicit, whether it induces profound alterations in psychological and physiological functioning or has only very mild effects, the reliance upon chemical substances to alleviate problems identifies a certain character type. The greater the use of unusual drugs, the more probable the use of ordinary ones (9, p. 114). Among those who tend toward the greatest use of legal nonprescription drugs are nervous mothers, firstborn children, and people who are above average in visits to physicians (45), and these same characteristics (plus others) apply to users of illicit substances.

Brehm and Back (11) asked students in an introductory psychology class to answer a questionnaire on their willingness to try various drugs. Those who were most willing to use social stimulants (tobacco, alcohol, and caffeine-containing beverages) were also most willing to use illicit drugs (amphetamines, hallucinogens, and opiates). For men, and to a lesser extent for women, there was also a relationship between willingness to use sedatives (e.g., sleeping pills), and willingness to use both social stimulants and illicit

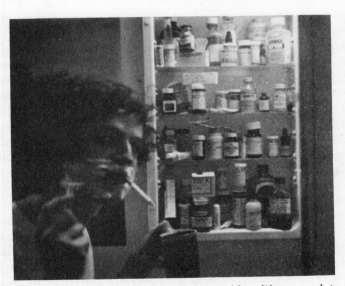

Figure 5–1 "Me smoke pot? You must be crazy. I love life too much to ever get hooked on drugs."

drugs. For both sexes, students who indicated the greatest willingness to use drugs were judged to be the most insecure, regardless of the type of drug. Curiosity was a powerful motivator for those who were willing to try illicit drugs. Those who were most willing also expressed least fear of losing control of themselves.

Blum et al. (10) showed that there is no sharp line of demarcation between users of licit and illicit drugs. They interviewed 200 people in the San Francisco Bay region, and asked them to describe their drug experiences. They then divided the respondents, on the basis of their answers, into four groups:

1. Two people had had no experience with any drug type.

2. Twenty-eight people had used one or more of the following: aspirin or related substances, alcoholic beverages, tobacco, pain killers, and laxatives.

3. One hundred and thirty-five people had used one or more of the above plus any of the following: drugs for control of anxiety, sleep aids, health and appearance aids, wake-ups and stay-awakes, drugs for allergy, birth control drugs, weight control drugs, amphetamines, and antidepressants.

4. Thirty-four people had used one or more drugs from each of the other two groups, plus any of the following: marijuana, proprietary remedies for kicks, heroin, cocaine, hallucinogens, volatile intoxicants, and drugs for altering sexual desires.

Table 5.1 lists the various drugs and indicates that experience with certain types is associated with a wide variety of drug experiences. For example, from Table 5.1 it can be seen that among people who had tried marijuana at least once, the *minimal* number of drug experiences was seven.

Those respondents who reported heavy or high drug usage may be labeled H, comprising groups 3 and 4. Groups 1 and 2 may be labeled together as L, for low or light usage of drugs. The differences between H and L in Blum's study are worth noting. Subjects in groups 3 and 4 (H) reported that they kept more drugs at home, and had more faith in the curative powers of drugs when they were sick than did the respondents in groups 1 and 2 (L). H reported more serious childhood illnesses, more medication during childhood, and also more advantages to being sick than did L. The present subjective states of health were equivalent for H and L, but H visited their doctors more frequently. H had less favorable home environments as children. Their parents were more often disliked, and tended to react negatively to outbursts of excitement or anger. H also had less favorable adult personality traits; they were more dissatisfied than L with self, job, and relations with others. H more often reported cravings for love, emotion, and for particular foods. They

TABLE 5.1 Minimal Number of Other Drug Experiences Reported by Persons Using Each Drug on the Inquiry Spectrum*

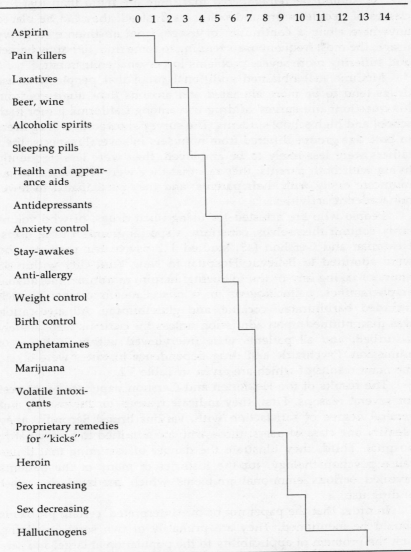

	0	1	2	3	4	5	6	7	8	9	10	11	12	13	14
Aspirin															
Pain killers															
Laxatives															
Beer, wine															
Alcoholic spirits															
Sleeping pills															
Health and appearance aids															
Antidepressants															
Anxiety control															
Stay-awakes															
Anti-allergy															
Weight control															
Birth control															
Amphetamines															
Marijuana															
Volatile intoxicants															
Proprietary remedies for "kicks"															
Heroin															
Sex increasing															
Sex decreasing															
Hallucinogens															

*From Blum, R., Braunstein, L., and Stone, A. Normal drug use: an exploratory study of patterns and correlates. *In* Cole, J., and Wittenborn, J. (eds.), *Drug Abuse* (Springfield: Charles C Thomas, 1969), p. 71.

had more frequent extreme dislikes of particular foods and activities. They had more past and present eating problems. Overall, the respondents grouped as H tended to be younger, went to church less frequently, and were better educated than L. In summary, however, it should be remembered that there are more than just two classes of people, users and nonusers. Instead, they can be placed anywhere along a continuum of usage, from abstinence to heavy usage, the most frequent users tending to come from unhappy homes and suffering more severe problems in personal adjustment.

McCune (54) obtained additional proof that people who use drugs tend to be more alienated and anxious than nonusers from his questionnaire survey of drug use among California junior high school and high school students. The survey showed that drug users in both age groups differed from nonusers in several respects: their fathers were less likely to be employed; they were less frequently living with both parents; they felt that they were less able to communicate easily with their parents; and they participated in fewer nonacademic activities.

People who are arrested for using illicit drugs, or who voluntarily commit themselves, constitute a special group of drug users. Hekimian and Gershon (43) studied 112 psychiatric patients who were admitted to Bellevue Hospital in New York City within 48 hours of taking any of the following: heroin, morphine, marijuana, amphetamines, hallucinogens, or a miscellaneous category which included barbiturates, cocaine, and glutethimide. All medication was discontinued upon admission unless the patients were acutely disturbed, and all patients were interviewed within 24 hours of admission. Psychiatric and drug dependence histories were taken, the main results of which are given in Table 5.2.

The results of the Hekimian and Gershon paper are of interest for several reasons. First, they indicate reasons for the use of, and general degree of satisfaction with, various drugs. Secondly, they identify one class of users: those who are admitted to a psychiatric hospital. Third, they illustrate the danger of assuming that drugs cause psychopathology, for the histories of many of the patients revealed serious emotional problems which predated the onset of drug use.

In order that the paper not be overinterpreted, certain problems should be mentioned. They are primarily of two sorts, involving first the problem of applicability to the population at large, and second the source of the information. As regards the first, generalizations about personality characteristics of typical drug takers should not be attempted; the Hekimian and Gershon sample is nonrandom, for only a small proportion of people who take illicit drugs are ever apprehended or commit themselves as a result. It is not surprising that psychiatrists estimated that most of the subject patients had be-

TABLE 5.2 Data on Psychiatric Patients Admitted to Bellevue Hospital for Drug Abuse*

A. – HISTORY AND PREADMISSION DATA

Patient Group, No.	Mean Age, Yr	Sex M	Sex F	Family History of Drug Abuse or Psychiatric Treatment	Patient's Reason for Taking Drug				Other Drugs Taken by	Previous Psychiatric Treatment	Predrug Psychiatric Diagnosis			
					Desire for Euphoria	Influenced by Friends or Environment	Curiosity	Other Reasons or None			Schizophrenia	Sociopath Personality	Other Personality Disorder	Depression, Neurosis, or Other
Heroin 22	29.5	21	1	†	†	†	†	†	19	†	2	11	2	7
10	29.9	10	0	2	6	2	2	0	9	7	0	3	2	5
Marijuana 8	24.4	6	2	1	3	4	0	1	6	7	6	0	1	1
Amphetamine 22	24.8	18	4	5	12	4	2	4	18	13	9	4	2	7
Hallucinogen 47	22.0	34	13	12	19	9	12	7	40	24	23	6	10	8
Miscellaneous 13	31.3	5	8	0	8	3	1	1	12	11	3	3	2	5

†Complete data was not obtained.

(Table continued on following page.)

TABLE 5.2 Data on Psychiatric Patients Admitted to Bellevue Hospital for Drug Abuse* (*Continued*)

B. – ADMISSION AND POSTDRUG INGESTION DATA

Patient Group, No.	Patients' Subjective Effects or Responses		Effect of Drug Ingestion on Admission		Criminality Associated With Drug Abuse	Final Psychiatric Diagnosis				Disposition	
	Favorable	Unfavorable	Psychosis or Increase of Psychopathology	Symptoms Relieved or No Effect		Schizophrenia	Sociopath Personality	Other Personality Disorder	Depression, Neurosis, or Other	Hospitalization	Home
Heroin											
22	†	†	†	†	†	3	15	1	3	4	18
10	10	0	9	1	7	1	6	1	2	2	8
Marijuana											
8	5	3	7	1	0	6	0	1	1	4	4
Amphetamine											
22	16	6	22	0	4	11	5	2	4	8	14
Hallucinogen											
47	15	32	43	4	6	32	6	4	5	16	31
Miscellaneous											
13	10	3	13	0	4	3	5	0	5	2	11

†Complete data was not obtained.

(Table continued on opposite page.)

TABLE 5.2 Data on Psychiatric Patients Admitted to Bellevue Hospital for Drug Abuse* (Continued)

C. — PROMINENT FEATURES OF EACH DRUG GROUP

Patient Group, No.	Patients' Reason for Taking Drug (%)	Other Drugs Taken by (%)	Previous Psychiatric Treatment (%)	Predrug Psychiatric Diagnosis (%)	Patients' Subjective Response to Drug (%)	Psychosis or Increased Psychopathology Due to Drug (%)	Criminality Associated with Drug (%)	Final Psychiatric Diagnosis (%)	Disposition (%)
Heroin 22	Desire for euphoria 60	87	70	Sociopathic personality 50	Favorable 100	90	70	Sociopathic personality 68	Home 82
Marijuana 8	Friends or environment 50	75	88	Schizophrenic reaction 75	Favorable 63	88	0	Schizophrenic reaction 75	Home 50
Amphetamine 2	Desire for euphoria 55	82	59	Schizophrenic reaction 41	Favorable 73	100	18	Schizophrenic reaction 50	Home 64
Hallucinogen 47	Desire for euphoria 40	85	51	Schizophrenic reaction 49	Unfavorable 68	66	13	Schizophrenic reaction 68	Home 66
Miscellaneous 13	Desire for euphoria 62	93	85	Depression or other 38	Favorable 77	100	31	Sociopathic personality 31 Depression or other 31	Home 85

†Complete data was not obtained.
*From Hekimian, L., and Gershon, S. Characteristics of drug abusers admitted to a psychiatric hospital. J.A.M.A., 1968, 205: p. 127. Copyright 1968, American Medical Association.

come more seriously psychopathic because of the drugs; after all, their psychopathy was the reason for their admittance.

The second problem concerns the actual sources of the study data. Much of the information came from patients who were in psychotic states, and who could hardly have been expected to be reliable witnesses. For example, one patient claimed to have taken 400 doses of 1500 μg LSD over a period of two years. The dose is extremely large, since an average dose is 100 to 350 μg. In addition, tolerance to LSD develops rapidly, so that an administration schedule of more than every other day would greatly reduce the effects of the drug. The patient's claim invites doubt, and of course another reason for distrusting the testimony of all the patients is that they may have been deceived as to the drug which they had ingested (see Chap. 4).

An additional problem concerns the procedure of grouping patients according to the drug responsible for their admission. Most were taking other drugs (see Table 5.2), and some had taken the drug for which they were admitted only once or twice. Thus the patients could with considerable justification have been assigned differently.

Finally, psychiatric diagnosis is not an unassailable procedure. The reliability and validity of diagnoses have been the subject of much criticism (51, 62).

Simmons and Winograd (73) developed a different perspective on youthful drug users, at least of the California variety. They asserted that users regard excitation of the senses and the emotions as among the most meaningful of all experiences, and that drugs are valued as catalysts for such experiences. Simmons and Winograd described the emergence of a "hang-loose" ethic among users, characterized by rejection of traditional American values such as those of hard work, devotion, and respect for institutions. Suchman (78) further elaborated upon these views. He surveyed students from a West Coast university and found that drug use was associated with nonconformist behavior, reading of underground newspapers, opposition to the Vietnam War, mass protests, and atheism. While the data are nice to have, as data are always more valuable than intuitions, the results should have come as no surprise. The drugs which were being studied are illegal. Users break the law. Therefore, it would be expected that most users are people who have no great respect for the law, or at least feel that some laws are bad and should not be followed blindly. By virtue of the fact that use of the drugs is criminal, they may come to regard themselves as criminals, opposed to the values espoused by most members of their society. Since liberal politicians have tended to advocate relaxation of penalties against drugs, youthful users would be expected to embrace a liberal philosophy.

MARIJUANA

Zinberg and Weil (87) compared nonusers of marijuana with those who had used the drug at least once and those who were chronic users. One finding, which is consistent with others which have already been cited, is that use of hard drugs varied directly with marijuana use. On the other hand, most chronic marijuana users rarely partook of alcohol, and among occasional users drinking varied inversely with marijuana usage. Chronic users were more radical politically than were members of the other two groups. They had had more serious family disturbances, and these were reflected in current personality aberrations. Several of the chronic users scored beyond the normal range on a personality scale which had compulsivity at one end and hysteria at the other; they also evidenced greater anxiety and paranoia. Nonusers tended to be the most compulsive of the three groups (compulsivity measured the desire for control over life situations, especially emotions, and the maintenance of emotional distance from others). The scores of occasional users ranged toward hysteria (indicating ready access to emotions and more direct relationships with others, but at the expense of the ability to organize one's life and resist suggestion).

Robins et al. (66) studied long-term adjustments of marijuana users and nonusers. Again, users had increased difficulty in adjusting to society. Compared to nonusers, users were less likely to have graduated from high school (a finding at odds with Blum's, that high drug users tended to be better educated), were less faithful to their spouses, had more illegitimate children, more frequently required financial aid, had adult records for nondrug criminal offenses, and were more likely to become violent. Students who use marijuana have more criminal convictions than nonusers (reported in Ref. 61). In the Robins et al. study, marijuana users drank more than nonusers, which indicates that the relationship between marijuana and alcohol use is complex.

King (48, 49) submitted questionnaires on drug use to Dartmouth College students and graduates. Of the respondents, 16.7 percent reported that they had used marijuana but not LSD; another 3.7 percent had used both drugs; and 79.7 percent had used neither. The primary difference between users and nonusers was that the former were more strongly opposed to any form of external control. This was shown by their greater opposition to regulations, whether in the form of college curfews, prohibitions against sexual intercourse, or bans on cigarette advertising. Users and nonusers did not differ on college entrance examinations scores or grade point averages. Their personalities, as assessed by the Minnesota Multiphasic Personality Inventory, were similar.

TOBACCO

Tobacco firms did not accept passively the Surgeon General's report on the adverse health consequences of smoking. They sponsored research aimed at uncovering differences between smokers (S) and nonsmokers (N) which predated the onset of smoking. Several such differences were found between nonsmokers and the 70 million Americans who smoke more than 550 billion cigarettes per year. In fact, differences were shown to exist between cigarette, cigar, and pipe smokers (2). More men smoke than women (3), and men have more favorable attitudes toward smoking than do women, even when the sexes are equated for amount of smoking (3). Not surprisingly, attitudes of N were least favorable to smoking, while present S were more favorable than former S. Present S were also less inclined to believe that smoking causes cancer. In general, people who scored highest on college entrance examinations had the most favorable attitudes toward smoking, whether they themselves smoked or not (3).

The statistical analyses in Baer's experiments are questionable on two counts. First, he tested a great many measures, and some would be expected to be significant by chance alone. Secondly, he used one-tailed tests, which always may be inappropriate (13), but are certainly so when there is no prior reason for expecting differences between groups to be in a particular direction.

Eysenck (33) suggested that extroverts smoke more than introverts. Smith (76), however, noted that the experiments upon which Eysenck based his conclusions actually revealed extremely small differences between S and N; the differences reached significance because very large numbers of subjects were used. Kanekar and Dolke (47) found a more substantial relationship between extroversion scores and smoking, as did Smith. Kanekar and Dolke also found that S were more neurotic than N.

Smith found several self-report measures which discriminated between S and N. The most powerful was "order." S had less need for or interest in maintaining order and organization in their activities. The accuracy of classification for "order" scores was 59 percent. That is, when individuals were given a test which measured "order," and those who scored above the mean were classified as N, and those below the mean as S, 59 percent of the subjects were correctly assigned. S were also less deferent than N, and scored higher on a measure of heterosexuality, according to their own self-reports. When rated by their peers, S were found to be less adaptable than N, along with being less tender, self-effacing, trusting, and good-natured; they were more prone to jealousy, more assertive, attention-seeking, and demanding. In sum, they were judged to be less agreeable to their peers than were N. S were also judged to have less strength of character, and to be more tense, easily upset, and emotional. They were rated as being more crude and unmannerly. The accuracy of classification of S versus N, when several factors (agreeableness, extroversion, strength of character, emotionality, and refinement) were combined, was 68 percent; for N versus heavy smokers, the accuracy was 76 percent.

There is considerable evidence that S and N differ physically. Brown (12) showed that EEG patterns were different, S having a higher frequency EEG than that of N. High frequency EEG is generally accompanied by nonrhythmic, low amplitude waves, but the wave form for the EEG of S is rhythmic and of high amplitude. EEG responses to photic stimulation were also different in the S and N groups. S breathe more slowly than N (42), and have a reduced pulmonary capacity (37). Smokers' heart rates both during rest and after vigorous exercise are higher (19). Their cholesterol levels are also higher than those of nonsmokers (80).

Seltzer (70) claimed that many of the differences between S and N antedate the onset of smoking. He studied college sophomores, many of whom, he argued, had not yet begun smoking. Those who subsequently began to smoke were found to be taller and heavier than the others who did not smoke. There were some other small differences in bodily dimensions between the groups.

Seltzer's results were challenged by Livson and Stewart (52). One criticism was that 40 to 55 percent of male smokers have already begun smoking by the age at which Seltzer's subjects were tested. Moreover, despite having a large number of subjects (922), when N were compared separately with each of three groups of "pure" smokers (cigarettes only, pipe only, cigars only), some of the differences were no longer significant. Pure cigarette smokers differed least from N (despite the fact that death rates are highest for cigarette smokers). Livson and Stewart suggested that all of the observed differences might have resulted from one primary one, that cigarette smokers were heavier. They made an important observation for those who would use Seltzer's data to invalidate the claim that smoking causes lung cancer: the more one smokes, the greater one's risk of getting cancer; if it were not smoking, but inherited constitutional factors such as tendency to large body size which contributed to cancer, then heavy smokers would be tallest. However, in Seltzer's study the moderate smokers were taller and heavier than both nonsmokers and heavy smokers.

Livson and Stewart collected their own data. They found no differences for any anthropometric measurement of subjects tested at ages 12 and 18 who eventually did and did not become smokers. Baer (2) also found no differences in the weight or ponderal index (a ratio of body weight to stature) of smokers and nonsmokers. Moderate smokers were shorter than heavy smokers, a difference in the opposite direction from that found by Seltzer.

Despite the criticisms of Seltzer's study, there *is* abundant evidence that S and N differ genetically. Fisher (34, 35) employed a paradigm which is valuable for separating genetic from environmental influences, namely, the comparison of identical with fraternal twins. The rationale for the comparison is that differences in environment are approximately equal for pairs of identical twins and pairs of fraternals; therefore, if identical twins are more similar in some trait than are fraternals, the reason must be that only the identical twins have the same heredity. Fisher found that identical twins were much more similar in smoking habits than were fraternal twins.

Carney (15) and Carney et al. (16) analyzed the amount of sex chromatin in buccal (cheek) smears and blood neutrophils (mature white blood cells) of S and N. Sex chromatin is an extra bit of chromosomal material which had been believed to occur in over 25 percent of buccal cells of normal females, but not in the cells of normal males (56). However, the two Carney studies found that sex chromatin was highest in people who had at any time smoked regularly, whether they did so currently or not. Among women, heavy smokers had more sex chromatin than light smokers, but men who were heavy smokers had less sex chromatin than men who were light smokers. It is possible but unlikely that smoking affects sex chromatin, and more likely that amount of sex chromatin affects predisposition to smoke, so the results suggest a genetic basis for smoking. However, because most authorities claim that normal men do not have sex chromatin, the results should be regarded with caution.

Cohen and Thomas (20) found that people with blood type B were less likely to be heavy smokers than were people with other blood types, and the same authors reported that a higher proportion of S than N can taste phenylthiourea (81). The capacity to taste phenylthiourea has a well-established genetic basis.

It should be emphasized that although constitutional factors may influence smoking behavior, they do not by themselves account for the poor health of smokers. It has been firmly established that chronic smoking is hazardous. One type of confirmatory evidence is that animals exposed to cigarette smoke develop malignant growths (57, 71); a second is that the mortality risk of people who stop smoking, compared with others of their same age who continue, is reduced, and the discrepancy between the two groups increases with duration of time discontinued (27).

PSYCHOTROPICS

Parry (63) defined all of the following as psychotropic drugs: sedatives, such as barbiturates and nonprescription drugs that help

TABLE 5.3 Proportions of Demographic Groups in a National Sample Who Used Psychotropic Drugs in Past 12 Months*

Groups	Number of Respondents (unweighted)	Percent Using Any Type	Seda-tives	Tran-quilizers	Stimu-lants
TOTAL U.S. SAMPLE	2,071	24	11	15	7
Sex					
Men	991	15	7	9	3
Women	1,080	31	13	20	9
Age (years)					
18–20	95	25	4	12	14
21–29	408	26	9	15	9
30–39	417	26	11	16	9
40–49	417	26	12	16	7
50–59	347	18	7	14	4
60 years or over	452	23	14	14	2
Education					
Less than high school completed	899	23	10	15	5
High school completed	641	25	10	15	9
Some college	512	24	12	15	7
Occupation					
Professional	254	24	11	15	7
Managerial	215	31	12	15	10
Clerical, sales	208	25	9	15	7
Craftsman, foreman	391	25	9	17	9
Other manual, service	505	20	9	13	5
Farmer, farm laborer	134	19	8	10	4
Population of home town					
Rural	589	25	12	15	7
2,500–99,999	412	26	13	15	7
100,000–999,999	468	24	10	15	7
1,000,000 or over	602	22	8	14	6
Region					
Northeast	510	21	11	13	5
North Central	651	24	11	12	8
South	602	27	12	19	5
West	308	23	7	14	9
Income					
Under $5,000	640	22	12	14	4
$5,000–$6,999	519	20	9	11	5
$7,000–$9,999	437	24	11	14	7
$10,000 or over	445	31	10	20	11
Race					
White	1,703	26	11	16	7
Negro	211	13	7	8	2
Religion					
Protestant	1,294	23	10	15	6
Catholic	474	24	10	13	8
Jewish	43	47	21	36	8

*From Parry, H. Use of psychotropic drugs by U.S. adults. Public Health Report 1968, *83*: p. 119.

TABLE 5.4 Proportion of Adults in California and in Selected Subgroups Reporting Frequent Use of One or More of Three Drug Types— Stimulants, Sedatives, and Tranquilizers*

	STIMULANTS %	SEDATIVES %	TRANQUILIZERS %	ANY OF THE THREE %	BASE FOR PERCENT
All Adults	6	7	10	17	1,026
Sex					
Male	4	5	6	12	527
Female	8	8	14	22	499
Age					
21–29	8	3	7	13	210
30–39	10	4	12	21	197
40–49	6	7	11	17	230
50–59	4	8	11	18	161
60+	2	11	8	16	228
Marital Status					
Married	6	6	10	16	813
Single	7	7	3	14	73
Widowed	4	14	10	20	80
Separated-divorced	8	10	18	27	60
Race					
White	6	7	9	17	909
Negro	5	10	15	19	78
Other	5	5	13	15	39
Education					
Grade school graduate	4	8	10	16	315
High school graduate	5	6	9	16	287
Some college	9	6	9	19	255
College graduate or more	7	6	11	17	169
Family Income†					
$3,000	5	10	10	19	122
$3–5,000	6	5	8	14	118
$5–7,000	6	8	9	18	171
$7–10,000	6	5	11	16	227
$10–15,000	7	5	8	16	238
$15,000 or more	5	8	11	20	134
Respondent's Occupation					
Professional, technician, etc.	8	6	8	17	192
Clerical	8	10	9	18	79
Sales	9	9	10	22	67
Skilled craftsmen	5	4	2	9	97
Service and semi-skilled	3	1	9	12	98
Laborers	0	0	3	3	37
Males not in labor force	1	11	8	16	118
Females not in labor force	7	7	14	21	338

*Reprinted from *California's Health*, Feb., 1969, 26:8, p. 6, with permission of California State Department of Health.

†Omitted from this table were 16 persons for whom income data were not ascertained.

one fall asleep; tranquilizers, such as diazepam, chlordiazepoxide, and Compoz; and stimulants, such as amphetamines and NoDoz. The nationwide use of these drugs was detailed by Parry (from two surveys, with a total sample size of about 6500 people), and are summarized in Table 5.3. The findings may be contrasted with those of Table 5.4, which summarizes the results of a survey of adults in California (31, p. 30). Two items on which both surveys agree are that more women use psychotropics than do men, and that tranquilizers are more widely used than stimulants. The sex difference contrasts with the findings of Blackford (8) on drug use among California students from the seventh grade through high school. Boys used more marijuana, alcohol, and LSD (and other hallucinogens), than did the girls, but amphetamine and tobacco use were distributed evenly among the boys and girls. It is possible that higher proportions of boys than girls "mature out" of drug habits. Blackford also found that use of all drugs was greater in 1969 than in 1968. Perhaps attitudes relating to drug use are changing, so that although there may have been the same number of users in both years, they may have been more ready to acknowledge their habits in 1969 than in 1968.

AMPHETAMINES

Psychiatric patients who used amphetamines reported their sexual adjustment as being poor or perverse much more frequently than did nonusers in the same setting (67). The results confirm those of Bell and Trethowan (6) on disturbed sexuality in the majority of chronic amphetamine users. This study also showed that none of the addicts had had what the authors regarded as a normal home life (6, see also 64). The majority of people who react badly to amphetamine have been found to have had personality disorders prior to initial use, and to have had few friends (30). Though high proportions of people who are dependent on amphetamines have criminal records (40), amphetamine abuse is not restricted to any social class; unlike narcotic addiction, it is found in all strata of society (74, p. 22).

HALLUCINOGENS

Edwards et al. (29) advertised for people who had taken LSD at least 50 times, and matched the respondents with control subjects on several variables judged to be important. (The two groups were also dissimilar in some ways which may have been important; for example, more drug subjects were living on their own.) Several personality tests were administered to both groups. There were only a few differences between them which were significant: drug users were less dependent, less conforming, and more hostile. The authors suggested that the hostility scores indicate that comments like "Make love, not war," may not be valid indices of the true natures of LSD users. On the other hand, people who are genuinely passive may express very hostile attitudes toward a society which they regard as warlike and which persecutes them for their use of drugs.

McGlothlin et al. (55) reported that LSD users are more introverted and more artistically inclined than nonusers. Kleckner (50) compared scores of psychedelic drug users and nonusers on a popular personality test. The users tended to be more aloof, anxious, paranoid, dominant, intelligent, creative, and accident-prone.

People who volunteer for studies on hallucinogenic drugs differ in many ways from nonvolunteers, even if they have not actually experienced the drugs. In one study, about one-third of the volunteers were judged to be in need of psychiatric care (32). This provides further evidence of the danger in assuming that differences between users and nonusers are caused by the drug.

Blum and his associates (9) conducted a very extensive study of drug use on five college campuses. They used interviews, batteries of tests, student diaries, and records of various agencies such as school and police. Their work was reported in two large volumes, and any summary statement is clearly inadequate. Nevertheless, in Table 5.5 an attempt is made to describe some of the more salient points.

OPIATES

Not all opium addicts are morally depraved and physically wasted. In fact, physicians and nurses number more heavily in the addict population than any other occupational group (7, p. 167). Still, most addicts are maladjusted. Gerard and Kornetsky (36) found that all of 32 adolescent male drug addicts whom they studied had personality disorders. They were dysphoric, had difficulties in dealing with others, and had problems of sexual identification. Many addicts have criminal records prior to drug use (28). Zimmering et al. (86) and Toolan et al. (82) found that heroin addicts are extremely passive, nonaggressive, fearful of new situations, and unable to enter into meaningful personal relationships with others.

Chein et al. (18) compared characteristics of New York City neighborhoods where narcotics use was epidemic with nonepidemic areas. The epidemic areas had higher proportions of underprivileged

TABLE 5.5 Personality and Life History Correlates of College Student Drug Users*

	TOBACCO	MARIJUANA	ALCOHOL	LSD	AMPHETAMINES	TRANQUILIZERS AND SEDATIVES	OPIATES
Sex	male	male	equal	male	equal	female	equal
College major	(A/H),† social sciences	A/H, social sciences	A/H	A/H	A/H, biological sciences	general studies, A/H	A/H
Family income	students from families with annual income in excess of $25,000 report greatest experience with all listed drugs except opiates, where greatest users are from lowest income bracket (less than $5,000 per year)						
One or both parents dead	no differences for any drug groups						
Religion	NA†	NA	NA	NA	NA	Jewish	NA
Religious participation	those for whom religious participation is unimportant report more experiences with all drugs						
Political beliefs	the more leftist one's political views, the greater the use of all classes of drugs						
Satisfaction with school	the more dissatisfied, the greater the use of all classes of drugs						
Grade point average§	lower	lower	lower	higher	higher	higher	higher
Attitudes toward future	pessimism toward future was higher than optimism in all classes of drug use						
Experience with general anesthesia and/or medical use of painkillers	greater use of all classes of drugs						
Caffeine—daily use	high	high	high	high	high	high	–
Was there an advantage to being sick as a child?	yes	yes	yes	yes	yes	yes	yes

*Summarized from Blum, R., et al. *Students and Drugs II* (San Francisco: Jossey Bass, 1969). The characteristics cited for each drug indicate those most frequently reported.
†Arts and humanities.
‡No affiliation.
§The differences were very small.

minority groups, overcrowding, poverty, and low educational attainment. Family life was more often disrupted, and the family groups of addicts had greater proportions of adult women and teenagers. Noble (60) and Noble and Barnes (61), working in London, did not detect a link between conditions of poverty and addiction; however, as in the Chein et al. study, the addicts did tend to come from broken homes, and to have received poor parental care.

Chein et al. described several differences between users and nonusers within a given neighborhood. Nonusers more frequently had adult models whom they wished to emulate, the models possessing personality attributes such as courage or kindness which were viewed as desirable. Nonusers also had more stable and intimate friendships. Users preferred material things, like wealth or skills.

The likelihood that a heroin experience will be perceived as pleasurable changes with age. The balance of positive to negative reactions is most favorable at about age 16 (18, p. 153). Users were most apt to have begun experimenting with drugs at about this age. The most susceptible age has probably changed downward during the last few years.

Only 17 percent of users, and 79 percent of nonusers, reported having heard any deterrent information about drugs. The data suggest that widespread informational campaigns may be effective deterrents to the use of opiates.

Table 5.6 indicates questionnaire items for which addict and control answers were quite different.

Drug abusers are often indiscriminate in their use. Richard Ratner, who spent a year as an Army psychiatrist in Vietnam, emphatically stated the point. He said (65) that men addicted to heroin would, when it was not available, swallow unknown pills, steal medication of all sorts from other patients, and inject peanut butter and mayonnaise into their veins. A related finding is that about one-third of narcotics addicts also use barbiturates excessively (39).

ALCOHOL

Jellinek (46) argued that the term "alcoholism" is too broad, and suggested instead that alcoholics be described as belonging to one of five types: alpha, beta, gamma, delta, or epsilon. The alpha type continually relies upon alcohol to relieve physical or emotional pain, but is able to abstain; alpha alcoholics retain control over themselves, rarely progressing to more serious kinds of alcoholism. Beta alcoholics are not dependent upon alcohol; their drinking is unfortunately often combined with an improper diet, and as a result,

TABLE 5.6 Selected Single Items on Which Addict and Control Family Backgrounds Were Highly Contrasted*

ITEM	ADDICTS	CONTROLS
	Percentages	
1. Boy experienced an extremely weak father-son relationship (30, 29)	80	45
2. For a significant part of early childhood, boy did not have a father figure in his life (29, 29)	48	17
3. Some father figure was cool or hostile to boy (23, 24)	52	13
4. Father had unrealistically low aspirations for the boy (late childhood and early adolescence) (16, 22)	44	0
5. Some father figure was an immoral model (early childhood) (26, 24)	23	0
6. Marked impulse orientation in father figure (23, 23)	26	0
7. Father had unstable work history during boy's early childhood (28, 28)	43	14
8. Father was unrealistically pessimistic or felt that life is a gamble (17, 19)	47	11
9. Lack of warmth or overtly discordant relations between parents (30, 29)	97	41
10. Mother figure was more important parent in boy's life during late childhood period (30, 29)	73	45
11. Some mother figure cool or hostile to boy (early childhood) (30, 28)	23	0
12. Some mother figure cool or hostile to boy (late childhood) (30, 29)	37	3
13. Boy experienced extremely weak mother-son relationship (30, 29)	40	7
14. Mother did not trust authority figures (29, 29)	38	10
15. Mother had unrealistically low aspirations for boy (late childhood and early adolescence) (29, 28)	31	0
16. Mother was unrealistically pessimistic or felt that life is a gamble (29, 29)	31	7
17. No clear pattern of parental roles in formation of disciplinary policy (adolescence) (30, 29)	23	0
18. Parental standards for boy were vague or inconsistent (early childhood) (29, 28)	55	4
19. Parental standards for boy were vague or inconsistent (adolescence) (30, 29)	63	3
20. Boy was overindulged, frustrated in his wishes, or both (30, 29)	70	10

*From Chein, I., Gerard, D., Lee, R., and Rosenfeld, E. *Narcotics, Delinquency, and Social Policy* (London: Tavistock, 1964), pp. 272–273.

they suffer many of the sicknesses common to alcoholics. Gamma alcoholism has, as the defining characteristic, physical dependence; in addition, there is loss of control, so that the person finds it extremely difficult to stop once he has had even a single drink. Delta alcoholics, as are found in countries where many families take wine with every meal (as in France), are also physically dependent. However they drink small amounts continually rather than going on enormous binges. Delta alcoholics rarely get drunk. Epsilon alcoholics have long periods of abstinence, which are interrupted by periodic sprees.

The characteristic common to virtually all alcoholics is anxiety, which can be relieved only by alcohol. The alcoholic feels inadequate socially, and almost invariably has sexual problems (14). He believes that alcohol will help him regain his self-esteem, and that under its influence he will become more socially adept. Yet, sadly, the invariable outcome is just the reverse; self-esteem is reduced during bouts of drinking (83).

Chafetz (17), on the basis of his clinical experiences, listed what he felt were the primary reasons for excessive drinking:

1. Many drink as a means of combating depression. If they succeed, they become fearful of stopping; if, on the other hand, alcohol deepens the depression, they keep drinking in hopes of eventually finding surcease.

2. Some drink to block awareness of socially unacceptable impulses, or to allow expression of the impulses while absolving themselves of responsibility. Chafetz gave the example of a man who did not acknowledge his homosexual impulses but who, while drunk, engaged in homosexual activity. He blamed the liquor for his actions.

3. Some alcoholics act out forbidden desires, then, upon recovery, claim to have no recollection of their actions.

4. Drinking is regarded as a means to reduce those inhibitions which impair performance. Thus liquor is regarded as an ally in overcoming stagefright, improving salesmanship, reducing anxiety in sexual situations, and so forth. Social inhibition is also reduced. Alcohol is considered valuable at parties because it promotes relaxation and fosters a sense of intimacy. Though a type of alcoholism, such drinking as this is not as serious as the types above.

5. By contrast, some severely disturbed people drink to attain oblivion. They have strong self-destructive tendencies.

6. Some people drink because of social pressures. Chafetz described a situation which is frequently observed: an alcoholic is subtly pressured into continuing the drinking habit by a nonalcoholic spouse, because cure of the alcoholic would expose previously hidden problems in the other.

In sum, alcoholism is a complex disease with a variety of manifestations, supported by varying motives. It would be surprising if there were a common etiology. Many theories have been proposed about why people become alcoholics. Some feel that the primary cause is a character disorder; others emphasize cultural factors; still others have talked about metabolic or nutritional deficiencies, allergy, or genetic determinants. While all of the factors may be relevant, none have been demonstrated to be critical to the development of alcoholism. A few of the suggestive experiments are briefly described below.

Genetic Component

McClearn and his colleagues have shown that strains of mice differ in their preferences for alcohol (53); by selective breeding, they were able to increase the disparity between groups until there was no overlap between them. The experiments suggested that predisposition toward alcoholism may have, at least in part, a genetic basis. A different kind of evidence comes from a series of experiments by Cruz-Coke and Varela (22–25). They found links between cirrhosis of the liver and color blindness, and between alcoholism and color blindness. Color blindness is a recessive X-linked characteristic, and the findings suggested that the same genes which produce color blindness might favor the development of alcoholism. However, Smith and Brinton (77) showed that the defective color vision of alcoholics is secondary to their poor nutritional status. Smith and Brinton found that 65 of 172 male alcoholics and 13 of 33 women had poor red-green color vision, a defect present in only three to four percent of men (and even fewer women) in the general population. After receiving nutritionally balanced diets with vitamin supplements, the number of men and women with defective color vision was reduced to 17 and 5, respectively.

Nutritional Deficiencies

Beerstecher et al. (5) fed rats diets deficient in various vitamins. Several diets were without effect, but those deficient in thiamine, riboflavin, pyridoxine, or pantothenate led to increases in alcohol consumption. Williams (85) believes that alcoholism can be effectively treated by proper attention to nutritional factors, and further evidence that a metabolic defect might underlie alcoholism is that, following ethanol loading, alcoholics show plasma amino acid patterns different from those of normal individuals (72).

A problem general to most of the dietary studies is the failure to consider that vitamin-deficient animals are unable to properly metabolize certain foods, and therefore do not get enough calories. Alcohol provides calories, so is chosen in preference to water when those are the only alternatives available. Greenberg and Lester (38) showed that the presentation of other substances, e.g., fat or sugar, reduced the alcohol intake of vitamin-deficient rats. Therefore, although vitamin deficiencies may lead to increased alcohol intake in rats restricted to a choice between alcohol and water, the relevance of the findings to alcoholism in man is limited.

Stress

Myers and his colleagues (58, 59) have studied the effects of stress on the alcohol intake of laboratory rats. When the animals were exposed to daily unavoidable electric shocks, their alcohol intakes did not change. However, when they were able to avoid the shocks by pressing a lever (a stress-inducing factor), they increased their consumption. Crowding produces another kind of stress. Veale and Myers (84) studied the alcohol intake of a group of rats in an experiment wherein rats were added to the group while living space was kept constant.* As more and more rats were added, alcohol intake increased. Strains of mice differ in their reactions to the stress of increased population density; for instance, grouping reduces alcohol consumption in mice of the C57 strain but does not affect RIII mice (79). Smart (75), in a study which might conceivably be related to the effects of grouping, found that alcoholics tend to come from large families.

CONCLUSIONS

References in the news media to the "drug culture," which implies a homogeneous group of people united by their use of drugs, may convey the false impression that they are united in other ways as well. Such is not the case, and people who use drugs come from all social classes, from both urban and rural areas, and from a wide range of professions. Moreover, people who have similar preferences for a particular class of drugs tend to be more similar to each other than to people who prefer drugs of a different class. Nevertheless, there are some characteristics which show up per-

---

*Rogers and Thiessen (68) did not find that alcohol intake of rats was affected by group size. However, they were interested in group size per se, and not in overcrowding, so that they increased the floor space to accommodate additional rats.

sistently in surveys of chronic drug users. Users tend to be politically liberal; highly curious and adventurous; less accepting than abstainers of the American way of life, with its emphasis on religion, hard work, and accumulation of material goods; and, perhaps as a consequence of the aforementioned, but also because of unsatisfactory early family lives, more unhappy in and dissatisfied with the society in which they find themselves.

REFERENCES

1. Baer, D. Height, weight, and ponderal index of college male smokers and nonsmokers. J. Psychol., 1966, 64:101–105.
2. Baer, D. Scholastic aptitude and smoking attitude and behavior of college males. J. Psychol., 1966, 64:63–68.
3. Baer, D. Sex differences in smoking attitude, behavior, and beliefs of college students. J. Psychol., 1966, 64:249–255.
4. Bakan, D. The test of significance in psychological research. Psychol. Bull., 1966, 66:423–437.
5. Beerstecher, E., Reed, J., Brown, W., and Berry, L. The effects of single vitamin deficiencies on the consumption of alcohol by white rats. U. Texas Pub. No. 5109, 1951.
6. Bell, D., and Trethowan, W. Amphetamine addiction and disturbed sexuality. Arch. Gen. Psychiat., 1961, 4:74–78.
7. Bier, W. (Ed.) Problems in Addiction. New York: Fordham, 1962.
8. Blackford, L. Trends in student drug use in San Mateo County. California's Health, 1969, 27:3–6.
9. Blum, R. et al. Students and Drugs II. San Francisco: Jossey-Bass, 1969.
10. Blum, R., Braunstein, L., and Stone, A. Normal drug use: an exploratory study of patterns and correlates. In Cole, J., and Wittenborn, J. (Eds.) Drug Abuse. Springfield, Ill.: Charles C Thomas, 1969.
11. Brehm, M., and Back, K. Self image and attitudes toward drugs. J. Person., 1968, 36:299–314.
12. Brown, B. Some characteristic EEG differences between heavy smoker and nonsmoker subjects. Neuropsychologia, 1968, 6:381–388.
13. Burke, C. A brief note on one-tailed tests. Psychol. Bull., 1953, 50:384–387.
14. Campbell, R. Background and Special Problems of Alcoholism. 1. The etiology and background. In Bier, W. (Ed.) Problems in Addiction. New York: Fordham, 1962.
15. Carney, R. Sex chromatin, body masculinity, achievement motivation and smoking behavior. Psychol. Rep., 1967, 20:859–866.
16. Carney, R., Feldman, H., and Loh, W. Sex chromatin, body masculinity and smoking behavior. Psychol. Rep., 1969, 25:261–262.
17. Chafetz, M. Clinical syndromes of liquor drinkers. In Popham, R. (Ed.) Alcohol and Alcoholism. Toronto: Univ. Toronto, 1970.
18. Chein, I., Gerard, D., Lee, R., and Rosenfeld, E. Narcotics, Delinquency, and Social Policy. London: Tavistock, 1964.
19. Chevalier, R., Bowers, J., Dondurant, S., and Ross, J. Circulatory and ventilatory effects of exercise in smokers and nonsmokers. J. Appl. Physiol., 1963, 18: 357–360.
20. Cohen, B., and Thomas, C. Comparison of smokers and nonsmokers II. The distribution of ABO and Rh (d) blood groups. Bull. Johns Hopkins Hosp., 1962, 110:1–7.
21. Connell, P. Proceedings of the Leeds Symposium on Behavioural Disorders. Dagenham: May and Baker Ltd., 1965.
22. Cruz-Coke, R. Association between opportunity for natural selection, color blind-

ness and chronic alcoholism in different human populations. Arch. Biol. Med. Exper., 1966, 3:21–26.

23. Cruz-Coke, R. Colour-blindness and alcohol addiction. Lancet, 1965, 2:1348.

24. Cruz-Coke, R. Colour-blindness and cirrhosis of the liver. Lancet, 1964, 2:1064–1065.

25. Cruz-Coke, R. and Varela, A. Inheritance of alcoholism. Its association with colour-blindness. Lancet, 1966, 2:1282–1284.

26. Davis, J., and Miller, N. Fear and pain: their effect on self-injection of amobarbital sodium in rats. Science, 1963, 141:1286–1287.

27. Doll, R. and Hill, A. Mortality in relation to smoking: 10 years' observations of British doctors. (Concluded.) Brit. Med. J., 1964, 1:1460–1467.

28. D'Orban, P. Heroin dependency and delinquency in women — a study of heroin addicts in Holloway Prison. Brit. J. Addict., 1970, 65:67–78.

29. Edwards, A., Bloom, M., and Cohen, S. The psychedelics: love or hostility potion? Psychol. Rep., 1969, 24:843–846.

30. Ellinwood, E. Amphetamine psychosis: Description of the individuals and process. J. Nerv. Ment. Dis., 1967, 144:273–283.

31. Epstein, S. (Ed.) Drugs of Abuse. Cambridge, Mass.: MIT Press, 1971.

32. Esecover, H., Malitz, S., and Wilkens, B. Clinical profiles of paid normal subjects volunteering for hallucinogen drug studies. Am. J. Psychiat., 1961, 117:910–915.

33. Eysenck, H. Smoking, Health, and Personality. New York: Basic Books, 1965.

34. Fisher, R. Cancer and cigarettes. Nature, 1958, 182:108.

35. Fisher, R. Cancer and smoking. Nature, 1958, 182:596.

36. Gerard, D. and Kornetsky, C. Social and psychiatric study of adolescent opiate addicts. Psychiat. Quart., 1954, 28:113–125.

37. Goldsmith, J., Hechter, H., Perkins, N., and Borhani, N. Pulmonary function and respiratory findings among longshoremen. Am. Rev. Resp. Dis., 1962, 86:867–874.

38. Greenberg, L., and Lester, D. Vitamin deficiency and the etiology of alcoholism. In Himwich, H. (Ed.) Alcoholism. Pub. No. 47, AAAS, Wash., D.C., 1957.

39. Hamberger, E. Barbiturate use in narcotic addicts. J.A.M.A., 1964, 189:366–368.

40. Hawks, D., Mitcheson, M., Ogborne, A., and Edwards, G. Abuse of methylamphetamine. Brit. Med. J., 1969, 1:715–721.

41. The Health Consequences of Smoking. Pub. Health Service Review, 1967.

42. Heath, C. Differences between smokers and nonsmokers. Arch. Int. Med., 1958, 101:377–388.

43. Hekimian, L., and Gershon, S. Characteristics of drug abusers admitted to a psychiatric hospital. J.A.M.A., 1968, 205:125–130.

44. Hill, H., Haertzen, C., and Davis, H. An MMPI factor analytic study of alcoholics, narcotic addicts and criminals. Quart. J. Stud. Alcohol, 1962, 23:411–431.

45. Jeffreys, M., Brotherston, J., and Cartwright, A. Consumption of medicine on a working class housing estate. Brit. J. Prev. Soc. Med., 1960, 14:64–76.

46. Jellinek, E. The Disease Concept of Alcoholism. New Haven: Rillhouse, 1946.

47. Kanekar, S. and Dolke, A. Smoking, extraversion, and neuroticism. Psychol. Rep., 1970, 26:384.

48. King, F. Marijuana and LSD usage among male college students: prevalence rate, frequency, and self-estimates of future use. Psychiat., 1969, 32:265–276.

49. King, F. Users and nonusers of marijuana: some attitudinal and behavioral correlates. J. Am. Coll. Health Assoc., 1970, 18:213–217.

50. Kleckner, J. Personality differences between psychedelic drug users and nonusers. Psychol., 1968, 5:66–71.

51. Lee, S., and Temerlin, M. Social class, diagnosis, and prognosis for psychotherapy. Psychother.: Theory, Res., Pract., 1970, 7:181–185.

52. Livson, N., and Stewart, L. Morphological constitution and smoking. J.A.M.A., 1965, 192:806–808.

53. McClearn, G., and Rodgers, D. Differences in alcohol preference among inbred strains of mice. Quart. J. Stud. Alc., 1959, 20:691–695.

54. McCune, D. A study of more effective education relative to narcotics, other harmful drugs, and hallucinogenic substances. Progress Report submitted to California Legislature, 1970.
55. McGlothlin, W., Cohen, S., and McGlothlin, M. Personality and attitude changes in volunteer subjects following repeated administration of LSD. Excerpta Med. Int. Cong. Rep., 1966, 129:425–434.
56. Mittwock, U. Sex Chromosomes. New York: Academic Press, 1967.
57. Mori, K. Enhancement of experimental lung cancer in mice by inhalation of cigarette smoke. Gann; Japanese J. Cancer Res., 1966, 57:537–541.
58. Myers, R., and Carey, R. Preference factors in experimental alcoholism. Science, 1961, 134:469–470.
59. Myers, R., and Holman, R. Failure of stress of electric shock to increase ethanol intake in rats. Quart. J. Stud. Alc., 1967, 28:132–137.
60. Noble, P. Drug-taking in delinquent boys. Brit. Med. J., 1970, 1:102–105.
61. Noble, P., and Barnes, G. Drug taking in adolescent girls: factors associated with the progression to narcotic use. Brit. Med. J., 1971, 2:620–623.
62. Norris, V. Mental Illness in London. London: Chapman and Hall, Ltd, 1959.
63. Parry, H. Use of psychotropic drugs by U.S. adults. Pub. Health Rep., 1968, 83: 799–810.
64. Prison and Borstal After-Care. Ann. Rep. Council Cent. After-Care Assoc., H.M.S.O., 1963.
65. Ratner, R. Drugs and despair in Vietnam. U. Chic. Mag., 1972, 64:15–23.
66. Robins, L., Darvish, H., and Murphy, G. The long-term outcome for adolescent drug users: a follow-up study of 76 users and 146 non-users. In Zubin, J., and Freedman, A. (Eds.) Psychopathology of Adolescence. New York: Grune and Stratton, 1970.
67. Rockwell, D. Amphetamine use and abuse in psychiatric patients. In Cole, J., and Wittenborn, J. (Eds.) Drug Abuse. Springfield, Ill.: Charles C Thomas, 1969.
68. Rodgers, D., and Thiessen, D. Effects of population density on adrenal size, behavioural arousal, and alcohol preference of inbred mice. Quart. J. Stud. Alc., 1964, 25:240–247.
69. Rosenberg, C. Young drug addicts: background and personality. J. Nerv. Ment. Dis., 1969, 148:65–73.
70. Seltzer, C. Constitution and heredity in relation to tobacco smoking. Ann. N.Y. Acad. Sci., 1967, 142:322–330.
71. Severi, L. (Ed.) Lung Tumors in Animals. Perugia, Italy: U. Perugia, 1966.
72. Siegel, F., Roach, M., and Pomeroy, L. Plasma amino acid patterns in alcoholism: the effects of ethanol loading. Proc. Nat. Acad. Sci., 1964, 51:605–611.
73. Simmons, J., and Winograd, B. It's Happening: A Portrait of the Youth Scene Today. Santa Barbara: Marc-Laird, 1966.
74. Sjoqvist, F., and Tottie, M. (Eds.) Abuse of Central Stimulants. New York: Raven, 1969.
75. Smart, R. Alcoholism, birth order, and family size. J. Ab. Soc. Psychol., 1963, 66: 17–23.
76. Smith, G. Personality correlates of cigarette smoking in students of college age. Ann. N.Y. Acad. Sci., 1967, 142:308–321.
77. Smith, J., and Brinton, G. Color-vision defects in alcoholism. Quart. J. Stud. Alc., 1971, 32:41–44.
78. Suchman, E. The "hang-loose" ethic and the spirit of drug use. J. Health Soc. Behav., 1968, 9:140–155.
79. Thiessen, D., and Rodgers, D. Alcohol injection, grouping, and voluntary alcohol consumption of inbred strains of mice. Quart. J. Stud. Alc., 1965, 26:378–383.
80. Thomas, C. Characteristics of smokers compared with nonsmokers in a population of healthy young adults, including observations on family history, blood pressure, heart rate, body weight, cholesterol and certain psychologic traits. Ann. Int. Med., 1960, 33:697–718.

81. Thomas, C., and Cohen, B. Comparison of smokers and nonsmokers I. A preliminary report on the ability to taste phenylthiourea (PTC). Bull. Johns Hopkins Hosp., 1960, *106*:205–214.

82. Toolan, J., Zimmering, P., and Wortis, S. Adolescent drug addiction. N.Y. State J. Med., 1952, *52*:72–74.

83. Vanderpool, J. Self-concept differences in the alcoholic under varying conditions of drinking and sobriety. Unpublished Ph.D. dissertation, 1966, Loyola U.

84. Veale, W., and Myers, R. Increased alcohol preference in rats following repeated exposures to alcohol. Psychopharmacologia, 1969, *15*:361–372.

85. Williams, R. *Alcoholism, The Nutritional Approach.* Austin: U. Texas, 1959.

86. Zimmering, P., Toolan, J., Safrin, R., and Wortis, S. Drug addiction in relation to problems of adolescence. Am. J. Psychiat., 1952, *109*:272–278.

87. Zinberg, N., and Weil, A. A comparison of marijuana users and non-users. Nature, 1970, *226*:119–123.

CHAPTER 6

THERAPY FOR DRUG ABUSE

Any therapy for drug abuse, to be completely successful, must deal with three separate problems. The first is that termination of use may induce abstinence symptoms. While these may be mild, as after chronic smoking or amphetamine use, some withdrawal symptoms are very painful and prolonged—even threatening to life, as observed in some alcoholics and narcotic and barbiturate addicts. Patients must be handled very carefully during withdrawal from drugs. Even once they have been withdrawn and are no longer physically dependent, former drug addicts remain highly susceptible to readdiction. This susceptibility is the second problem which therapy must confront, and during the postwithdrawal phase it is important to attempt to eliminate or replace the rewarding properties of the drug. Finally, any character disorder which might underlie compulsive drug use should be treated. It is a reasonable assumption that character disorders underlie virtually all instances of compulsive drug use. There are no known drugs which are invariably addicting; drug addiction is caused by people, not drugs. Fewer than 10 percent of people who drink become alcoholics (3), and even heroin, the most infamous drug of addiction, may entrap only about one half of the people who try it (11, p. 159). In essence, the ideal cure for addiction would involve considerably more than symptomatic treatment; the addict would also receive extensive psychotherapy, vocational guidance, and job placement.

THE WITHDRAWAL PERIOD

Opiates

Jaffe (30) described studies in which patients who were physically dependent upon morphine were withdrawn by replacing it with either a placebo or some other drug. The only agents which prevented or relieved withdrawal symptoms were those which were cross-tolerant with morphine and which produced morphine-like dependence. Some non-opiates were useful because they relieved anxiety during withdrawal, and others, such as chlorpromazine, reduced vomiting. Still others — reserpine and related drugs — only exacerbated the symptoms.

The current drug of choice for relief of withdrawal symptoms is methadone, a synthetic narcotic analgesic which has pharmacological actions that differ only quantitatively from those of morphine. In 1971, procedures were initiated in New York State for more than 20,000 addicts to receive methadone treatment (15). The rationale for its use is that, when administered in high doses, it reduces the intensity of heroin withdrawal symptoms, although it also prolongs them.

Casriel and Amen (10, p. xvii) claimed that the non-narcotic drug Perse virtually eliminates withdrawal symptoms, and the later physiological need for heroin. However, physicians have remained unconvinced of the merits of Perse.

CNS Depressants

Alcohol and barbiturates are cross-tolerant, and each can suppress abstinence symptoms induced by the other. In fact, meprobamate, glutethimide, chlordiazepoxide, paraldehyde, and other depressants are also interchangeable in that anyone can suppress the withdrawal symptoms of any other (18). The drug of choice for treating withdrawal from any of the above is pentobarbital. The basis for its superiority is that the dose-response curve has a flatter slope than most other CNS depressants; hence the proper dose (that which prevents convulsions and deliria while inducing only slight intoxication) can be determined with the greatest safety.

POSTWITHDRAWAL MODIFICATION OF THE REWARDING PROPERTIES OF DRUGS

The Problem

Physical dependence, although dramatized in newspapers and films, is a relatively minor aspect of narcotic addiction. For example,

Nichols (42) estimated that as high as one percent of all physicians are addicted to morphine, yet their patients who receive morphine for relief of pain have a much lower incidence of addiction. Yet the physiological reactions to the drug, and the physical dependence produced by it, are the same for doctors and their patients. Nichols recognized that a critical difference between the two groups is that doctors actively self-administer morphine, whereas patients are passive recipients. (Of course there are other differences which may be important. One such is that the doctors risk less in developing a morphine habit, because only they can be sure of a continuing, trouble-free supply). He tested with rats his idea that the active vs. passive distinction is an important one. Rats were given a choice between tap water and water in which was dissolved 0.5 mg morphine per cc. The rats overwhelmingly chose water. Then he made them physically dependent on morphine via daily injections for 25 days, but they still preferred water to morphine. Nichols used the injection procedure to make more rats physically dependent, and then deprived one half of them of unadulterated water during withdrawal; they were able to obtain water only by drinking the morphine solution. The rest of the rats were allowed to drink unadulterated water, but they too received morphine, being injected with the drug in amounts equal to that which was drunk by rats in the other group. Thus the two new groups were equated for morphine intake, but differed in the way the drug was obtained. When they were then given additional preference tests, rats which had *actively* drunk morphine preferred it to water. The other rats maintained their preference for water.

Further proof that morphine addiction is not maintained solely by physical dependence is shown by work with monkeys. Schuster and Woods (cited in 52) required monkeys to bar press for injections of morphine, and obtained an inverted U-shaped dose-response curve. That is, response rates were greatest for the middle dose ranges (about 100 μg/kg), and were less for doses of 10 or 1000 μg/kg. During extinction sessions, when saline was substituted for morphine, monkeys at the lowest dosage promptly stopped responding, while those at the highest dosage greatly increased their rates of responding. The authors concluded that monkeys in the high dosage group had been physically dependent, and those in the low dosage group had not. Yet despite differences in physical dependence, those in the low dose group had maintained slightly higher rates of responding prior to extinction.

When monkeys which had learned to respond for morphine were given the amount they had stabilized on, but in a divided dose, they never underwent withdrawal, yet they continued to bar press for morphine (cited in Ref. 52).

Finally, some drugs which produce physical dependence, such as the narcotic antagonists, are not abused. Others, such as cocaine, do not produce dependence but are abused. These findings might seem to invalidate the author's unwillingness to accept the concept of psychological dependence (see Chap. 4). However, all they really show is the nonessentiality of physical dependence for drug abuse. They do not establish any unique features of drugs which set them apart from other aspects of life which give pleasure, such as friends, sex, television, or books. These do not produce physical dependence, but in some people are indulged in to excess. The argument presented in Chapter 4, that any experience which is pleasurable (whether pharmacological or otherwise) will evoke a desire for repetition, still holds.

Although physical dependence per se is neither necessary nor sufficient for the development of addiction, a history of physical dependence is relevant. Weeks and Collins (57) established this when they compared rates of self-administration of morphine in three groups of rats. Group (a) learned to prevent withdrawal symptoms by bar pressing for morphine while physically dependent on it; group (b) learned to bar press for water as a reward, and received periodic injections of morphine so that the rats became physically dependent. Group (c) bar pressed for water, and was not made physically dependent on morphine. After having been drug-free for four weeks, and presumably no longer physically dependent, the rats were retested. Those in group (a) bar pressed for morphine the most, those in group (c) the least. One cautionary note on interpretation: the animals may have been physically dependent even after four drug-free weeks; in man, there are persistent changes following morphine withdrawal for at least six months (39).

Kumar and Stolerman (32) confirmed the importance of a history of physical dependence. They trained rats to drink a morphine-quinine solution, then withdrew them from morphine for 110 days. When then tested for a morphine or water preference, the rats selected morphine on a greater percentage of trials than did naive (unconditioned) controls. Rats given a choice between quinine (which is normally aversive) and water were intermediate in their preferences. In other words, the prior association of quinine with morphine had altered the innate aversion of the rats toward quinine.

Branchey et al. (8) showed that experiential factors are important where alcohol is considered. For three weeks rats were given a liquid diet containing substantial amounts of alcohol. The procedure induced physical dependence, i.e., when the alcohol was removed, the rats had withdrawal symptoms. Two weeks later, both the ex-addicts and a control group received alcohol for four days. Fifty percent of the previously addicted group experienced severe withdrawal when the alcohol was taken away, but none of the controls exhibited such a response.

The degree of similarity between environmental stimuli during initial addiction to and withdrawal from a drug, and subsequent exposure to it, greatly influences the outcome of the later exposures. For example, rats which were readdicted to morphine in the same environment in which the original self-administration response was learned drank much more morphine than rats which were readdicted in a new environment (54). Moreover, their characteristic withdrawal response, which includes sudden brief body twitches, increased in frequency when they were placed in the cages in which they were originally addicted, even though they had been drug-free for several months (59).

Goldberg and Schuster (24) injected morphine-dependent rats with doses of nalorphine, a narcotic antagonist which precipitates withdrawal symptoms in addicted individuals. The injections were paired with the sound of a buzzer. After several trials, withdrawal symptoms were induced merely by sounding the buzzer. These experiments make more comprehensible the common observation that heroin addicts, even after long periods of hospitalization or imprisonment, report experiencing withdrawal when they return to the environments in which they had formerly become addicted.

Some Solutions

The preceding section emphasized that drug addiction is not at all synonymous with physical dependence. Therefore, methods of treatment which focus exclusively on control of withdrawal symptoms are doomed to failure. Goldberg (23) specified that any treatment program for drug addiction should involve exposure of the patients to their original drug-taking environment. In addition, the patients should be allowed to self-administer their drugs, but the effects should be blocked by antagonists. Certain pharmacological approaches to the problem of drug dependence satisfy these two criteria.

Pharmacological Approaches to the Treatment of Drug Addiction

METHADONE MAINTENANCE FOR NARCOTIC ADDICTS.   There is an appealing simplicity about the idea of using a drug to cure a drug habit. Thus, disulfiram has long been used in the treatment of alcoholism, lobeline is prescribed for people who wish to stop smoking, and methadone is offered to heroin addicts. The approach is not without its hazards; when Sigmund Freud prescribed cocaine to a friend who was addicted to morphine, the friend became the first known cocaine addict of modern times (25, p. 367). Heroin is another drug which at one time was substituted for morphine; in fact, its name derives from "hero" because of its alleged heroic powers in curing both morphine and opium addiction (13, p. 71). These early failures should merely encourage caution, not lead to total abandonment of all further attempts.

Dole and Nyswander (16) developed methadone as a therapeutic tool for the treatment of narcotic addiction. The drug has several virtues; among them are that it is long-acting, inexpensive, and effective when taken orally, and it produces neither sedation nor impairment of mental function. Most importantly, it is cross tolerant with heroin, blocking its euphoric effects. The craving for heroin is also blocked. The major drawback of methadone is that it is itself addicting, although less so than heroin and morphine.

Methadone treatment has been reserved primarily for long-standing addictions which have been refractory to other forms of treatment. Application for treatment is on a purely voluntary basis. In the experience of Dole and Nyswander (16), about 17 percent leave the program and become readdicted. However, none of the more than 2000 who remained became readdicted; many of them are now working or attending school.

Jaffe (29) has also reported favorable experiences with methadone. He randomly assigned addict volunteers to high or low dose treatment. Those on low dose were told that the methadone was merely serving as preparation for other therapy and therefore might be discontinued after only a short period of time. Despite the fact that Jaffe did not exclude anyone from participation in the experiment for reasons of ill health or psychiatric problems, the cure rate was extremely high; seven months after the study's inception, 75 percent of the patients who had started were still in treatment and making satisfactory progress; only 15 percent of those who remained in treatment showed positive on tests of urine samples for illicit drugs. Jaffe's study was important in showing that methadone maintenance could be effective even when the drug was administered in low doses.

Methadone maintenance has been criticized on several counts, both moral and empirical. The primary moral consideration is that maintenance involves nothing more than the substitution of one form of drug dependency for another (35). The objection seems to be a frivolous one, if the alternative to methadone is a life of hopeless despair, unproductiveness, and crime.

On the empirical side, there are disagreements about the safety of methadone, and about its ability to produce euphoric effects.

Lennard et al. (35) stated that chronic methadone maintenance produces many side effects: patients tire easily, are more somnolent, are frequently constipated, and often report sexual impotence. The withdrawal from methadone may be intense. Ausubel (2) claimed that methadone is a euphoriant, and Freedman et al. (22) reported incidents of mild euphoria after high doses. Lennard et al. have taken the position that the extent of euphoria is determined more by the route of administration than by the actual narcotic used, and that in any event neither heroin nor methadone has a very strong euphoric effect once tolerance develops. Moreover, they noted, methadone-treated addicts continue to abuse a wide variety of drugs for which the euphoric action is not blocked. One additional point is that sufficiently high doses of heroin can overcome the blocking effects of methadone. Lennard et al. feel that the foregoing considerations sufficiently blur the distinction between heroin and methadone to make continued use of the latter indefensible.

The strongest rebuttal to the arguments by Lennard and his colleagues is that methadone maintenance works. Addicts do not continue to take heroin; they take methadone orally rather than intravenously; the euphoria, if it appears, is of a different order of magnitude from heroin-induced euphoria, and in fact many addicts are unable to distinguish between the active and inactive stereoisomers of methadone until the onset of withdrawal symptoms (17); above all, methadone enables heroin addicts to live relatively normal, healthy lives.

Despite the claims of Lennard et al., the side effects do not frequently appear, and in any event are of the nuisance variety rather than being of great seriousness. Many patients have been maintained on methadone for several years and have reported no side effects. Nyswander (43) claimed that methadone does not impair reaction time, intellectual capacity, affect, or vigilance. More to the point, the physical and emotional problems which *are* encountered are much less than those found with heroin use.

Lennard and his associates raised the point that uncritical acceptance of methadone maintenance might lead to the assignment of addicts to drug programs when other forms of rehabilitation might be more suitable; further, methadone maintenance might retard the development of new programs. These dangers are probably real, and it would be a mistake if physicians began prescribing methadone indiscriminately to all addicts. However, it has proved its effectiveness, even though its use has been restricted largely to patients who were believed to have small likelihood of ever overcoming their addictions. For many it may represent the only chance for a normal life.

NARCOTIC ANTAGONISTS FOR NARCOTIC ADDICTS. An alternative pharmacological strategy involves the use of narcotic antagonists. These are drugs which compete with heroin or morphine for receptor sites, thereby preventing or reversing their actions while having little or no morphine-like effects. Nalorphine was the first well-described morphine antagonist. It induces withdrawal symptoms in individuals physically dependent on morphine, and it promptly abolishes the latter's effects, euphoric or otherwise. Nalorphine is short acting and produces very unpleasant subjective effects, giving it little clinical utility. However, when its mode of action became publicized, an intense search was begun for other narcotic antagonists. Among the several which have been tried with some measure of success are naloxone, pentazocine, and cyclazocine. The latter appears most promising. It has weak analgesic and psychotomimetic actions, to which tolerance develops. Tolerance does not develop to the narcotic blocking action, however. Jaffe (28) reported mixed success with cyclazocine. Volunteers who were accepted in his clinic were first given methadone for withdrawal. Then cyclazocine was given on an individualized basis, with dosage schedules ranging from every day to every third day. His patients reduced their use of illicit narcotics over the course of a year, but none of them stopped entirely. Many developed techniques for thwarting the actions of cyclazocine. For example, they took the entire amount in one dose just before bedtime, thus making the blockade minimal by the next evening; under such circumstances, heroin produces euphoria but no physical dependence.

DETERRENTS TO SMOKING. The pharmacological approach has been promoted as a means of helping people stop smoking. The preparations which have been marketed can be classified into three general types, depending on their active ingredients. For two of these types—astringents and local anesthetics—there is no obvious rationale for use, nor any experiments on which to base claims of efficacy. Compounds of the third type, such as Bantron and Nikoban, contain lobeline. The rationale for use of lobeline to reduce the need to smoke is roughly analogous to that for methadone and heroin. Lobeline is cross-tolerant with and similar to nicotine, although less potent in physiological effects.

Rapp and Olen (48) and Rapp et al. (47) reported that Bantron was effective in reducing the urge to smoke. (The latter project was sponsored by a grant from the manufacturers of Bantron.) In the first study, many smokers quit entirely, and in the second, they reduced their daily number of cigarettes. Subsequent research by other experimenters (4, 41) has not been confirmatory. Two general findings have been that placebos are just as effective deterrents to smoking as lobeline preparations, and that the relapse rate of quitters is very high.

Conditioning Therapies

SMOKING. Conditioning therapies, also called behavioral modification techniques, attempt to change behavior by employing the
findings from psychological laboratories on laws of learning. Conditioning therapies for drug abuse have been applied almost exclusively to smokers and alcoholics. In 1968 Keutzer et al. (31) reviewed the literature on behavioral modification approaches to
smoking, and concluded that they were no more effective than traditional forms of therapy. Since then, there have been several promising developments, most of which involve the use of punishment.
The experiments cited are only a small sample of the many ingenious
techniques which have been tried.

Whaley et al. (58) required their patients to carry a special cigarette case which delivered shock when opened. The technique
represents a significant methodological advance, because patients
were punished for using their own cigarettes whenever and wherever
they chose to do so. In previous work, the laboratory had been the
sole site for conditioning, and the carryover to other situations was
small. Whaley et al. found that 5 of 10 people who entered into the
treatment program were abstinent 18 months after the program's
termination.

Lublin and Joslyn (38) required their patients, most of whom
were heavy smokers, to smoke at a rapid rate while a special machine
blew hot smoke at them. Of 99 who started treatment, 21 dropped
out after three sessions or less. Forty of the remaining group temporarily stopped smoking, 15 remained abstinent for at least one
year, and 16 others had reduced their smoking by more than 50 percent. Lichtenstein (reported in 36) used a similar procedure, and
obtained equally impressive results. He also added a control group
which received warm, mentholated air instead of hot smoke. They,
too, stopped smoking. If the latter results hold up, they have important implications. After all, the number of people who are willing
to be shocked whenever they attempt to smoke, or to have hot smoke
blown in their faces, must be only a small percentage of the total
number of smokers. As a result, conditioning therapies are greatly
limited. However, if a nonaversive procedure proves to be effective
in curbing smoking, many more people are likely to try to quit.

Resnick (50) devised a technique which has aversive components, but which is extremely simple in both concept and application. He randomly assigned his patients to one of three groups,
instructing group (1) to smoke their normal amounts of cigarettes
for one week, group (2) to double their smoking rate for one week
and group (3) to triple their rate for one week. At the end of the
week, all patients were instructed to stop smoking. No attempt was

made to determine if the members assigned to each group complied with the instructions. Nevertheless, the results were impressive. After four months, 20 percent of the first group and 63 percent of the other two were no longer smoking.

Elliott and Tighe (19) utilized a technique which did not involve physical unpleasantness. College students paid $65 at the start of treatment, and were required to announce their participation in the campus newspaper. They were asked to read several powerful statements against smoking. During the next 16 weeks they reported on their smoking, and were rewarded for periods of abstinence by having portions of their money refunded. Eighty-four percent claimed not to have smoked for the duration of the experiment, and 38 percent remained abstinent for follow-up periods ranging to 17 months. Of course, the temptations to lie in order to be paid back were great. In addition, the impact of the antismoking material by itself was not assessed. The procedure is intriguing in that it does not depend on a client-therapist relationship. If its effectiveness can be more firmly established, it might easily be adopted for use by any two smokers. They could make small wagers with each other about their ability to stop smoking.

ALCOHOLISM.   Conditioning therapies aimed at stopping excessive drinking also employ aversive techniques. The best known of these entails the use of disulfiram. Although disulfiram is a drug, it is described here, rather than in the section on pharmacological approaches to therapy, because the basis of disulfiram therapy is that it makes drinking alcohol exceedingly unpleasant. Unlike methadone, which suppresses the desire for heroin, or lobeline, which is touted as a substitute for smoking, disulfiram has few independent effects and does not alter the wish for alcohol. However, the ingestion of alcohol causes people who have taken disulfiram (for up to five days previously) to react violently. The heart begins pounding, a severe headache develops, blood pressure first rises and then falls precipitously, and the patient becomes weak, nauseous, and fearful.

The first description of disulfiram-alcohol interaction was given by Hald and Jacobsen (26), and its therapeutic value quickly became apparent. The strategy was to give the patients disulfiram tablets, then to give them alcohol. Competent medical personnel were generally kept in attendance, but there were nevertheless several serious and even fatal reactions (1). In addition, several patients complained of side effects from the disulfiram alone. Fox (20) used much smaller doses, which largely eliminated the side effects and reduced the severity of the reaction to alcohol. She has treated about 2300 patients and has reported great success (though she did not state her criteria for success).

An interesting aspect of the disulfiram treatment is that the rationale on which it is based is probably invalid. That is, it was originally believed that the aversive consequences of drinking following the ingestion of disulfiram would condition dislike for alcohol. However, disulfiram therapy generally continues for weeks, and often years, which suggests that the patient still craves alcohol, but abstains because he is cognizant of its acquired toxicity.

Franks (21) reviewed the history of behavior modification techniques with alcoholics, and noted that many of the frequently cited early failures were poorly conceived in that the investigators did not understand how to apply the principles of conditioning. Yet there have been some impressive successes, most notably that of Lemere and Voegtlin (34). They treated more than 4000 patients, and reported that 51 percent of them abstained from drinking for at least two years, and 23 percent remained abstinent for at least 10 years. (Note that even after two years of abstinence there is still a substantial relapse rate, which shows that therapists have no business reporting "cures" after treatment of only a few weeks or months duration; this applies not only to alcoholism, but to treatment of smoking and narcotic addiction as well.) Lemere and Voegtlin treated their patients by injecting them with apomorphine, which is an emetic, prior to having them ingest alcohol. The patients then became nauseous shortly after taking the alcohol. The procedure was given a sophisticated twist by Raymond (49). First he produced aversion to alcohol by the use of apomorphine. Then he intermixed trials of apomorphine and alcohol with choice situations, wherein patients were injected with saline instead of apomorphine, and given a choice between alcohol and various soft drinks. Since they had already been conditioned to avoid alcohol, they invariably chose the soft drinks. This was followed by praise, and by assurance to the patient that he would not be ill. Thus, by the time the patients had finished treatment, they had been punished for drinking alcohol, and rewarded for selecting alternatives to it.

Many related forms of behavior therapy have been developed, one of which is discussed below. (The reader interested in a review of alcoholism and therapy is referred to Fox's *Alcoholism* [20].)

Lovibond and Caddy (37) patterned the first phase of their approach on the principles of biofeedback. They accepted for treatment all individuals who were not overtly psychotic and who were willing to accept electric shock as part of the treatment. Their patients were instructed on the behavioral and subjective effects associated with different blood levels of alcohol. Then they drank pure alcohol mixed with fruit juice, in sufficient quantity to raise their blood alcohol concentrations (BAC) to 0.08 percent. During the session, which lasted about two hours, they were asked to estimate their BAC at 15 to 20 minute intervals. They were given immediate feedback by being allowed to observe a reading of the actual BAC on a meter in front of them. In the second and subsequent sessions, which also lasted about two hours, patients were required to drink and to estimate BAC. They were told that when concentrations exceeded 0.065 percent, a level which is associated with minimal learning impairment, they would receive periodic shocks, but they were required to continue drinking.

The schedule of shocks was designed to maximize uncertainty. Once the critical level was reached, shock was given on most but not all trials; moreover, both the duration and intensity of the shocks were varied, and they were administered at different stages of the drinking sequence, from picking up the glass to actually swallowing.

Patients were seen for 6 to 12 sessions, while otherwise continuing normal work and living routines. Where possible, a member of the patient's family also attended the sessions, and his or her support was enlisted. A control group was used, whose members were treated identically except for the schedule of shocks; they received their first shocks before BAC reached 0.065 percent, and later shocks during periods when they were not drinking. While it is hoped that individuals were randomly assigned to treatment and control groups, the authors did not so state.

Subjects were able to estimate their BAC to a high degree of accuracy. Of 13 control subjects, only 5 completed at least three sessions, compared with 28 of 31 treatment subjects. Of those who finished, the controls showed transient declines in alcohol consumption while the experimental subjects continued to have reduced intake even after 50 weeks. Far more significant is the reduction, in the experimental group alone, in the frequency of having BAC exceed 0.07 percent. The pretreatment figure for the frequency of excess BAC was 3.5 times per week, and the post-treatment figure only about 0.5 times per week. Thus, although they were not abstinent, the conditioned subjects were able to control their drinking. The authors regarded 21 of their 28 patients as complete successes, and claimed that their overall functioning had greatly improved.

Although the results are impressive and seem to offer hope to alcoholics, the study should be repeated with better control procedures. The experimenters made no mention of having conducted the treatment as a blind study, and probably conveyed to the control subjects the expectation that they would fail. They may have conducted themselves differently toward the two groups, in subtle and probably unintentional ways. That experimenter bias does intrude in such situations has been amply demonstrated (51), and its likelihood of occurrence in the Lovibond and Caddy study is attested to by the unwillingness of the control subjects to continue in the experiment. Were they told that they were not likely to be cured?

A general problem with studies on the treatment of smoking and alcoholism is that experimenters have relied on questionnaire replies from patients for estimating drug use. (The problem does not arise with patients who are being treated for heroin addiction, because they have generally been required to submit to urine analyses.) The patients responding to a questionnaire are undoubtedly frequently motivated to comply with expectations and hopes of the experimenters (45) and, as a result, probably substantially underestimate their use of drugs. Bias which is prejudicial to favorable outcomes would be greatest when the criteria are subjective, such as in estimation of BAC.

RESTRUCTURING OF PERSONALITY

Psychotherapy

Most drug addicts have favorable attitudes toward drugs. Pescor (46) reported that only 27 percent of hospitalized addicts strongly condemned drugs, while 71 percent thought that they were beneficial. Hence, addicts cannot be expected to voluntarily initiate or continue any form of treatment as long as there is no great difficulty in obtaining a regular supply of drugs. The problem applies to all forms of therapy for addicts, but may be most acute in traditional psychotherapy, where hostility on the part of the patient may create an insurmountable barrier between himself and the therapist. In addition, most addicts who are seriously enough ill to require treatment, regardless of the drug they use, have inadequate personalities. Narcotic addicts tend to be withdrawn and poor at communication — significant obstacles, since communication between patient and therapist is the essence of traditional psychotherapy. Therefore, Jaffe's claim (11, p. 554) that "psychotherapeutic techniques to prevent relapse have been spectacularly unsuccessful" should occasion no great surprise.

Therapeutic Communities

Alcoholics Anonymous

Alcoholics Anonymous, which was founded in 1935 by the late William Griffith, is a good example of a therapeutic community. Its membership is open to all who genuinely desire to stop drinking. Treatment is based upon 12 steps and 12 traditions which emphasize the member's helplessness against alcohol and the belief that faith in a higher power, whether it be God or the organization itself, is the key to the fight for sobriety. The members are enjoined to never again drink alcohol. They are encouraged to practice introspection in order to understand particular defects of their character which led to alcoholism, and to share their understanding with at least one other member of the group. They are asked to atone for the grief which they have caused others because of their sickness, and to help other alcoholics. Alcoholics Anonymous is completely self-supporting, and now has about 500,000 members. It has proved its worth as a means of rehabilitation for alcoholics who are highly motivated to quit. It has also provided inspiration for formation of other groups, such as those formed for stopping smoking or losing weight. Other live-in therapeutic communities, such as Phoenix House, Odyssey House, Synanon, and Daytop Village, created for the purpose of curing narcotic addicts, have been patterned after Alcoholics Anonymous. These organizations share the philosophy that the addict is most likely to recover if he is allowed to share his experiences with other addicts in a supportive, noncondemnatory atmosphere. Daytop Village, in New York State, is an appropriate model.

Daytop Village

Whereas Synanon is self-supporting, Daytop receives considerable support from state funds. Addicts come voluntarily, and must go through withdrawal without the aid of drugs. Others within the house offer distraction during the withdrawal period, and give comfort when needed. The result is a relatively pain-free withdrawal, at least in contrast with that which is normally observed in jails and hospitals (10).

Only two rules are enforced: no physical violence, and no drugs. The addicts are assigned to seven- or eight-member groups, balanced by sex and personality characteristics. The composition of the groups changes regularly, so that all members in the house eventually get to know each other. The groups meet for two hour sessions, three times per week. Members are encouraged to speak honestly and intensely about day to day living. No attempts are made to probe early childhood experiences.

Members also hold periodic meetings for intensive exploration of problems of general concern, such as prejudice or homosexual fear. These may last up to 12 hours. Marathon sessions which last 30 to 50 hours are held every few months, and have as their goal the direct experience of pain, fear, anger, and love.

Addicts are encouraged to participate in daily seminars on philosophical issues. In this way, it is believed, they will begin to realize the existence of many sources of stimulation and diversion which are offered by society. The residents do all the daily housekeeping, and are rewarded for good work by promotions in status. After about 12 months at Daytop, residents can begin helping in one of three storefront facilities which operate in areas where drug abuse is high. For the first time since entering Daytop, the addicts face the temptations of outside society. They interview prospects for Daytop, and conduct lectures and seminars. If deemed ready after about two months of such work, they are permitted to take jobs or continue their education, while still living at Daytop. After about six months they are once again evaluated and, if they pass the hurdle, are given the choice of leaving Daytop or applying for a position on its staff. Even those who leave are encouraged to stay involved.

Daytop has enjoyed great success. As of February, 1971, 158 of 176 graduates had remained free of drugs (10, p. xv). Although the program is too new for many of them to have reached the five year criterion of abstinence, the prognosis is favorable. (Consider the rapidity of the appearance of readdiction: Hunt and Odoroff [27] reported that 92 percent of patients who were discharged from Lexington and who became readdicted did so within the first six months after discharge.) On the negative side, only slightly more than 50 percent of the people who started in the Daytop program remained to completion (10, p. xvi). Altogether, less than one half of an initially very select addict population, namely those who voluntarily came for treatment, have had successful outcomes. Therapeutic villages have also been criticized for substituting one dependency, narcotics, for another—their program. In the case of Daytop, as of 1971, 75 percent of their graduates were doing staff work at Daytop or other therapeutic communities, (10, p. xvi). This indicates that therapeutic communities do not offer the ultimate solution, but it should be obvious that they are preferable alternatives to addiction.

Transcendental Meditation

Transcendental meditation (TM) has become popular throughout the country, especially on college campuses. Approximately 40,000 people have paid for the brief course in TM, which entails little more than soundlessly repeating one's mantra twice a day for about 15 minutes. Despite its simplicity, TM induces many physiological changes, including profound alterations in blood pressure and oxygen consumption (56). Recently, Benson and Wallace (5) tested the hypothesis that TM might be an aid to reducing drug use. They sent questionnaires to 1950 people who had practiced TM for at least three months, and received 1862 replies. The results were encouraging: total drug use declined with time spent in TM (up to 21 months, which was the longest period spent in TM). The extent of heavy use of drugs during a period six months prior to beginning TM is compared with that 21 months afterwards in Table 6.1.

The results, once again, should be interpreted cautiously. In the first place, prospective transcendental meditators are asked to abstain from all drug use for 15 days prior to starting meditation. As a result, people with very strong dependence on drugs would not qualify for the program. Secondly, the figures in Table 6.1 refer only to people who had practiced TM for at least three months; the drop-out rate is not given. Perhaps some people attended initially because they wanted to find an alternative to drugs, and stopped meditating because it did not work. Their number is unknown, and they are not included in the sample.

It must be assumed that those who did successfully complete at least three months of training had both an emotional and a monetary investment in TM, and may have falsified answers to questionnaire items. The likelihood that answers were falsified is substantial, since those who practice TM are assured that faithful meditators do not need drugs. The commitment to meditation would, of course, increase with time spent in the program (and the memory for extent of drug use six months prior to entry into the program would become increasingly subjected to upward distortions).

A final point is that no control group was employed. Perhaps people who tried TM did so because they had become dissatisfied with the effects they were receiving from drugs; for them, any alternative may have worked.

The Benson and Wallace study has been strongly criticized. It is hardly definitive. Yet, readers should not overlook the impressive changes which were reported by the population sampled. The results may be real, and further research is certainly warranted.

TABLE 6.1 **Percentages of Heavy Users of Various Drugs Before and After Starting the Practice of Transcendental Meditation (as Reported by Themselves)***

Drug	6 Months Before TM (%)	21 Months After TM (%)
Marijuana	28	0.1
LSD	14	0
Other hallucinogens	0.3	0
Narcotics	0.6	0
Amphetamines	1.6	0
Barbiturates	1.0	0
Hard liquor	2.7	0.4
Tobacco	27.0	5.7

*Adapted from Benson, H., and Wallace, K. Decreased drug abuse with transcendental meditation—a study of 1862 subjects. In Zarafonetis, C. (ed.), *Drug Abuse* (Philadelphia: Lea & Febiger, 1972).

CONCLUSIONS

Prognosis for Drug Addicts

A person who uses a drug to excess — whether it be narcotics, barbiturates, alcohol, nicotine, caffeine, or some other — is unlikely to be permanently cured by any known method of treatment. There are no sure-fire cures, and most of the many apparent successes have been only temporary, or, in the case of therapeutic communities, have been achieved at the price of total dependency on the community of ex-addicts. The most extensive information on long range outcomes has been collected for narcotic addicts. Some of the research is described below.

The morbidity of heroin addiction is high. O'Donnell (44) reported that more than one half of addicts discharged from the federal facility at Lexington, Kentucky had died within 12 years of discharge. The death rate for male addicts was 2.7 times that of the same age group in the general population, while that for female addicts approximated the non-addict death rate. James (cited in 60, p. 203) reported that among British addicts obtaining drugs from illicit sources, the death rate was 20 times the expected rate. The findings indicate that the most popular programs for treating drug addiction have not met with great success. A few additional statistics bolster the point. Pescor (46) found that about one-half of patients released from Lexington begin using drugs immediately upon discharge, and another 20 percent relapse within a month. Hunt and Odoroff (27) found that after six months from the time of discharge, the recidivism rate was 83 percent. Vaillant (55) found that about 95 percent of discharged addicts eventually returned to drug use. Casriel (10) claimed that the criterion of five years total abstinence is attained by fewer than five percent of people treated at the federal facilities at Lexington and Fort Worth, or through the Rockefeller program in New York State.

Langenauer and Bowden (33) studied addicts who had been discharged from Lexington. During their stays, they had received job training, opportunities for continuing education, group therapy sessions, and vocational counseling. Upon discharge, each ex-addict was assigned to an agency which provided therapy, and occasional job placement. Yet in the first month of aftercare, 45 percent of the ex-addicts used opioids at least once, and another five percent used other drugs. In the ensuing seven months, the number who used opioids at least once in any given month ranged from 42 to 57 percent. By the end of the sixth month only 14.4 percent remained totally abstinent, and by the eighth month 42 percent had been recommended for recommitment.

Age may be the best cure for narcotic addiction. Zimmering et al. (62) noted that onset of addiction parallels the appearance of adolescent conflicts, and that many addicts voluntarily stop taking drugs upon reaching an age when the conflicts have subsided. Winick (61) analyzed records held by the Federal Bureau of Narcotics on known addicts. He found that the length of addiction averaged 8.6 years, and that it varied inversely with the age of starting. He suggested that those who become addicted at earlier ages probably have the most severe problems.

The British System

The British handle their narcotics problem in a manner much different from American procedures. The British system regards drug addiction as a medical rather than a law enforcement problem. Therefore, physicians in Britain were at one time empowered to administer morphine or heroin to registered addicts who were deemed otherwise capable of leading normal lives, but who suffered severe disruption when deprived of drugs. Some physicians abused their privilege and dispensed heroin with abandon. As a result the number of addicts increased dramatically: from 1959 to 1964, the number of known heroin addicts in England increased from 68 to 342 (7, p. 69); and from 1961 to 1967, the number of those known to be addicted to morphine and morphine-like drugs (including heroin) increased from 470 to 2100. (The increase further accelerated in the early part of 1968 [60, p. 375]). Moreover, there is evidence (14) that these figures are gross underestimates. The British were understandably alarmed and formed a committee under the chairmanship of Sir Russell Brain to advise on possible courses of action. The following recommendations were made, and were implemented by 1968:

1. Where addiction is in doubt, physicians should seek expert advice.

2. Addicts should be identified.

3. Treatment centers should be established which, if necessary, could serve as detention centers.

4. The sanction to prescribe heroin and cocaine should be limited to doctors at the treatment centers, and the amounts prescribed should be restricted.

It should not be concluded from the above that British policy is to blame for the rise in drug addiction. The problem is worldwide. In the United States, the Bureau of Narcotics in 1965 had on file 52,793 active cases of heroin addiction and, as with the British, these records probably underappraise the actual number by a substantial margin (60, pp. 188–189). In California, in 1965, the number of listed heroin addicts grew by about 100 per month (60, p. 189).

The British system has much to commend it. By decriminalizing drug addiction, the need for a vast law enforcement apparatus, with the attendant enormous expense to the citizenry, is eliminated. Stachnik (53) has suggested several other benefits of decriminalization, pointing out just what the illegal status of addiction can entail. Consider three of Stachnik's observations:

1. If an addict has a $50 per day habit, and if the police are able to successfully close down his source, he will seek his supply elsewhere. But, the laws of supply and demand being operative, the reduced supply will eventuate in higher prices. Consequently the same habit might increase in cost to $70 per day, a distressing rise, since most or all of the addict's money is obtained through criminal activities.

2. The law is not a very effective deterrent to drug use. In a survey of high school students which Stachnik cited, it was found that only 7.1 percent of nonusers were stopped because of fear of criminal penalties.

3. The illegality of heroin may actually serve to increase the number of addicts. Addicts must raise large sums of money to keep themselves supplied, and do so by resorting to criminal activities. Some crimes entail less risks than others, and, as selling illicit drugs is a relatively safe crime, the addict recruits others to whom he can supply drugs.

One of the surprising failures of the British system is that it has not resulted in any substantial improvement in the health or productivity of the addicts, as compared with their American counterparts. In fact, their morbidity rates are higher, and infectious diseases, suicide, and overdose are all commonly found(6).

A Proposed Policy Toward Drugs

Brecher, in collaboration with the editors of Consumer Reports, has written an excellent, important book on the drug problem (9). Brecher offered several policy recommendations. They are outlined below as a fitting conclusion to this chapter, but without the wealth of documentation which Brecher used to support his case.

1. *Drugs should not be proscribed by law.* Prohibition leads to an increase in the price of drugs, and a concomitant increase in crime. Proscription leads to contaminated drugs, *and* to more powerful preparations (because they are less bulky and hence more easily smuggled and marketed).

2. *Do not use scare publicity.* Sensationalist campaigns which

depict the horrors of drugs are often counterproductive, actually serving to recruit users.

3. *Minimize the damage done by drugs.* This may be accomplished by attempting to stop the flow of contaminated drugs; by removing restrictions on the sale of drug paraphernalia such as hypodermic syringes, so that addicts are not forced to share needles and thereby spread communicable diseases; and by warning addicts of specific, easily avoidable dangers (e.g., warning that heroin and alcohol may interact in a dangerous fashion).

4. *Stop misclassifying drugs.* Alcohol and nicotine are drugs, and government officials should treat them as such. Officials should not classify marijuana and heroin together. Nor should they set up an artificial dichotomy between licit and illicit drugs. These classifications are harmful: they probably serve to increase the use of licit although hazardous drugs, and they interfere with efforts to educate the public about dangers of drugs.

5. *The drug problem should be dealt with on local rather than national levels.* A solution which works in one part of the country may not work in another part.

6. *Eradication of all illicit drug use is not a realistic goal.* The result of campaigns to stamp out drug use is often an increase in use, an increase in the damage done by drugs, or a shift of usage from one drug to another (sometimes more dangerous) one. A more sensible program would aim at reducing usage through education.

REFERENCES

1. Alha, A., Hjelt, E., and Tamminen, V. Disulfiram-alcohol interaction, investigation of five fatal cases and the chemical determination of disulfiram and blood acetaldehyde. Acta Pharmacol. Toxicol., 1957, 13:277–288.
2. Ausubel, D. The Dole-Nyswander treatment of heroin addiction. J.A.M.A., 1966, 195:949–950.
3. Bacon, S. Social settings conducive to alcoholism. N.Y.S. J. Med., 1958, 58:3494–3495.
4. Bartlett, W., and Whitehead, R. The effectiveness of meprobamate and lobeline as smoking deterrents. J. Lab. Clin. Med., 1957, 50:278–281.
5. Benson, H., and Wallace, K. Decreased drug abuse with transcendental meditation—a study of 1,862 subjects. *In* Zarafonetis, C. (ed.) *Drug Abuse.* Lea and Febiger, 1972.
6. Bewley, T. Heroin addiction in the United Kingdom. Brit. Med. J., 1965, 2:1284–1286.
7. Blachly, P. (Ed.) *Drug Abuse.* Springfield, Ill.: Charles C Thomas, 1970.
8. Branchey, M., Rauscher, G., and Kissin, B. Modifications in the response to alcohol following the establishment of physical dependence. Psychopharmacologia, 1971, 22:314–322.
9. Brecher, E. *Licit and Illicit Drugs.* Boston: Little, Brown & Co., 1972.
10. Casriel, D., and Amen, G. *Daytop: Three Addicts and Their Cure.* New York: Hill and Wang, 1971.
11. Chein, I., Gerard, D., Lee, R., and Rosenfeld, E. *Narcotics, Delinquency, and Social Policy.* London: Tavistock, 1964.

12. Clark, W., and Del Guidice, J. (Eds.) *Principles of Psychopharmacology.* New York: Academic, 1970.
13. Cohen, S. *The Drug Dilemma.* New York: McGraw Hill, 1969.
14. De Alarcon, R., and Rathod, N. Prevalence and early detection of heroin abuse. Brit. Med. J., 1968, 2:549–553.
15. Dole, V. Methadone maintenance treatment for 25,000 heroin addicts. J.A.M.A., 1971, 215:1131–1134.
16. Dole, V., and Nyswander, M. A medical treatment for diacetylmorphine (heroin) addiction. J.A.M.A., 1965, 193:646–650.
17. Dole, V., Nyswander, M., and Kreek, M. Narcotic blockade. Arch. Int. Med., 1966, 118:304–309.
18. Eddy, N., Halbach, H., Isbell, H., and Seevers, M. Drug dependence: its significance and characteristics. Bull. WHO, 1965, 32:721–733.
19. Elliott, R., and Tighe, T. Breaking the cigarette habit: effects of a technique involving threatened loss of money. Psychol. Rec., 1968, 18:503–513.
20. Fox, R. Disulfiram (Antabuse) as an adjunct in the treatment of alcoholism. *In* Fox, R. (Ed.) *Alcoholism.* New York: Springer, 1967.
21. Franks, C. Behavior modification and the treatment of the alcoholic. *In* Fox, R. (Ed.) *Alcoholism.* New York: Springer, 1967.
22. Freedman, A., Fink, M., Sharoff, R., and Zaks, A. Cyclazocine and methadone in narcotic addiction. J.A.M.A., 1967, 202:191–194.
23. Goldberg, S. Relapse to opioid dependence: the role of conditioning. *In* Harris, R., McIsaac, W., and Schuster, C. (Eds.) *Drug Dependence.* Austin: U. Texas, 1970.
24. Goldberg, S., and Schuster, C. Conditioned suppression by a stimulus associated with nalorphine in morphine-dependent monkeys. J. Exp. Anal. Behav., 1967, 10:235–242.
25. Goodman, L., and Gilman, A. *The Pharmacological Basis of Therapeutics.* New York: Macmillan, 1965.
26. Hald, J., and Jacobsen, E. Drug sensitising organism to ethyl alcohol. Lancet, 1948, 2B:1001–1004.
27. Hunt, G., and Odoroff, M. Follow-up study of narcotic drug addicts after hospitalization. Pub. Health Rep., 1962, 77:41–54.
28. Jaffe, J. Cyclazocine in the treatment of narcotic addiction. Curr. Psychiat. Ther., 1967, 7:147–156.
29. Jaffe, J. Further experience with methadone in the treatment of narcotic addicts. Int. J. Addict., 1970, 5:375–389.
30. Jaffe, J. Psychopharmacology and opiate dependence. *In* Efron, D. (Ed.) *Psychopharmacology: A Review of Progress.* U.S. PHS No. 1836, 1968.
31. Kreutzer, A. C., Lichtenstein, E., and Mees, H. Modification of smoking behavior: a review. Psychol. Bull., 1968, 70:520–533.
32. Kumar, R., and Stolerman, I. Resumption of morphine self-administration by ex-addict rats. J. Comp. Physiol. Psychol., 1972, 78:457–465.
33. Langenauer, B., and Bowden, C. A follow-up study of narcotic addicts in the NARA program. Am. J. Psychiat., 1971, 128:41–46.
34. Lemere, F., and Voegtlin, W. An evaluation of the aversion treatment of alcoholism. Quart. J. Stud. Alc., 1950, 11:199–204.
35. Lennard, H., Epstein, L., and Rosenthal, M. The methadone illusion. Science, 1972, 176:881–884.
36. Lichtenstein, E. and Kreutzer, C. Modification of smoking behavior: a later look. Adv. Behav. Ther., 1971, 61–75.
37. Lovibond, S., and Caddy, G. Discriminated aversive control in the moderation of alcoholics' drinking behavior. Behav. Ther., 1970, 1:437–444.
38. Lublin, I., and Joslyn, L. Aversive conditioning of cigarette addiction. Paper read at Am. Psychol. Assoc. Convention, 1968.
39. Martin, W., and Jasinski, D. Physiological parameters of morphine dependence in man—tolerance, early abstinence, protracted abstinence. J. Psychiat. Res., 1969, 7:9–17.
40. Methadone in the management of opiate addiction. The Med. Letter, 1969, 11:97–99.

41. Miley, R., and White, W. Giving up smoking. Brit. Med. J., 1958, *1*:101.
42. Nichols, J. How opiates change behavior. Sci. Am., 1965, *212*:80–88.
43. Nyswander, M. Methadone therapy for heroin addiction: Where are we? Where are we going? Drug Ther., 1971.
44. O'Donnell, J. A follow-up of narcotic addicts. Mortality, relapse and abstinence. Am. J. Orthopsychiat., 1964, *34*:948–954.
45. Orne, M. On the social psychology of the psychological experiment: with particular reference to demand characteristics and their implications. Am. Psychol., 1962, *17*:776–783.
46. Pescor, M. Follow-up study of treated narcotic drug addicts. Pub. Health Rep., 1943, Supp. No. 170.
47. Rapp, G., Dusza, B., and Blanchet, L. Absorption and utility of lobeline as a smoking deterrent. Am. J. Med. Sci., 1959, *237*:287–292.
48. Rapp, G. and Olen, A. Critical evaluation of lobeline based smoking deterrent. Am. J. Med. Sci., 1955, *230*:9–14.
49. Raymond, M. The treatment of addiction by aversive conditioning with apomorphine. Behav. Res. Ther., 1964, *1*:287–291.
50. Resnick, J. The control of smoking behaviour by stimulus satiation. Behav. Res. Ther., 1968, *6*:113–114.
51. Rosenthal, R. On the social psychology of the psychological experiment: the experimenter's hypothesis as unintended determinant of experimental results. Am. Sci., 1963, *51*:268–283.
52. Schuster, C., and Villareal, J. The experimental analysis of opioid dependence. *In* Efron, D. (Ed.) *Psychopharmacology: A Review of Progress.* U.S. PHS No. 1836, 1968.
53. Stachnik, T. The case against criminal penalties for illicit drug use. Am. Psychol., 1972, *27*:637–642.
54. Thompson, T., and Ostlund, W. Susceptibility to readdiction as a function of the addiction and withdrawal environments. J. Comp. Physiol. Psychol., 1965, *60*:388–392.
55. Vaillant, G. A twelve year follow-up study of New York narcotic addicts. Am. J. Psychiat., 1966, *122*:727–737.
56. Wallace, K. Physiological effects of transcendental meditation. Science, 1970, *167*: 1751–1754.
57. Weeks, J., and Collins, R. XXII. Patterns of intravenous self-injection by morphine-addicted rats. Res. Pub. Ass. Res. Nerv. Ment. Dis., 1968, *46*:288–298.
58. Whaley, D., Rosenkrantz, A., and Knowles, P. Automatic punishment of cigarette smoking by a portable electric device. Adv. Behav. Ther., 1971, 61–75.
59. Wikler, A. Conditioning factors in opiate addiction and relapse. *In* Wilner, D. and Kassebaum, G. (Eds.) *Narcotics.* New York: McGraw-Hill, 1965.
60. Wilson, C. (Ed.) *Adolescent Drug Dependence.* London: Pergamon, 1968.
61. Winick, C. Maturing out of narcotic addiction. Bull. Narcot., 1962, *14*:1–7.
62. Zimmering, P., Toolan, J., Safron, R., and Wortis, S. Drug addiction in relation to problems of adolescence. Am. J. Psychiat., 1952, *109*:272–278.

CHAPTER 7

PSYCHOPHARMACOTHERAPY

Mental illness may be America's most serious health problem. More than half of the patients seen by physicians, both in routine office practice and in the hospital, are being treated for psychiatric illness. The cost is staggering. In 1962, newly admitted psychiatric patients lost an estimated 293 million dollars in wages, and the total expenses for state and country exceeded one billion dollars (52). Although there is no known treatment which produces total remission of symptoms for the vast majority of the mentally ill, the continuing development of psychotropic drugs offers encouragement for the future. Kline (37) cited an incredible statistic: "In the 175-year history of public mental hospitals in the United States there had always been (until 1956) more patients in the hospitals at the end of any single year than there were at the beginning. This total had then reached the staggering number of 750,000, i.e., three-quarters of a million patients with an estimated cost to our economy of some four billion dollars a year." The reason for the reversal of the trend toward an ever-increasing patient population was the discovery and widespread use of just a few drugs.

OVERVIEW

The use of drugs to modify behavior often produces quite positive results. For controlling schizophrenic behavior, pharmacotherapy is more beneficial and entails fewer risks than electroconvulsive shock therapy (48). Drugs are also valuable, when used as adjuncts to psychoanalysis, in the treatment of anxiety and depression

147

(55). Some researchers claim that drugs eliminate the need for psycho-analysis or other psychotherapy altogether (48). Yet, as Irwin (29) has noted, drugs change behavior only temporarily. Real, perma-nent improvement of symptoms results from favorable experiences with the environment which shape behavior so that it can persist in the absence of drugs. The benefit of a drug which temporarily permits normal functioning by relieving anxiety or facilitating com-municativeness, is that it may indirectly lead to long-range improve-ments. For a detailed comparison of the relative merits of drugs and other forms of psychotherapy, see May (46).

DRUGS USED TO COMBAT PSYCHOSES

Chlorpromazine

The phenothiazine derivatives, of which chlorpromazine (CPZ) is by far the best known, are the most popular agents for treatment of psychotic behavior. CPZ will be discussed as the prototype of the class. CPZ was introduced into psychiatric practice in 1952. Within ten years, it had been given to about 50 million patients worldwide (2). CPZ reduces responsiveness to external stimuli, decreases initiation of activity, and diminishes anxiety, yet it has minimal effect on intellectual functioning. Hallucinations and delusions are reduced in frequency or completely eliminated. Initially, CPZ has sedating effects, but tolerance to these effects develops rapidly; however, even after long periods of usage, spon-taneous motor activity is reduced. CPZ has a very long duration of action, and various metabolites of the drug can be found in the urine for as long as 12 months after administration is discontinued.

CPZ is a strong adrenergic and a weak peripheral cholinergic blocker. It has a high therapeutic index and is not addicting. The frequencies of various ANS effects of CPZ and other phenothiazines are listed in Table 1.8. (ANS side effects of many other drugs dis-cussed in this chapter are listed in Tables 1.6 to 1.10). Several types of side effects have been noted, the most troublesome of which is postural hypotension. This is rarely a problem after the first few days of treatment. Other side effects include palpitation, reduction in the number of white cells in the blood, tremor and rigidity, jaundice, skin reactions, and ocular reactions.

Courvoisier et al. (9) developed a test which clearly differentiated between CPZ and barbiturates. After receiving CPZ, rats did not heed a previously learned warning signal which preceded the onset of shock, even though the shock obviously caused them pain; they escaped as soon as the shock began. Rats given barbiturates avoided the shock, and stopped avoiding only at doses which also impaired their escape behavior. Courvoisier's study can be taken as evidence that CPZ diminishes anxiety.

In a study of 400 schizophrenic patients, investigators at the National Institute of Mental Health (53) reported that 75 percent showed substantial improvement within six weeks of treatment with CPZ or other phenothiazines. The corresponding figure for patients who received placebos was 23 percent. There was an impressive interaction between drug and illness: fluphenazine was most effective in treating withdrawn, suspicious patients, whereas thioridazine worked best with withdrawn, periodically agitated patients (34).

Cole and Davis (8) reviewed studies comparing CPZ with placebos in the treatment of schizophrenia. With doses equal to or less than 400 mg per day, CPZ was clearly superior in only 14 of 33 studies. At doses greater than 500 mg per day, CPZ was superior in all of 23 studies. Cole and Davis further showed that no phenothiazine is clearly superior to CPZ, although some may be as effective. CPZ has also proved to be useful in the treatment of depressed and anxious patients (16).

Reserpine

Reserpine, the active principle of the plant *Rauwolfia serpentina*, was introduced into psychiatric practice at about the same time as was CPZ. However, the root of the plant had been used as a folk medicine for centuries before that, for hypertension and psychotic behavior. Many of the effects of reserpine are similar to those of CPZ. It too is a calming agent which produces indifference to environmental stimuli. However, CPZ is far preferable to reserpine in the treatment of psychoses, primarily because of the toxicity of the latter. Reserpine causes slowing of the heart, drowsiness, excess salivation, nausea, diarrhea, and postural hypotension. The most serious side effect, the one which has caused it to fall into disfavor, is depression. Patients who are maintained on reserpine often become suicidal. Nevertheless, reserpine has uses as an antihypertensive agent, and for patients who are refractory to phenothiazines and other antipsychotic drugs.

Megavitamin Therapy

Hoffer and Osmond (23–25, 27, 54) have long been advocates of the use of nicotinic acid and nicotinamide in the treatment of schizophrenia. They initiated their research in 1952 at a general hospital in Saskatchewan, Canada, accepting for treatment all patients who were diagnosed as schizophrenic. Patients were assigned, in a double blind study, to one of three groups — placebo, nicotinic acid, or nicotinamide — and all patients received psychotherapy. The results indicated a clear superiority, which extended for at least three years after discharge, for the groups given megavitamin therapy in addition to psychotherapy. Several other studies have convinced Hoffer that the vitamins are most effective when given early in the course of sickness and when combined with other forms of treatment. A problem with many of the later studies is that they did not employ double blind control groups.

Nicotinamide adenine dinucleotide (NAD) has also been claimed by Hoffer to be useful for treating schizophrenia (23). Kline et al. (38) found no improvement in patients treated with NAD. The contrary findings may be explained by two other studies: McComb and Gay (49) reported that commercial preparations of NAD differ in physical and chemical characteristics; and Pfeiffer, after comparing the EEG effects of the NAD used by Hoffer with that of Kline, concluded that Kline's preparation was relatively inactive (reported in 23).

Megavitamin therapy is safe (25). The chief side effect, which is usually restricted to the initial phase of treatment, is flush throughout the upper part of the body. Gastrointestinal symptoms such as nausea and diarrhea are occasionally reported. Skin reactions and headaches are infrequent occurrences.

DRUGS USED IN THE TREATMENT OF DEPRESSION

Many lines of evidence have converged to suggest to several scientists that mood is dependent upon the functional state of brain catecholamines. (Epinephrine, norepinephrine, and dopamine are all catecholamines.) They believe that reduced catecholamine activity is associated with depression, and hyperactivity with mania. Some of the evidence pointing to such relations has been summarized by Weil-Malherbe (67), and follows:

1. Severe stress, which often precipitates depression, reduces brain catecholamines.

2. Reserpine, which also depletes catecholamines, frequently precipitates depressions (and consequently has fallen into disfavor as an antipsychotic drug). Both alpha-methyl-dopa, which depletes brain stores of norepinephrine; and propranolol, which blocks adrenergic receptors, also cause depression.

3. MAOI's, imipramine, and amphetamine are used as antidepressant drugs, and all three facilitate adrenergic functioning.

4. Electroconvulsive shock therapy, which is an effective treatment for depression, produces a massive output of catecholamines.

Poschel and Ninteman (58) proposed that the integrity of the "reward system" of the brain depends on sufficient levels of brain norepinephrine, deficient levels being associated with depression. The hypothesis is useful because it makes meaningful the similarity in therapeutic action of several drugs which otherwise seem unrelated; moreover, it suggests directions for future research. For further reading on brain catecholamines and mood, see References 10 and 62 and the discussion of electrical stimulation of the brain in Chapter 16.

There are three classes of drugs which have been employed against depression: stimulants, MAOI's, and imipramine-like drugs. Berger (4) questioned the rationale for the use of stimulants (e.g., amphetamine), warning that "depression has characteristics of exhaustion, so administration of stimulants to a depressed patient is like flogging a tired horse" (p. 101). In addition, there is often a rebound depression following a period of amphetamine administration.

Monoamine Oxidase Inhibitors (MAOI's)

MAOI's irreversibly inactivate MAO, which is of major importance in the metabolism of epinephrine, norepinephrine, dopamine, and serotonin. Following the administration of MAOI's, there is an increase in the concentration of the catecholamines and serotonin in both the brain and other tissues.

MAOI's produce minimal changes in most measures of animal behavior. In man, they act as strong mood elevators and have long-lasting effects. Unfortunately, the mood-elevating effects are not manifested for several weeks, and toxic effects may appear much sooner; toxicity with chronic usage of MAOI's is more serious than with any other group of therapeutic drugs (31). The most serious consequence of prolonged administration is liver damage, and the drugs should not be given to patients with liver or kidney disease. Postural hypotension, headache, weakness, and fatigue have been reported. The MAOI's are notorious for their interactions with other drugs and with many common foods, such as aged cheeses, chopped liver, broad beans, schmalz pickled herring, and yogurt. The interactions have precipitated dangerous hypertensive crises.

Imipramine

Imipramine is probably the drug of choice against depression. Unlike the MAOI's, it does not produce euphoria in normal individuals, but it does elevate mood in depressed patients. Imipramine produces several relatively minor side effects, most of which are related to its atropine-like actions, i.e., dry mouth, constipation, and blurred vision. Tolerance develops to these effects.

Investigators have tried to determine whether certain types of patients are more responsive to imipramine-like drugs or to MAOI's. In 1958, Kuhn (40) claimed that imipramine is most effective in patients for whom the onset of depression has not been precipitated by obvious external causes, and whose premorbid personality is non-neurotic. Less likely to be helped by imipramine is the patient with a pattern of depression characterized by primary symptoms of anxiety, tension, and insomnia. Subsequent research (60) has called into question the usefulness of the dichotomy between the two types of depressions. It is probable that imipramine and its congeners are most effective in cases of severe depression, while MAOI's are best when anxiety is a major component of the depression.

Lithium

Lithium salts have been promoted for the treatment, and possibly the prevention, of both mania and depression in individuals who have recurring episodes of mania and/or depression. Lithium is especially useful in cases of prolonged mania. Even in the most severe cases, lithium often causes symptoms to disappear after a few weeks of treatment, and Schou (64, p. 659) claimed that 70 to 80 percent of manic patients show distinct improvement within two weeks. The major drawback of lithium is that it produces some toxicity, especially at the beginning of treatment. Among the many side effects are gastrointestinal irritation and nausea, muscular weakness and tremor, a dazed feeling, and perhaps nontoxic goiter (64, p. 655). In order to protect against these, the dosage schedule must be very carefully regulated, which entails weekly check-ups and several laboratory tests.

Effectiveness of Antidepressant Drugs

Electroconvulsive shock therapy (ECT) was introduced in 1938 as a treatment for depression. ECT is still widely used, but it is a dangerous procedure (68), and the development of a truly effective drug against depression would be most welcome. At present, the best that can be said is that there is little difference in antidepressant activity between drugs and ECT, but it is probable that ECT is somewhat superior (11).

In 1969 Smith et al. (65) published a very important analysis of research on antidepressant drugs during the period from 1955 through 1966. Their examination of research methodology produced results which are frightening in their implications for the whole field of psychopharmacotherapy, and probably for other forms of therapy as well. Table 7.1 indicates the level of sophistication in the research designs of the 490 studies covered in the Smith project. When Smith and his associates surveyed research techniques over the twelve-year period, they noted an apparent trend toward better designs, but even in the best year only 64 percent of the studies employed control groups, and 54 percent used blind techniques. In only 34 percent of the cases was the median age of the patient sample reported. In 55 percent of the studies the time limits were not reported, and those in which time limits were indicated varied in duration from eight hours to more than five years. The living arrangements for the patients—whether they were institutionalized or in an outpatient setting—were mentioned in 65 percent of the studies. The sex composition of the patients was indicated in 71 percent of the studies. In over 80 percent of the studies no mention was made of concurrent use of other therapies such as ECT or psycho-

TABLE 7.1 Drugs Studied and Research Sophistication*†

Drug	Times Drug is Studied	Times Control Group is Used		Times Blind Technique is Used	
		Number	Percent	Number	Percent
Imipramine	148	100	68	70	47
Amitriptyline	68	45	66	31	46
Phenelzine	48	37	77	18	38
Tranylcypromine	46	29	63	15	33
Iproniazid	40	27	68	12	30
Nialamide	39	22	56	8	21
Isocarboxazid	35	24	69	11	31
Desipramine	34	12	35	9	26
Trifluoperazine	26	7	27	4	15
Perphenazine	18	8	44	5	28
Nortriptyline	17	9	53	4	24
Pheniprazine	15	9	60	3	20
Dextroamphetamine	14	9	64	6	43
Meprobamate	14	10	71	6	43
Methylphenidate	13	6	46	2	15
Benactyzine	12	5	42	3	25
Chlordiazepoxide	12	8	67	3	25
Etryptamine	12	5	42	4	33
Protriptyline	10	5	50	4	40

*Only drugs studied 10 times or more are included in this table.
†From Smith, A., Traganza, E., and Harrison, G. Studies on the effectiveness of antidepressant drugs. Psychopharm. Bull., 1969, Special Issue, p. 3.

therapy, although drugs are rarely administered alone. In 67 percent of the studies the investigator knew which drug each patient was receiving. Furthermore, there was no uniform procedure for dosage schedule (see Table 7.2), and few investigators commented on the appearance of side effects.

Smith and his colleagues tried to ascertain the extent to which each of the neglected factors contributed to the likelihood of a particular type of outcome. They pooled all studies, regardless of the particular drug under consideration, and then isolated each variable individually. They emphasized that a factor would have had to exert very powerful effects in order to be shown to influence outcome under these circumstances. Several, as indicated in the next few paragraphs, were sufficiently powerful.

One influential variable was severity of illness, which was presumed to be reflected by inpatient or outpatient status. Improvement rates were significantly lower in inpatients, who were probably more severely ill at the start of drug administration. Study design was likewise a powerful variable: the highest rates of improvement were reported in studies in which there was no control group, while the lowest rates were seen in studies which employed both control groups and blind techniques. In percentage terms, 58 percent of the uncontrolled studies reported improvement rates of at least 70 percent, while only 33 percent of the controlled, blind studies did so. The criterion for improvement was not the same in all the studies; those where conclusions were based on statistical analyses of data reported high improvement rates less frequently than those where conclusions were based on the clinical judgment of the evaluator.

When all studies were considered, the median improvement

TABLE 7.2   Dosage Schedule*

Dosage schedule used for patients in the studies	Number of studies reporting dosage schedule
Fixed (one dose) throughout	93
Fixed initial with fixed increments and decrements	80
Fixed initial with adjustments according to patients conditions	32
Fixed initial only, no regulation thereafter	53
Limits imposed, free to regulate within	52
No regulations imposed	148
Other	29
Not reported	3
Total	490

*From Smith, A., Traganza, E., and Harrison, G. Studies on the effectiveness of antidepressants drugs. Psychopharm. Bull., 1969, Special Issue, p. 8.

rate for all drugs was 70.13 percent. Studies in which placebos were used reported improvement rates for placebo-treated patients which averaged 39.5 percent. If only those two facts were known, it would appear that antidepressant drugs were considerably better than the placebos. However, the apparent advantage dwindled upon further analysis: the median improvement rate for all drugs in studies with both placebo controls and blind techniques was only 61.1 percent; in the same studies, the improvement rates for placebo-treated patients was 46.3 percent.

When the various antidepressant drugs were compared without regard to research design, differences in efficacy among them were negligible. When design was considered, and only those studies counted in which control groups and blind techniques were used, imipramine and related drugs were significantly better than MAOI's.

ANTIANXIETY DRUGS

The antianxiety drugs, or minor tranquilizers, are unlike the major tranquilizers in that they are of little use in the treatment of psychotic behavior. The most popular antianxiety drugs are meprobamate and the two benzodiazepine derivatives, chlordiazepoxide and diazepam. Barbiturates and alcohol also relieve anxiety, but they are insufficiently selective. At doses which relieve anxiety both produce several undesirable side effects. (At other doses they may produce effects ranging from excitement and delirium to sleep and even surgical anesthesia.)

Meprobamate

Meprobamate is similar in many respects to the barbiturates. Like them, it has anticonvulsant properties, and withdrawal from meprobamate is often accompanied by convulsive seizures. Meprobamate is a muscle relaxant, and it has been suggested that both the tranquilizing and muscle relaxant effects may be secondary to sedation (13). As with all the antianxiety agents, meprobromate produces drowsiness as a major side effect (43). The hypnotic effect of meprobamate is comparable to that of the barbiturate drug phenobarbital (41). There are data indicating that meprobamate, like the barbiturates, impairs performance of passive avoidance and digit-symbol substitution tasks in man (30). On most tasks, it does not produce performance decrements (5).

Berger (5) emphasized the differences between meprobamate and barbiturates. Only the latter depress motor areas of the cortex and the midbrain reticular formation. Barbiturates produce much greater decrements in perceptual and intellectual performance than meprobamate. Both phenobarbital and meprobamate reduce activity in mice, but the depression of activity is preceded by a stimulant phase only in the case of phenobarbital. Meprobamate does not affect alertness except at doses which are so high as to produce substantial motor incoordination, while phenobarbital reduces alertness even at doses which leave motor performance intact.

Berger concluded that the differences between the drugs have important implications for therapy. Barbiturates are most useful for reducing a patient's awareness of external stimuli, and thus promoting sleep. Meprobamate reduces emotional hyperexcitability and anxiety arising from neurotic conflicts.

The most extensive review of the efficacy of meprobamate was conducted by Ayd (3), who cited 65 double blind studies. The evidence clearly favored meprobamate over barbiturates or placebos for the treatment of tension and anxiety. Ayd estimated that in the decade from 1954 to 1964, 80 million patients had been given meprobamate.

Chlordiazepoxide and Diazepam

Chlordiazepoxide was introduced into psychiatric practice in 1960, and diazepam in the following year. Both are very similar to meprobamate: they are muscle relaxants and anticonvulsants, and are characterized by barbiturate-like withdrawal. Their toxicity is low, but greater than that of meprobamate (31, p. 189). Like all of the antianxiety drugs, chlordiazepoxide and diazepam stimulate appetite, often resulting in weight gain. Both drugs reduce aggression in laboratory animals in doses which do not produce motor impairment; in contrast, the muscle relaxant dose of meprobamate is less than the dose which blocks fighting. Both benzodiazepine derivatives are also more powerful anticonvulsants than meprobamate, and are of some use in the treatment of epilepsy. Although no antianxiety drug has been demonstrated to be clearly superior to the others, it is nevertheless true that by 1965, one third of all prescriptions for psychoactive drugs outside of hospitals were for chlordiazepoxide (22).

Propranolol

Pitts (56) described the symptoms of anxiety neurosis, a disorder which afflicts about ten million Americans. The symptoms resemble those following physical exertion: shortness of breath, heart palpitation, chest pain, dizziness, trembling, and faintness. In addition, there are feelings of tension, apprehension, and severe anxiety. Pitts cited evidence which showed that the concentration of lactate in the blood, which normally rises somewhat during exercise, is excessively elevated in anxiety neurotics by exercise. At the same time, exercise often precipitates attacks in susceptible patients. Pitts studied the effects of lactate infusions on both anxiety neurotics and control subjects, and found that the infusions brought on severe attacks in the patient group, with symptoms lasting for as long as three days. Control subjects experienced mild symptoms after the lactate infusions.

Pitts suggested that anxiety neurotics may owe their illness to excessive production of epinephrine, which acts on cells to initiate the process which converts glycogen to lactate. Propranolol is a drug which blocks the actions of epinephrine at these and other sites. Propranolol has been shown to reduce the severity of anxiety symptoms, and even block them entirely.

Drugs Used as Adjuncts to Behavior Therapy for Anxiety

Behavior therapy is a fairly recent and controversial development which involves several related strategies for treating neurotic behavior. Behavior therapists consider neurotic behavior to be learned, and they believe that application of the laws of learning will enable neurotic responses to be eliminated. An excellent summary of behavior therapy techniques is found in Reference 57. Perhaps the most popular behavioral approach is systematic desensitization, in which patients are instructed to relax and imagine scenes which are capable of provoking varying degrees of anxiety. The rationale is that relaxation and anxiety are incompatible responses: if the anxiety provoked by a scene is not great, the relaxation will counteract it. If successful, the patient imagines another scene which originally aroused even greater anxiety than the first. The procedure continues through gradual increments in the intensity of the scenes until even the most vivid images no longer elicit anxiety.

The most time-consuming aspect of behavior therapy is training patients how to relax properly. Several drugs have proved useful in this respect, among them the phenothiazines and barbiturates — especially the short-acting barbiturate methohexital (7). Friedman (19) reported that methohexital eliminates the need for training voluntary relaxation, and actually induces a much more profound relaxation. As a result, the number of training sessions is generally reduced by one third or more. The value of drugs in behavior therapy has not been entirely settled, for Davison and Valins (12) have argued that drug-induced relaxation may not produce permanent changes in behavior.

LSD AS A THERAPEUTIC DRUG

In 1936 Guttman and Maclay (21) suggested that mescaline could be a valuable adjunct to psychotherapy. Since that time several psychedelic drugs, primarily LSD, have been regarded by some psychiatrists as the universal remedy, and have been used to treat schizophrenics, neurotics, alcoholics, autistic children, and people suffering from sexual disorders or phobias. Well over 2000 scientific publications have appeared extolling the therapeutic potentials of LSD. An international conference on the use of LSD in psychotherapy was held in New York in 1965, and attracted 46 registered participants, most of whom were prominent researchers or clinicians. They described many hundreds of successful outcomes of LSD therapy (1).

The rationale for such therapy has been given by Mogar (50), who claims that LSD can be used in two ways: as an adjunct to psychotherapy, it helps patients to reduce their defensiveness, relive childhood experiences, gain greater access to unconscious material, and increase their emotional expression; LSD can also foster rapid personality change by providing a transcendent experience that can bring about a resynthesis of basic values and beliefs and change relationships between self and environment. Mogar stated that the LSD experience results in an alteration of basic belief systems away from the material and toward the esthetic and religious. Mogar and Savage (51) reported that LSD therapy compares favorably with more traditional, longer term therapies. The significance of the last statement is questionable, since many psychologists have argued that traditional therapy is ineffectual (69).

LSD therapy, perhaps in part because it is such a radical departure from orthodox therapies, has attracted many critics. For example, in a conference on the value of psychedelic therapy, Unger stated that "not a single, methodologically-acceptable controlled study of psychedelic drug-assisted psychotherapy has yet been performed" (1, p. 366). Since then, there have been a few controlled studies which have yielded positive results, but careful evaluation remains sparse. Many of the best designed studies have yielded negative results. Johnson's work (32) on the use of LSD in alcoholism may be taken as representative. He randomly assigned 95 alcoholics who were free from serious organic disease to one of four treatment groups:

1. Patients were given LSD; a nurse was present throughout the experience, but the patients' therapists were not.

2. LSD was given in the presence of both nurse and therapist.

3. A combination of amobarbital and methamphetamine was given, with nurse and therapist present throughout.

4. Patients received routine clinical care.

The patients who received drugs got split doses, with the second dose being adjusted according to the response of the patients and the assessment of the therapist. The procedure ensured that each patient received an optimal dose, something which is unfortunately rarely achieved in double blind studies. The results indicated substantial improvement on several measures, such as degree of abstinence, and the effects that patients experienced when they did drink. The changes persisted for at least one year after the LSD experience. However, patients in every group improved, and *there were no significant differences among the groups on any measure.* LSD was effective, but no more so than conventional therapy, or the alteration in consciousness induced by the amobarbital-methamphetamine combination.

The United States government has imposed controls on LSD research which are much more stringent than those found in most other countries. This is unfortunate, as it reduces the probability that the many enthusiastic reports of its efficacy will receive proper scrutiny. Some scientists, including Hoffer and Osmond (26) and Mogar (50), feel that its value in clinical practice is already firmly established.

DRUGS USED IN THE TREATMENT OF HYPERKINETIC BEHAVIOR OF CHILDREN

The hyperkinetic syndrome is a common problem among children who are performing poorly in school, and includes as symptoms hyperactivity, short attention span, ready distractability, impulsivity, and poor coordination. In 1937, Bradley (6) published the startling and paradoxical finding that amphetamine is extremely useful in subduing the behavior of hyperactive children without causing them to lose interest in their surroundings. One benefit deriving from this effect was that the children's performance in school was greatly improved. In the ensuing years, there have been many studies on treatment of children who are diagnosed as hyperkinetic (see 14, 17, 18). The studies clearly demonstrate that stimulants are effective in treating hyperkinetic children; they neither pep up nor sedate, but allow more efficient organizing and focusing of behavior. The anticonvulsant drug diphenylhydantoin (44) and several phenothiazines (17) are also useful, while the barbiturates actually increase the severity of the symptoms.

Laufer and his colleagues (42) developed a screening test for hyperkinetic children. The test employed a combination of stroboscopic light and the convulsant drug pentylenetetrazol, which together induce abnormal EEG responses and twitching of the forearms. The dependent variable was the dose of pentylenetetrazol necessary for the induction of the response. Hyperkinetic children who required hospitalization for their disorders were found to be different in two respects from others in the hospital who had different forms of emotional disturbance. The hyperkinetic children initially required lower doses of pentylenetetrazol to induce the abnormal responses, and amphetamine reduced their susceptibility. Laufer et al. speculated that the site of action of amphetamine is the subcortical area of the brain. Amphetamine is most effective where there is obvious organic impairment (14). Still, not all hyperkinetic children have histories of organic brain dysfunction, and methylphenidate, which is very effective in treating the disorder, is equally useful in the treatment of hyperkinetic children who are not suffering from discernible brain damage (39). In short, the drugs work, but their mechanism is obscure.

A panel chaired by Freedman was convened in 1971 to discuss the role of stimulant drugs in the treatment of hyperkinetic children (61). The members of the panel concluded that stimulant medication is beneficial in somewhat more than half the cases, and that stimulants are the drugs of choice in treating the hyperkinetic syndrome. The panel members argued against the claim that childhood dependence on drugs in these special cases increases the hazard of later drug abuse. They noted that no such association has become evident in the 30 years that the drugs have been used. Whether or not the medication does increase the risk of adult drug abuse, the effect appears to be a small one, especially when weighed against the obvious benefits of the drug therapy.

WITHDRAWAL FROM DRUGS

As noted at the beginning of the chapter, drugs by themselves do not permanently alter behavior; they only facilitate the learning of new responses to replace maladaptive ones. Thus, work on state dependent learning (see Chap. 11), which shows that learning which takes place while an individual is drugged does not fully transfer to the nondrugged state, is highly relevant for drug therapy. The phenothiazines, for example, have been shown to produce dissociative learning. Hunt (28) induced fear in rats by pairing a clicking sound with electric shock, then extinguished the fear after the rats had been given chlorpromazine. When the drug was discontinued, the fear response to the clicks reappeared. The implications for therapy soon became apparent, and there followed a substantial literature which indicated serious danger of relapse upon withdrawal of psychotherapeutic drugs. Gross et al. (20) reported a relapse rate of 73 percent when drugs were withdrawn from psychotic patients.

Prien and Cole (59) also observed high relapse rates. Kamano (33) reviewed the literature in 1966, and identified many of the relevant variables. He noted that the length of treatment prior to drug withdrawal has not been shown to influence relapse rate. Dosage of drug is important, with the greatest transfer decrements arising after the highest dosages of drug. Kamano therefore questioned the practice of maintaining patients on the highest doses which do not produce serious side effects; he suggested that lower doses, although producing smaller initial results, would more readily enable patients to discontinue usage.

Clinicians are thus confronted with a serious problem. They may either maintain patients permanently on drugs, which is not only costly but also greatly increases the likelihood that the patients will suffer side effects; or they may terminate the drug and risk relapse. The choice is complicated by the variable time of onset of the symptoms of relapse, for in the studies cited by Kamano, the range was one to six months after discontinuation.

Davison and Valins (12) addressed themselves to the problem. They hypothesized that subjects who are tricked into believing that changes in their own behavior result not from a drug, but from some internal change, would be more likely to maintain the changes upon withdrawal. Using placebos rather than drugs, Davison and Valins devised an ingenious procedure for testing their hypothesis. Volunteers who agreed to participate in two ostensibly independent experiments were told that for the first they would be given a drug which might affect skin sensitivity. Sensitivity, measured by the threshold of tolerance to electric shock, was first determined before any "drug" was administered. Then all subjects were given the placebo. The threshold determinations were then repeated, but the shock intensities were secretly halved by the experimenters. Thus, the subjects were deceived into thinking that the pill had increased their capacity to tolerate shock. Next, half of the subjects were told that they had actually received placebo; the rest were assured that the drug effects would wear off in another minute. All were thanked for their participation, after which came the crucial part of the experiment.

The second experimenter arrived, and explained that he was conducting his experiment in tandem with the first only because it too involved determinations of sensitivity to shock. The beleaguered subjects were then exposed to a third series of shocks, and the two groups differed significantly in their performance. Subjects who attributed their changes during the second series of shocks to the effects of a drug tolerated less than they did during the initial series; subjects who believed that their improvement in performance during series two was not due to a drug improved on series three.

The study by Davison and Valins suggests one strategy for withdrawing patients from drugs, namely, convincing them that they have actually been receiving placebos. However, the problem of relapse following termination is almost surely more complex. For one thing, the long periods of time which elapse between termination and the renewed onset of symptoms indicate that a patient's beliefs concerning the mechanism by which his change in behavior is effected may not be very important. Otherwise, the drug-free period of normalcy would be sufficient to insure relatively permanent cures. Secondly, the literature on state dependent learning, most of which deals with animals, demonstrates that changes in state affect transfer of learning independently of a subject's knowledge of drug condition.

A possible alternative strategy would be to have therapists reduce dosage gradually and surreptitiously, leaving the appearance of the medication unaltered. Then, only after the patient was fully withdrawn from the drug would he be told that withdrawal was about to begin. He could then be given a (fictitious) schedule of progressively weaker doses. This two-stage procedure would separate pharmacological from psychological withdrawal.

NON-SPECIFIC FACTORS WHICH INFLUENCE DRUG THERAPY

Klett and Moseley (36) attacked the implicit assumption of many drug researchers ". . . that drugs of a given class have more or less the same kind of effect on all patients and that the only important parameters are dosage and side effects." They analyzed data from a study of a large number of hospitalized schizophrenics who had been randomly assigned to receive chlorpromazine, fluphenazine, or thioridazine. Pretreatment scores of the patients in 10 separate diagnostic categories were available, as well as post-treatment outcomes. The authors developed equations which described therapeutic outcomes as a function of the interaction between initial symptomatology and the particular drug used. No one drug was best for all patients. Then the equations were applied, on the basis of pretreatment scores, to a second large sample of patients for whom the same data were available, and who had also been treated with one of the three drugs. Patients were classified according to whether or not they had received the drug which would have been assigned had their therapists used the equations. Klett and Moseley found that those patients who had received the drug which would have been assigned on the basis of the equations showed superior outcomes. In other words, the title for their paper was justified; therapists should recognize the need to find "the right drug for the right patient."

The study by Klett and Moseley indicates that the personality of patients influences their responsiveness to the antipsychotic drugs. Individual differences also influence outcomes in the treatment of neurotic patients. Rickels (62) and Uhlenhuth et al. (66) have published excellent reviews of this subject. Patient characteristics associated with the most favorable response to the minor tranquilizers include chronic illness, previous experience with minor tranquilizers, male sex, high verbal ability, middle social class, high compliance, high ego strength, and low hypochondriasis. Patients who respond best to placebos tend to show these characteristics: low social class, low verbal I.Q., low anxiety, low psychopathology, low hypochondriasis, no previous drug treatment, brief duration of illness, and high ego strength.

Rickels and his colleagues identified three other important variables in addition to the personality of the patient: the treatment milieu, the nontreatment milieu, and the attitude and bearing of the physician. As regards the first, an appropriate set and therapeutic atmosphere are associated with favorable responses to minor tranquilizers. The nontreatment milieu is an important variable because unfavorable external events reduce the efficacy of both active drug and placebo. As for the attitude of the physician, the greatest differences between drug and placebo are found in patients of physicians who are supportive and encouraging.

A very important non-specific factor in therapy, which is influenced by all of the other variables, is the expectation of the patient. Lipman et al. (45) tested the consequences of modifying expectations by inducing a side effect in their patients and varying its meaning for them. A total of 24 groups of anxious neurotics was used, including four drug groups:

Group 1 received chlordiazepoxide and atropine, the latter in a dose which produces dry mouth in a large percentage of subjects.

Group 2 was given chlordiazepoxide alone.

Group 3 received atropine alone, in the same dose as given group 1.

Group 4 was given inert placebo.

Half of the patients in each group were told that a possible side effect of the medication would be that they might get a dry mouth, which would be a sign that it was working properly. The other half were told, "This medicine may make your mouth dry but this is nothing to worry about." These latter instructions were designed to convey neutral feelings toward dry mouth. The groups were further subdivided by assigning members to any of three participating clinics.

There was a significant drug effect. Patients who received chlordiazepoxide exhibited significantly greater improvement of symptoms than those who did not. Surprisingly, however, atropine reduced effectiveness, especially in those patients who were told that feelings of a dry mouth should be favorably interpreted. The authors speculated that patients who were told to expect a side effect focused on side effects; thus, they reported more atropine-related side effects than patients who had received neutral instructions. The results led the authors to question the advisability of using active placebos in drug studies, since they may be associated with poorer therapeutic outcome than inert placebos. Hence, the difference between drug and placebo might actually be magnified.

One additional finding was that the results varied reliably according to the clinic in which the drugs were administered. This is further evidence of the pervasiveness of non-specific factors in therapy.

SUMMARY

The psychopharmacological revolution has saved millions of people with emotional disorders from permanent internment in mental institutions, and has enabled many of them to lead relatively normal lives. The greatest advances are probably still to come. At present, the therapeutic drugs most commonly prescribed are probably as follows: for schizophrenia, chlorpromazine; for mania, lithium; for depression, imipramine or the closely related amitriptyline; for anxiety, meprobamate and chlordiazepoxide; for hyperkinetic behavior disorders of childhood, amphetamine and methylphenidate. Of course, it has now been firmly established that there is no single "drug of choice" for a particular type of disorder. An enormous number of factors contribute to determine the best drug for a particular patient.

Advances in psychopharmacotherapy will probably come as a result of research on two fronts. First, new drugs will be developed, and second, more powerful diagnostic tools will enable better matchings of patient with drug, physician, and adjunctive therapy. Already, new drug research has produced tybamate, which is structurally similar to meprobamate, and may eventually supplant it in the treatment of anxiety. In addition, the butyrophenone series, of which haloperidol is the prototype, and the thioxanthenes, of which chlorprothixene is most popular, may have valuable applications as antipsychotics.

REFERENCES

1. Abramson, H. (Ed.) *The Use of LSD in Psychotherapy and Alcoholism.* Indianapolis: Bobbs-Merrill, 1967.

2. Ayd, F., Jr. Chlorpromazine: ten years' experience. J.A.M.A., 1963, *184*:51–54.
3. Ayd, F., Jr. Meprobromate: a decade of experience. Psychosomatics, 1964, *5*:82–87.
4. Berger, F. Classification of psychoactive drugs according to their chemical structures and sites of action. *In* Uhr, L., and Miller, J. (Eds.) *Drugs and Behavior.* New York: Wiley, 1960.
5. Berger, F. The relation between the pharmacological properties of meprobamate and the clinical usefulness of the drug. *In* Efron, D. (Ed.) *Psychopharmacology: A Review of Progress.* U.S. PHS Pub. No. 1836, 1968.
6. Bradley, C. The behavior of children receiving benzedrine. Am. J. Psychiat., 1937, *94*:577–585.
7. Brady, J. Drugs in behavior therapy. *In* Efron, D. (Ed.) *Psychopharmacology: A Review of Progress.* U.S. PHS Pub. No. 1836, 1968.
8. Cole, J., and Davis, J. Clinical efficacy of the phenothiazines as antipsychotic drugs. *In* Efron, D. (Ed.) *Psychopharmacology: A Review of Progress.* U.S. PHS Pub. No. 1836, 1968.
9. Courvoisier, S., Fournel, J., Ducrot, R., Kolsky, M., and Koetschet, P. Properties pharmacodynamiques du chlorhydrate de chloro-3 (dimethylamino-3 propyl-phenothiazine (4560 RP). Arch. Int. Pharmacol. Ther., 1952, *92*:305–361.
10. Davis, J. Theories of biological etiology of affective disorders. Int. Rev. Neurobiol., 1970, *12*:145–175.
11. Davis, J., Klerman, G., and Schildkraut, J. Drugs used in the treatment of depression. *In* Efron, D. (Ed.) *Psychopharmacology: A Review of Progress* U.S. PHS Pub. No. 1836, 1968.
12. Davison, G., and Valins, S. Maintenance of self-attributed and drug-attributed behavior change. J. Person. Soc. Psychol., 1969, *11*:25–33.
13. Domino, E. Psychosedative drugs II: meprobamate, chlordiazepoxide, and miscellaneous agents. *In* DiPalma, J. (Ed.) *Drill's Pharmacology in Medicine.* New York: McGraw-Hill, 1965.
14. Eisenberg, L. The management of the hyperkinetic child. Develop. Med. Child Neurol., 1966, *8*:593–598.
15. Epstein, L., Lasagna, L., Conners, C., and Rodriguez, A. Correlation of dextroamphetamine excretion and drug response in hyperkinetic children. J. Nerv. Ment. Dis., 1968, *146*:136–146.
16. Fink, M., Klein, D., and Kramer, J. Clinical efficacy of chlorpromazine-procyclidine combination, imipramine and placebo in depressive disorders. Psychopharmacologia, 1965, *7*:27–36.
17. Freed, H., and Frignito, M. Tranquilizers in child psychiatry: current status on drugs, particularly phenothiazine. Penn. Psychiat. Quart., 1961, *1*:39–48.
18. Freeman, R. Drug effects on learning in children—a selective review of the past thirty years. J. Special Educ., 1966, *1*:17–37.
19. Friedman, D. A new technique for the systematic desensitization of phobic symptoms. Behav. Res. Ther., 1966, *4*:139–140.
20. Gross, M., Hitchman, I., Reeves, W., Lawrence, J., and Newell, P. Discontinuation of treatment with ataractic drugs. Rec. Adv. Biol. Psychiat., 1961, *3*:44–63.
21. Guttmann, E., and Maclay, W. J. Neurol. Psychopathol., 1936, *16*:193.
22. Himwich, H. Postgrad. Med., 1965, *37*:35.
23. Hoffer, A. Biochemical aspects of schizophrenia. Am. Schiz. Foundation, Comm. on Therapy. Meeting, Sept., 1968.
24. Hoffer, A. *Niacin Therapy in Psychiatry.* Springfield, Ill.: Charles C Thomas, 1962.
25. Hoffer, A. Safety, side effects and relative lack of toxicity of nicotinic acid and nicotinamide. Schizophrenia, 1969, *1*:78–87.
26. Hoffer, A. and Osmond, H. *The Hallucinogens.* New York: Academic Press, 1967.
27. Hoffer, A., and Osmond, H. Treatment of schizophrenia with nicotinic acid (a ten-year follow-up). Acta Psychiat. Scand., 1964, *40*:171–189.
28. Hunt, H. Some effects of drugs on classical (type S) conditioning. Ann. N.Y. Acad. Sci., 1956, *65*:258–267.
29. Irwin, S. Considerations for the pre-clinical evaluation of new psychiatric drugs: a case study with phenothiazine-like tranquilizers. Psychopharmacologia, 1966, *9*:259–287.
30. Janke, W., and Debus, G. Experimental studies on antianxiety agents with normal

subjects: methodological considerations and review of the main effects. *In* Efron, D. (Ed.) *Psychopharmacology: A Review of Progress.* U.S. PHS Pub. No. 1836, 1968.

31. Jarvik, M. Drugs used in the treatment of psychiatric disorders. *In* Goodman, L., and Gilman, A. (Ed.) *The Pharmacological Basis of Therapeutics.* New York: Macmillan, 1965.

32. Johnson, G. LSD in the treatment of alcoholism. Am. J. Psychiat., 1969, *126*:481–487.

33. Kamano, D. Selective review of effects of discontinuation of drug treatment: some implications and problems. Psychol. Rep., 1966, *19*:743–749.

34. Katz, M. A typological approach to the problem of predicting response to treatment. *In* Wittenborn, J., and May, P. (Eds.) *Prediction of Response to Pharmacotherapy.* Springfield, Ill.: Charles C Thomas, 1966.

35. King, P. Regressive ECT, chlorpromazine and group therapy in treatment of hospitalized schizophrenics. Am. J. Psychiat., 1958, *115*:354–357.

36. Klett, C., and Moseley, E. The right drug for the right patient. J. Consult. Psychol., 1965, *29*:546–551.

37. Kline, N. The challenge of the psychopharmaceuticals. Am. Philo. Soc., 1959, *103*: 455–462.

38. Kline, N., Barclay, C., Cole, J., Esser, A., Lehmann, H., and Wittenborn, J. Controlled evaluation of nicotinamide adenine dinucleotide. Brit. J. Psychiat., 1967, *11*:731–742.

39. Knights, R., and Hinton, G. The effects of methylphenidate (Ritalin) on the motor skills and behavior of children with learning problems. J. Nerv. Ment. Dis., 1969, *148*:643–653.

40. Kuhn, R. The treatment of depressive states with G 22355 (imipramine hydrochloride). Am. J. Psychiat., 1958, *115*:459.

41. Lasagna, L. A study of hypnotic drugs in patients with chronic diseases. J. Chron. Dis., 1956, *3*:122–133.

42. Laufer, M., Denhoff, E., and Solomon, G. Hyperkinetic impulse disorders in childrens' behavior problems. Psychosom. Med., 1957, *19*:38–49.

43. Lehmann, H. Differences in behavioral effects in humans. Excerpta Med., 1967, 215–221.

44. Lindsley, D., and Henry, C. The effect of drugs on behavior and the electroencephalograms of children with behavior disorders. Psychosomat. Med., 1942, *4*: 140–149.

45. Lipman, R., Park, L., and Rickels, K. Paradoxical influence of a therapeutic side effect interpretation. Arch. Gen. Psychiat., 1966, *15*:462–474.

46. May, P. Anti-psychotic drugs and other forms of therapy. *In* Efron, D. (Ed.) *Psychopharmacology: A Review of Progress.* U.S. PHS Pub. No. 1836, 1968.

47. May, P., and Tuma, A. Ataractic drugs and electroshock. Int. J. Neuropsychiat., 1965, *1*:84–89.

48. May, P., and Tuma, A. Treatment of schizophrenic. Brit. J. Psychiat., 1965, *3*:503–510.

49. McComb, R., and Gay, R. A comparison of reduced NAD preparations from four commercial sources. Clin. Chem., 1968, *14*:754–763.

50. Mogar, R. Current status and future trends in psychedelic (LSD) research. J. Human. Psychol., 1965, *2*:147–166.

51. Mogar, R., and Savage, C. Personality changes associated with psychedelic therapy. Psychother., 1964, *1*:154–163.

52. The National Health Education Committee, Inc. Facts on the major killing and crippling diseases in the U.S. today, 1964.

53. National Institute of Mental Health, Psychopharmacology Service Center Collaborative Study Group. Phenothiazine treatment in acute schizophrenia. Arch. Gen. Psychiat., 1964, *10*:246–261.

54. Osmond, H., and Hoffer, A. Massive niacin treatment in schizophrenia. Review of A Nine Year Study. Lancet, 1962, *1*:316–320.

55. Ostow, M. The complementary roles of psychoanalysis and drug therapy. *In* Solomon, P. (Ed.) *Psychiatric Drugs.* New York: Grune and Stratton, 1965.

56. Pitts, F., Jr. The biochemistry of anxiety. Sci. Am., 1969, *220*:69–75.

57. Porter, R. (Ed.) *The Role of Learning in Psychotherapy.* Boston: Little, Brown, 1968.

58. Poschel, P., and Ninteman, F. Excitatory (antidepressant) effects of monoamine oxidase inhibitors on the reward system of the brain. Life Sci., 1964, 3:903–910.
59. Prien, R., and Cole, J. High dose chlorpromazine therapy in chronic schizophrenia. Arch. Gen. Psychiat., 1968.
60. Raskin, A. The prediction of antidepressant drug effects: review and critique. In Efron, D. (Ed.) Psychopharmacology: A Review of Progress. U.S. PHS Pub. No. 1836, 1968.
61. Report of the conference on the use of stimulant drugs in the treatment of behaviorally disturbed young school children. Psychopharm. Bull., 1971, 7:23–29.
62. Rickels, K. Antineurotic agents: specific and non-specific effects. In Efron, D. (Ed.) Psychopharmacology: A Review of Progress. U.S. PHS Pub. No. 1836, 1968.
63. Schildkraut, J., and Kety, S. Biogenic amines and emotion. Science, 1967, 156:21–30.
64. Schou, M. Use of lithium. In Clark, W., and del Guidice, J. (Eds.) Principles of Psychopharmacology. New York: Academic Press, 1970.
65. Smith, A., Traganza, E., and Harrison, G. Studies on the effectiveness of antidepressant drugs. Psychopharm. Bull., 1969, Special Issue.
66. Uhlenhuth, E., Covi, L., and Lipman, R. Indications for minor tranquilizers in anxious outpatients. In Black, P. (Ed.) Drugs and the Brain. Baltimore: Johns Hopkins, 1969.
67. Weil-Malherbe, H. The biochemistry of affective disorders. In Clark, W., and del Guidice, J. (Eds.) Principles of Psychopharmacology. New York: Academic Press, 1970.
68. Will, O., Jr., Rehfeldt, F., and Neumann, M. A fatality in electroshock therapy. Report of a case and review of certain previously described cases. J. Nerv. Ment. Dis., 1948, 107:105–126.
69. Wolpe, J., Salter, A., and Reyan, L. (Eds.) The Conditioning Therapies: The Challenge in Psychotherapy. New York: Holt, Rinehart, and Winston, 1964.

CHAPTER 8

DEVELOPMENTAL ASPECTS

The action of a drug does not always terminate upon the discontinuation of its administration. Reserpine is a good example. It acts as an antipsychotic drug by depleting stores of catecholamines and serotonin in the brain. The neurotransmitters do not reattain their pre-drug levels until weeks after the reserpine is discontinued, and behavioral effects also persist well beyond the last administration.

The effects of some drugs persist even into the next generation. Friedler and Cochin (22, 23) reported that injections of morphine into female rats five days before they conceived their young led to differences in both physical development and response to morphine in the offspring. Gauron and Rowley (26) described an intriguing study along similar lines. They injected five-day-old rats daily with either saline or one of the major tranquilizers—chlorpromazine, trifluoperazine, or prochlorperazine—until the rats reached 55 days of age. The animals were then put aside until they were 75 days old, at which time they were tested in an avoidance conditioning apparatus. Saline-treated rats made the fewest errors. At 120 days of age the females were bred with males which had never received drugs. (The chlorpromazine-treated animals were poorer breeders than those from the other groups.) When the offspring reached 75 days, and without their having ever been exposed directly to drugs, they were tested in the conditioning apparatus. The offspring of the generation given trifluoperazine and prochlorperazine demonstrated inferior learning ability; they were also inferior in a competitive

168

test situation. The same two groups were also inferior to their mothers, who themselves were poor learners.

Drugs influence not only offspring still-to-be-conceived but also, to a far greater extent, developing fetuses and newborn infants. The thalidomide tragedy alerted people to the dangers of the administration of drugs to pregnant women. Very young organisms, too, are extremely susceptible to the effects of drugs. In fact, simple stimulation of any sort—handling, temperature change, electric shock, or shaking—permanently influences the behavior of rats. Changes can be detected in adult activity level, emotionality, perception, learning, physical maturation, and resistance to a wide variety of stressors (45). Other species besides rats, including humans, are also greatly influenced by early stimulation. Many of the effects are probably mediated by changes in rates of secretion of ACTH, corticosterone, and epinephrine. Therefore, it is not surprising that administration of any of the above named hormones, or drugs which influence their levels within the body, should affect development. Developmental processes are also affected by a great many other drugs which have less fully understood mechanisms of action.

TERATOGENIC EFFECTS OF DRUGS

Substances which produce malformed offspring are called teratogens. In Chapter 4, the teratogenic potential of LSD was considered, along with some of the difficulties encountered in laboratory research on teratogens. Among the many problems confronting the researcher are the following factors:

1. There are critical periods for effects of stimulation upon behavior. A fairly good generalization is that, the younger the animal, the greater the permanent effect of abnormal stimulation. However, in some instances an animal is susceptible at a late stage of development, but not at an earlier one. If a drug is not administered during the critical period, a potentially serious effect may go undetected in the laboratory.

2. The dosage is crucial. Too small a dose has no effect. Too large a dose may lead to an increase in fetal mortality and spontaneous abortions, but may not always be accompanied by an increase in the number of malformed liveborn. Thus, unless attention is paid to fetal deaths, potential teratogens may go undetected.

3. Many drugs may produce rare defects, which might not show up in small samples or which might be attributed to other causes.

4. The developing fetus is extremely sensitive to any unusual stimulus. Large doses of anything are likely to be dangerous.

5. Many malformations are not manifest at birth (Warkany and Kalter, cited in Ref. 16).

6. Species differences are very important. It cannot be said with certainty that a drug is or is not teratogenic in man, unless it is tested in man. The sedative thalidomide is an excellent case in point. Although thalidomide produces congenital malformations in man, the effects are difficult to produce in rats and mice (91, p. 204).

Some Specific Drugs

Narcotics

Most textbooks state that narcotic drugs readily cross the placental barrier, and that pregnant women who are physically dependent upon heroin are likely to transfer their dependency to the newborn. The infants are said to evidence respiratory depression and withdrawal symptoms. The likelihood of fetal death and infant mortality is believed to be greatly increased by opiates; in one study (36), 93 percent of untreated heroin-addicted infants died. Other complications may include premature birth (57), postpartum hemorrhage, breech presentation, and toxemia (toxic substances in the blood) (78). However, the data have recently been questioned. Blinick et al. (7) claimed that there is no good evidence to indicate placental transfer of narcotics; furthermore, after studying a series of 100 births to heroin addicts, they reported that the babies did not show withdrawal symptoms. Eighty-eight of the babies were healthy at birth, and the major problem of most of the remainder was low birth weight. In any event, the defects were most likely not caused by the drug itself, but rather by secondary consequences of such drug-related circumstances as the mother's poverty, inadequate diet, and poor general health care. In an even more recent study (65, p. 83), only 2 of 230 babies born to addicted mothers had congenital defects.

Nicotine

Children born to women who smoke during pregnancy are more often premature and of low weight than are babies of non-smoking mothers (60, 66, 94). However, even though low birth weight is usually associated with increased infantile mortality, babies of smokers tend to be small but as viable as those of nonsmokers (94). There is an increase in the number of abortions and stillbirths of smokers, so perhaps they also have a large percentage of weak fetuses who die before birth. The charge has been made (77) that maternal smoking may also be responsible for sudden unexpected deaths in infancy.

Ravenholt and Levinski (66) reported that the ratio of boys to girls is reduced among the offspring of mothers who smoke. Women who did not smoke during pregnancy averaged 52.8 boys per 100 births, while women who smoked in excess of 4000 cigarettes during pregnancy averaged 49.9 boys per 100. Lowe (47), however, disputed the findings, for two reasons: he felt that proper application of statistical tests showed Ravenhold and Levinski's data to be nonsignificant; moreover, his own data showed no trend toward increasing numbers of girls being born to smokers. The discrepancy between the two studies remains unresolved.

Sedatives and Tranquilizers

The best known teratogen, thalidomide, belongs to this group. Several hundred children were born malformed because physicians prescribed the drug for relief of anxiety and as an aid to sleep. Barbiturates have long been used for the same purposes. Although the barbiturates cross the placental barrier rapidly, they have few physical effects on the developing fetus. There have been a few reports of fetal death and reduced litter size in the offspring of rats, mice, and rabbits treated with barbiturates (13, 48, 59, 73).

Desmond et al. (19) reported on the treatment of pregnant women with reserpine for the amelioration of hypertensive states. Approximately 15 percent of the newborns had side effects such as nasal congestion, hypertonicity, and tremors; in rare cases, some of the effects persisted for months. The incidence of defects was considerably higher than that observed in the offspring of untreated mothers. In animals, reserpine increased the number of fetal deaths and abortions (11), and the liveborn were lighter than the offspring of untreated animals (24). Other sedatives and tranquilizers which increase the risk of stillbirth and fetal death in tests with animals are chlorpromazine, glutethimide, prochlorperazine, and meprobamate (12, 14, 68, 85). In contrast to these drugs, chlordiazepoxide appears safe (82, 101).

There have been two reports of alcohol withdrawal in the newborn (52, 70). Not only can alcohol dependence be transferred, but the symptomatology in the two cases described was much more severe in the infant than in the mother.

Stimulants

While amphetamines did not greatly influence the outcome of pregnancy in studies with rats and rabbits (11, 55), high doses of D-amphetamine increased cardiac problems and fetal deaths in descendants of treated mice (53). The stimulant methylphenidate also increased the number of fetal deaths in mice (82).

Monoamine Oxidase Inhibitors

The MAOI's are among the most popular antidepressant drugs. In experiments with rats and mice, iproniazid increased stillbirths and postnatal death (88), and isocarboxazid and phenelzine increased fetal death (64, 82). No untoward effects were described for tranylcypromine or nialamide (63).

Hormones

Though hormonal therapy is commonly prescribed for pregnant women, such treatment can be dangerous, as Delost has pointed out (18). Hormones injected during gestation have been shown to induce abortion in addition to producing retarded development and several different types of congenital malformations. The particular hormones implicated include thyroxine, corticosteroids, epinephrine, vasopressin, estrogens, and androgens.

Hallucinogens

Experiments on animals provide evidence that high doses of marijuana and mescaline increase fetal death (27, 28, 58). Several studies (again, involving animals) have shown an increased incidence of umbilical hernia in the offspring of marijuana-treated mothers (28, 58). No untoward effects have been mentioned in regard to harmaline (63) or psilocin (67). The possible teratogenic effects of LSD, the best studied hallucinogen, have been discussed in Chapter 4.

Antibiotics

This survey shall be concluded by mentioning that several antibiotic drugs induce growth disorders in the offspring of injected pregnant mice. The drugs include penicillin (9), streptomycin (10), and tetracycline (8).

THE BEHAVIORAL EFFECTS OF DRUGS

Three tranquilizing drugs — chlorpromazine, reserpine, and meprobamate — have received a preponderance of attention. An early study by Werboff and Havlena (89) established that high doses of all three, when administered to pregnant female rats, substantially increased neonatal mortality. The survivors were less active than controls, and meprobamate had the additional effect of impairing maze learning. Kletzkin et al. (43) repeated the experiment but used much smaller doses. They did not find any drug effects, and suggested that the survivors of the Werboff and Havlena experiment were probably unhealthy, which would account for their reduced activity.

Hoffeld and Webster (37, 38, 39) extended the work. A summary of their findings is presented in Table 8.1. As can be seen, the period during pregnancy when the drugs are administered is an important factor.

Young (99) added an additional twist to the study of chlorpromazine. He divided offspring of drugged mothers into two groups, one which received normal handling and the other extra stimulation. As earlier studies had shown, stimulated animals whose mothers had been injected with saline were more active and better maze learners than the unstimulated offspring of saline-treated mothers. However, stimulated offspring of chlorpromazine-treated mothers were equal in performance to unstimulated, undrugged rats. Young concluded that the action of chlorpromazine is to min-

TABLE 8.1 Drug Effects at Different Times of Pregnancy*

	Trimester of Pregnancy			Overall Drug Effect[†]
	1	2	3	
Adult body weight	$a = b > d > c$‡	$a > d > b$	$a > c$	$a > b = c = d$
Avoidance conditioning		$a = d > b$	$d > a$	
Trials to extinction	$d > a = b = c$	$d > b$	$d > a = b = c$	
Maze learning	$b = d > a$	$a > c = d$		
Activity wheel				$a = c > b = d$
Touching of electrified bars of cage (may be measure of activity)		$c = d > a = b$		$c = d > b$

*Summarized from data presented by D. Hoffeld and R. Webster (Nature, 1965, 205: pp. 1070–1072), and D. Hoffeld, R. Webster, and J. McNew (Nature, 1967, 215: pp. 182–183; Nature, 1968, 218: pp. 357–358).

†The symbol ">" signifies (respectively): increased body weight, more rapid avoidance conditioning, more trials to extinction, more rapid maze learning, more activity in wheel, and more activity in the electrified cage. Blanks in the table mean that there were no significant effects.

‡a = chlorpromazine
  b = meprobamate
  c = reserpine
  d = water

imize the effects of stimulation rather than to affect behavior directly. Lending support to his argument is Killam's (41) compilation of evidence indicating that chlorpromazine blocks the flow of sensory information into the arousal system of the brain. A study conducted by Doty et al. (20) was offered as further support. Doty and his colleagues injected rats daily, from ages 3 to 60 days, with chlorpromazine or saline. Half of the rats in the saline group received exposure to geometric forms which were later used for discrimination learning, and half did not. The chlorpromazine-treated animals were all exposed to the stimuli, and did as well as the nonexposed animals on the discrimination task. The saline-exposed group was superior to both of the others.

Despite the data just cited, the sensory reduction hypothesis is incomplete, because in the study by Young, unstimulated offspring of chlorpromazine-treated mothers showed greater deficits than unstimulated offspring of saline mothers. Therefore, in addition to affecting behavior by reducing the effects of stimulation, chlorpromazine must have other actions as well.

Woolley and van der Hoeven (93) have offered an alternative although not incompatible hypothesis regarding the learning deficits produced by chlorpromazine and reserpine. Their suggestion is that serotonin has some role in learning ability, and both drugs are known to deplete the brain's supply of serotonin. Serotonin deficiency has been postulated (by Woolley) as a possible cause of the inferior learning ability of children suffering from the disease phenylketonuria (93). Woolley and van der Hoeven found that learning deficits in chlorpromazine-treated mice could be eliminated by administration of the drugs melatonin or hydroxytryptophan, both of which have serotonin-like effects.

Jewett and Norton (40) injected female rats with chlorpromazine or reserpine during the first trimester of pregnancy. Offspring of the chlorpromazine-treated mothers were hypoactive and more susceptible to audiogenic seizures. The offspring of reserpine-treated animals did not differ from controls on either measure. Neither drug changed the LD_{50} of amphetamine. Ordy et al. (54) confirmed that offspring of chlorpromazine-treated mothers were hypoactive and less efficient learners. In addition, the rats slept longer after hexobarbital injection; since hexobarbital is metabolized in the liver while amphetamine is excreted largely unchanged, it is likely that chlorpromazine decreases the activity of hepatic enzymes.

The effects of pre- or neonatal chlorpromazine extend into adulthood. This was shown by Gauron and Rowley (25), who tested chlorpromazine and two other phenothiazines, prochlorphenazine and thioridazine, on five-day-old rats. The animals were injected daily with one of the drugs or with saline for 50 days. After a drug-free period of 20 days, they were given several tests. The groups did not differ in ability to learn an avoidance task. However, chlorpromazine reduced fertility and impaired performance when the rats competed for food. Neither of the other drugs affected fertility, and both enhanced competitive performance.

The effects of other CNS depressants have not been extensively studied. Learning deficits have been observed in the offspring of rats treated with sodium bromide (35), barbital, pentobarbital (1), phenobarbital (50), and alcohol (86).

There have been very few studies of the developmental effects of stimulant drugs. Le Boeuf and Peeke (44) tested the effects of daily doses of strychnine given to rats from age 21 days (when they were weaned) to 52 days. When the rats were 107 days old, they were tested in a complex maze. There was an interaction between drug and environment: strychnine facilitated learning of rats reared in a rich environment and produced decrements in the environmentally impoverished rats. (Enriched and impoverished environments are discussed in Chap. 11.) A follow-up study by Peeke et al. (56), with animals started on drugs at 51 days and continued for 20 days, soon appeared. When the rats were tested at 110 days, the results were very similar to those of the previous study. They illustrate the obvious but sometimes overlooked point that it is not safe to assume that permanent effects of a drug are confined to a critical period. Drug effects on adults may also be permanent.

Rosenzweig (84, p. 335) also showed that there are drug-environment interactions. He injected rats with either an excitant or depressant drug (neither specified by name), or with saline, and then placed the animals in either an enriched or impoverished environment. The saline-treated animals showed the usual effects of the condition of rearing, i.e., rats reared in the enriched environment had heavier brains. The excitant drug magnified the effects of rearing condition, and the depressant attenuated them.

INFLUENCES OF SEXUAL HORMONES

Sexual Behavior and Morphology

Despite what some members of the Women's Liberation Movement might say, some of the differences between men and women are not only anatomical, but physiological and behavioral as well. That they are due to gender per se, rather than to differences in socialization, is strongly indicated from work with laboratory animals. Even when reared under identical environmental conditions, male rats, hamsters, guinea pigs, and monkeys behave differently from the respective females in a wide variety of situations. Research pioneered largely by William Young and his colleagues at the Oregon Regional Primate Center established that the development of these sex-typical behavior patterns is dependent upon hormones secreted by the gonads. More specifically, during a critical period very early in life, the presence of male hormones called androgens, of which testosterone is the most important, is essential to the development of male characteristics. Absence of male hormones during the critical period causes femininization. The effects are independent of genetic sex.*

Females

The most thoroughly studied sex-typical characteristic is copulatory behavior itself. Dantchakoff (17) showed that the exposure of female guinea pigs to testosterone during the critical period of psychosexual differentiation resulted in females which, as adults, failed to display feminine sexual behavior. The loss of feminine behavior was complete, and was not restored by injections of estrogen. On the other hand, the females displayed considerable capacity for masculine behavior, although not as much as exhibited by normal genetic males. For example, they mounted sexually receptive female guinea pigs (untreated female guinea pigs also occasionally mount other females, but not nearly to the same extent). Surprisingly, large doses of estrogen, a hormone secreted by the ovaries, have some masculinizing effects when injected during the critical period. Female rats treated with large doses fail to ovulate and are thus sterile; they also have decreased sexual receptivity (90).

Early treatment of females with testosterone modifies morphology in addition to behavior. Androgenized female guinea pigs do not have external vaginal openings, and their clitorides are enlarged (61). Female monkeys exposed to androgen during the critical period develop masculinized external genitalia. The vaginal orifice is closed, the scrotum is empty but well-developed, and there is a small but complete penis (62).

Males

Male rats deprived of testosterone by castration at birth do not display normal male sexual behavior when they reach adulthood (5). By itself this finding is hardly startling, since castration of adults

---

*Mammals with an XY chromosome pair are genetically male, those with XX are genetically female.

also impairs sexual behavior. However, in the latter case, injections of testosterone can reverse the effects of castration and restore normal male behavior. But, when rats are castrated at birth, hormonal therapy does not restore normal male behavior. Their capacity for *female* sexual behavior, though, is retained, and can be elicited by injecting them with estrogen (33).

Male rats treated with estrogen during the critical period fail to develop an os penis (a slender bone located in the penis of many species of animals), and are incapable of ejaculation. Their accessory sexual organs atrophy, and they are infertile (42). Treatment of pregnant rats with the drug cyproterone acetate, which blocks the actions of testosterone on the fetus, also prevents the development of normal male external genitalia in the male offspring (51).

Gonadal Errors in Humans

At Johns Hopkins Hospital in Baltimore, physicians and scientists identify and treat several naturally occurring anomalies in

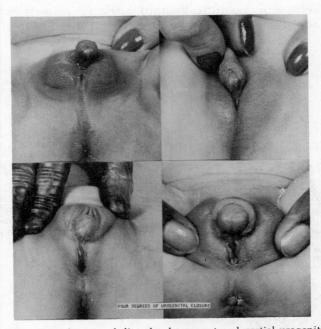

Figure 8–1 Four degrees of clitoral enlargement and partial urogenital closure, producing hermaphroditic ambiguity of appearance of the sex organs, in four cases of the masculinizing adrenogenital syndrome in genetic females. Exactly the same degrees of genital ambiguity may occur also in genetic males with incomplete masculinization. (From John Money and Anke A. Ehrhardt, *Man & Woman, Boy & Girl*, Baltimore: The Johns Hopkins University Press, 1972, p. 115.)

humans which result from atypical hormonal stimulation during development (49). Their work is mentioned because of their acknowledged debt to the laboratory research on early hormones and development.

FEMALES. In two conditions, the female fetus is exposed to an excess of androgen. One, called the congenital adrenogenital syndrome, is characterized by the production of excess fetal androgen. The other condition is called progestin-induced hermaphroditism, and was occasionally observed in the female offspring of mothers treated with the hormone progesterone for the purpose of preventing miscarriage; progesterone has many androgenic effects, and is administered with much more care now that the effects have been described. In both cases, although the newborn is genetically female, the external genitalia are masculinized; in extreme instances there is a normal-appearing penis and scrotum. The babies are often declared to be boys. (See Fig. 8–1.)

MALES. The corresponding condition in boys is called the testicular feminizing syndrome, and occurs when the cells of the body of a genetic male are unable to accept or use androgen. In such a case, the child is declared to be a girl and is raised as a girl. Such children encounter no difficulty until they reach puberty, when they fail to menstruate because they lack uteri. If they are then treated,

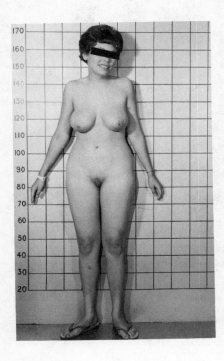

Figure 8–2 Genetic male who is insensitive to testosterone. (From Money and Ehrhardt, p. 116.)

both surgically and hormonally, they continue to live as women, and usually marry and adopt children. (See Fig. 8–2.)

Sexually Dimorphic Behaviors

Hormones administered during the neonatal period do not affect all behaviors, but they do affect those which are sexually dimorphic, i.e., different in the two sexes. For example, female rats are more active than males; their activity is increased by neonatal estrogen and decreased by testosterone (29). Aggressive behavior (21), exploration (79), body weight and length (81), stance during urination (3), and oxygen consumption (32) are also modified. Females, which normally show a much stronger preference for saccharin solution over water, have their preferences enhanced by estrogen and reduced by testosterone (87).

Young male rhesus monkeys have different patterns of play from those of females. The males have more rough and tumble play, threaten more, more frequently initiate play, and pursue more. When females were exposed to androgen during the critical period, their external genitalia were masculinized; in addition, their behavior was changed toward the male standard. On all four sexually dimorphic measures of play, their behavior more closely resembled that of males than that of females (62).

The Organization Hypothesis

At some stage in its development, the mammalian embryo has the capacity to form either a male or a female reproductive system. If sufficient androgen is present, a penis, seminal vesicles, and a prostrate gland develop; in the absence of androgen, an external vagina and feminine accessory structures derive from the same tissue. One set of structures develops at the expense of the other—the two cannot coexist.

Neonatal hormones also influence the brain. RNA synthesis and metabolism within the brain are affected (15, 74), as is pituitary function (which is regulated by the brain). The pituitary glands of males secrete hormones at a steady rate, whereas those of females function cyclically; the presence or absence of androgen at birth determines whether the pituitary functions acyclically or cyclically.

In 1959 Phoenix et al. (61) proposed that hormonal status during the critical period determines whether the CNS becomes masculinized or femininized. That is, from the observation that neonatal androgen gives rise to a male mating pattern, Phoenix and his associates inferred that it also produces a male CNS. Their idea, which has come to be known as the organization hypothesis, seemed a logical extension of the data on the role of androgens in masculinizing the reproductive structures and pituitary function. However, in a recent incisive article (4), Beach has shown that the hypothesis is unfounded. His arguments can be only briefly reviewed:

1. Neonatally castrated male rats mount receptive females as much as do other rats, but rarely achieve insertion of the penis into the vaginal opening. However, penis size is greatly reduced in such animals. The behavior of hormonally normal males which have had penis size reduced by surgical operation is indistinguishable from that of the day-1 castrates. Thus, penis size seems to be the crucial factor in the inability of day-1 castrates to achieve insertion.

2. Normal adult male rats are capable of showing female sexual behavior if they are placed on an appropriate hormone schedule.

3. Female rats treated early with testosterone retain the capacity for female behavior.

4. Untreated females retain the capacity for male behavior.

5. Early work by Goy et al. (31) with guinea pigs clearly demonstrated that hormonal treatments which had the greatest effects in augmenting masculine behavior correspondingly reduced feminine behavior to the greatest extent. However, since some animals retained the capacity for both male and female behavior, Goldfoot et al. (30) were encouraged to attempt systematically to produce bisexual animals. They injected androstenedione into castrated infant male rats. Androstenedione, like testosterone, is a hormone secreted by the fetal testis. Like testosterone, it offset the effects of castration, i.e., when androstenedione-treated rats were tested at maturity, after receiving injections of testosterone, they showed normal male sexual behavior. However, they also retained the capacity for female sexual behavior; injections of estrogen and progesterone elicited the appropriate female responses. The conclusion is that male and female systems develop independently.

If the organization hypothesis is incorrect, why does early hormonal exposure permanently influence behavior? Beach proposed in 1945 (2) that exposure acts to alter sensitivity to subsequent hormonal stimulation. The difference between the developmental processes proposed in the two hypotheses is that a neural system "organized" for maleness would never give rise to feminine behavior (just as the organization of undifferentiated tissue into a penis precludes the possibility of development of a vagina), whereas a system which is relatively insensitive to a particular hormone may nevertheless respond to large enough doses of the hormone.

Beach's position is supported by some recent work of Bell and Zucker (6). They found that rats injected neonatally with testosterone were more sensitive as adults to the weight-promoting effects of testosterone, and were less responsive to the weight-depressing combination of estrogen and progesterone. The effects of neonatal estrogen were similar to those of testosterone, for reasons still not understood.

Wade and Zucker (87) noted two additional ways in which early hormones may alter adult behavior: they may influence the pattern of adult secretions of sex hormones, and they may directly modify peripheral mechanisms such as taste receptors. In a relevant study, Hacik (34) showed that a single dose of testosterone modifies adult adrenal secretions—and the influence of adrenal function on aggressiveness and emotionality is well established. Thus, it is clear that early drug treatment may affect adult behavior in ways other than through direct action on the CNS.

EFFECTS OF OTHER HORMONES

Hormones other than estrogen and testosterone affect behavior. Administration of the thyroid hormone thyroxine caused permanent hypothyroidism in rats (46). Thyroxine advanced the time of appearance of evoked responses (ER's) to visual, auditory, and sensorimotor stimuli in infant rats (69),* and also accelerated the time of eye opening and the appearance of the startle reflex (72). Salas and Schapiro (69) suggested that thyroxine acts via a nonspecific stimulation of neural mechanisms.

Cortisol, secreted by the adrenal gland, had contrasting effects on maturation. Sensory ER's were delayed, even though cortisol-treated rats opened their eyes at an earlier age than did controls (69). Schapiro (71) showed that treatment of infants with either hormone may permanently influence behavior. Swanson and McKeag (80) found sex-dependent effects. They injected infant hamsters with large doses of cortisol. The adult activity of the females was elevated by the treatment, while that of the males was not.

When epinephrine is administered to pregnant rats, the activity, emotionality, and learning ability of the offspring are affected in complex ways. Thompson and Olian (83) reported that in mice, the direction of activity change from control levels was strain-dependent. Young conducted a series of experiments (95–100) in which he combined injections of epinephrine with various forms of postnatal stress. Errors on a maze learning task were consistently increased

---

*Evoked responses will be discussed in detail in Chapter 10.

by the drug. Its effects on activity and emotionality depended on environmental factors. Young and Klepinger (100) believe that epinephrine is a stressor, and that adult activity and emotionality are modified by infantile stress in a curvilinear fashion. The optimal environment contains some stress. Therefore, epinephrine has favorable effects when administered in an otherwise stress-free environment, but is detrimental when it acts to produce excess stress.

CONCLUSIONS

Some of the consequences of indiscriminate use of drugs during pregnancy are immediately and obviously tragic, but some may be very subtle. The full spectrum of effects of tranquilizers on human babies may never be known, but small deficits in learning, activity, and emotional responsiveness are likely. The most dangerous phase is probably the first trimester of pregnancy, but precautions are necessary throughout the entire period. In fact, the growing interest in natural childbirth may have a sound medical basis, as babies who are delivered from undrugged mothers are more alert than others (76). It has not been established whether any of the differences between babies of drugged and undrugged mothers are permanent.

Despite the extreme importance of developmental psychopharmacology, it is unlikely that the field will enjoy rapid advances of knowledge. Research on humans is severely restricted, primarily because of ethical considerations, but also because both patients and physicians do not accurately remember drug usage during pregnancy (75). In addition, a drug which appears harmless with respect to a particular behavior when given in a particular dosage regimen at a particular time of pregnancy may nevertheless have adverse consequences under other circumstances.

The field poses special difficulties to laboratory researchers. One problem concerns litter size. There is generally an effort to equalize the size of litters which undergo different treatments; this is achieved by discarding animals from oversized litters by means of procedures which are rarely described. In at least one instance (97), the first three males to be caught from each litter were retained for further testing. The animals which allow themselves to be caught are likely to be the least active and emotional; it is inappropriate to compare them with unselected animals from another group. Nonrandom selection is always dangerous, and may introduce sufficient bias into the system so that the experimenter may determine, by subtle variation in procedure, whether positive or negative results are obtained.

Animals within a litter are more similar to one another than they are to animals in other litters. Part of the difference is caused by differential mothering, and can be eliminated by the use of cross-fostering. For example, Ordy et al. (54) raised rat pups whose mothers had received chlorpromazine with mothers which had been given saline. The chlorpromazine effect was attenuated. However, even cross-fostering cannot eliminate genetic influences on behavior. As a result, significant differences among litters may be seen even in the absence of drug effects. Therefore, each litter which is given a drug treatment might best be regarded as a single unit, instead of counting each animal within the litter separately for statistical purposes. Such a procedure might make developmental studies unwieldy, but the implications are great enough to justify the effort.

Young organisms are inefficient in metabolizing drugs. Some drugs, such as reserpine, are extremely long-acting even in adults. The experimenter who is concerned with the permanence of neonatal drug effects must therefore wait a considerable length of time after administration before testing his subjects.

In many studies only one dose is used, generally a large one to ensure effects. Thus, fetal and neonatal mortality is high, with the feeblest animals suffering the heaviest tolls. The survivors are then compared with control groups which have not suffered selective mortality. Two possibilities arise from such experimental designs: the health of the offspring of drugged parents may be permanently damaged, thus impairing their performance on behavioral tests; or they may recover from the effects of the drugs and then, because they have been selected for hardiness, perform extremely well on the tests. The two effects oppose each other, but in a given experiment one may be more heavily weighted than the other.

The emphasis in laboratory research has been on CNS depressants, which constitute the drugs most likely to be prescribed by physicians. These drugs generally produce performance decrements. Little work has been done with stimulants such as caffeine, amphetamine, and methylphenidate. The few available reports indicate increased fetal mortality after high doses, but the possibility remains that smaller doses might enhance adult performance.

An important final point is that, in many of the studies, a dose-dependent response to hormones or other drugs was obtained. Therefore, the results have implications not just for pregnant women for whom drugs are prescribed, but for all prospective parents. Levels of circulating hormones naturally vary among women, and affect fetal development. Characteristics of the offspring may be modifiable in beneficial ways by judicious use of hormones, hormone antagonists, stimulants, depressants, or drugs which promote or reduce stress.

REFERENCES

1. Armitage, S. The effect of barbiturates on the behavior of rat offspring as measured on learning and reasoning situations. J. Comp. Physiol. Psychol., 1952, 45:146–152.
2. Beach, F. Bisexual mating behavior in the male rat: effects of castration and hormone administration. Physiol. Zool., 1945, 18:390–402.
3. Beach, F. Hormonal effects on socio-sexual behavior in dogs. In Gibian, M., and Plotz, F. (Eds.) Mammalian Reproduction. Berlin: Springer-Verlag, 1970.
4. Beach, F. Hormonal factors controlling the differentiation, development, and display of copulatory behavior in the ramstergig and related species. In Tobach, E., Aronson, L., and Shaw, E. (Eds.) The Biopsychology of Development. New York: Academic Press, 1971.
5. Beach, F., and Holz, A. Mating behavior in male rats castrated at various ages and injected with androgen. J. Exp. Zool., 1946, 101:91–142.
6. Bell, D., and Zucker, I. Sex differences in body weight and eating: organization and activation by gonadal hormones in the rat. Physiol. Behav., 1971, 7:27–34.
7. Blinick, G., Wallach, R., and Eulogio, J. Pregnancy in narcotics addicts treated by medical withdrawal: the methadone detoxification program. Am. J. Obstet. Gynec., 1969, 105:997–1003.
8. Boucher, D., and Delost, P. Développement post-natal de la Souris après traitement de la mère gestante et des descendants par les tetracyclines. C.R. Soc. Biol., 1967, 161:300–305.
9. Boucher, D., and Delost, P. Développement post-natal des descendants issus de mères traitées par la pénicilline au cours de la gestation chez la Souris. C.R. Soc. Biol., 1964, 158:528–532.
10. Boucher, D., and Delost, P. Développement post-natal des descendants issus de mères traitées par la streptomycine au cours de la gestation chez la Souris. C.R. Soc. Biol., 1964, 158:2065–2069.
11. Bovet-Nitti, F., and Bovet, D. Action of some sympatholytic agents on pregnancy in the rat. Proc. Soc. Exp. Biol. Med., 1959, 100:555–557.
12. Chambon, Y. Action de la chlorpromazine sur l'évolution et l'avenir de la gestation chez la rate. Ann. Endocr., 1955, 16:912–922.
13. Champakamalini, A., and Rao, M. Foetal resorption in barbital sodium treated pregnant rats. Curr. Sci., 1967, 36:3–5.
14. Clavert, J. Action of meprobamate on formation of the embryo. C.R. Soc. Biol., 1963, 157:1481–1482.
15. Clayton, R., Kogura, J., and Kraemer, H. Sexual differentiation of the brain: effects of testosterone on brain RNA metabolism in new-born female rats. Nature, 1970, 226:810–812.
16. Clegg, D. Teratology. Ann. Rev. Pharmacol., 1971, 11:409–424.
17. Dantchakoff, V. Rôle des hormones dans la manifestation des instincts sexuels. C.R. Acad. Sci., 1938, 206:945–947.
18. Delost, P. Fetal endocrinology and the effect of hormones on development. In Tobach, E., Aronson, L., and Shaw, E. (Eds.) The Biopsychology of Development. New York: Academic Press, 1971.
19. Desmond, M., Rogers, S., Lindley, J., and Moya, J. Management of toxemia of pregnancy with reserpine. II: the newborn infant. Obstet. Gynec., 1957, 10:140–145.
20. Doty, L., Doty, B., Wise, M., and Senn, R. Effects of postnatal chlorpromazine on discrimination in rats. Percept. Motor Skills, 1964, 18:329–332.
21. Edwards, D. Mice: fighting by neonatally androgenized females. Science, 1968, 161:1027–1028.
22. Friedler, G., and Cochin, J. Altered post-natal growth pattern of offspring of female rats chronically treated with morphine prior to mating. Pharmacologist, 1967, 9:230.
23. Friedler, G., and Cochin, J. Sensitivity and tolerance to morphine sulfate (MS)

in the rat as affected by neonatal thymectomy or MS-pretreatment of the mother. Pharmacologist, 1968, *10*:188.

24. Gaunt, R., Renzi, A., Antonchak, N., Miller, G., and Gilman, M. Endocrine aspects of the pharmacology of reserpine. Ann. N.Y. Acad. Sci., 1954, *59*:22–35.

25. Gauron, E., and Rowley, V. Behavioral effects of a chronic drug administration experience in infancy. J. Genetic Psychol., 1968, *112*:237–247.

26. Gauron, E., and Rowley, V. Effects on offspring behavior of mother's early chronic drug experience. Psychopharmacologia, 1969, *16*:5–15.

27. Geber, W. Congenital malformations induced by mescaline, lysergic acid diethylamide, and bromolysergic acid in the hamster. Science, 1967, *158*:265–267.

28. Geber, W., and Schramm, L. Effect of marijuana extract on fetal hamsters and rabbits. Toxic. Appl. Pharmacol., 1969, *14*:276–282.

29. Gerall, A. Effects of early postnatal androgen and estrogen injections on the estrous activity cycles and mating behavior of rats. Anat. Rec., 1967, *157*: 97–104.

30. Goldfoot, D., Feder, H., and Goy, R. Development of bisexuality in the male rat treated neonatally with androstenedione. J. Comp. Physiol. Psychol., 1969, *67*:41–45.

31. Goy, R., Bridson, W., and Young, W. Period of maximal susceptibility of the prenatal female guinea pig to masculinizing actions of testosterone propionate. J. Comp. Physiol. Psychol., 1964, *57*:166–174.

32. Goy, R., Mitchell, J., and Young, W. Effect of testosterone propionate on O_2 consumption of female and female pseudohermaphroditic guinea pigs. Am. Zool., 1962, *2*:525.

33. Grady, K., Phoenix, C., and Young, W. Role of the developing rat testis in differentiation of the neural tissues mediating mating behavior. J. Comp. Physiol. Psychol., 1965, *59*:176–182.

34. Hacik, T. Effects of a single dose of testosterone administered to rats in early postnatal period on the adrenal function in adult life. Arch. Int. Physiol. Biochim., 1966, *74*:1–8.

35. Harned, B., Hamilton, H., and Borrus, J. The effect of bromide administration to pregnant rats on the learning ability of offspring. Am. J. Med. Sci., 1940, *20*:846.

36. Henley, W., and Fisch, G. Newborn narcotic withdrawal associated with regional enteritis in pregnancy. N.Y. State J. Med., 1966, *66*:2565–2567.

37. Hoffeld, D., McNew, J., and Webster, R. Effect of tranquilizing drugs during pregnancy on activity of offspring. Nature, 1968, *218*:357–358.

38. Hoffeld, D., and Webster, R. Effect of injection of tranquilizing drugs during pregnancy on offspring. Nature, 1965, *205*:1070–1072.

39. Hoffeld, D., Webster, R., and McNew, J. Adverse effects on offspring of tranquilizing drugs during pregnancy. Nature, 1967, *215*:182–183.

40. Jewett, R., and Norton, S. Effect of tranquilizing drugs on postnatal behavior. Exp. Neurol., 1966, *14*:33–43.

41. Killam, K., and Killam, E. Drug action on pathways involving the reticular formation. In Jasper, H., Proctor, L., Knighton, R., Noshay, W., and Costello, R. (Eds.) Reticular Formation of the Brain. Boston: Little, Brown and Co., 1958.

42. Kincl, F., Floch Pi, A., and Herrara Lasso, L. Effect of oestradiol benzoate treatment in the newborn male rat. Endocrinol., 1963, *72*:966–968.

43. Kletzkin, M., Wojeiechowski, H., and Margolin, S. Postnatal behavioral effects of meprobamate injected into the gravid rat. Nature, 1964, *204*:1206.

44. LeBoeuf, B., and Peeke, H. The effect of strychnine administration during development on adult maze learning in the rat. Psychopharmacologia, 1969, *16*: 49–53.

45. Levine, S. The psychophysiological effects of infantile stimulation. In Bliss, E. (Ed.) Roots of Behavior. New York: Hoeber, 1962.

46. Levine, S., and Mullins, R. Hormonal influences on brain organization in infant rats. Science, 1966, *152*:1585–1592.

47. Lowe, C. Smoking during pregnancy. Lancet, 1965, *1*:1071.

48. McColl, J., Robinson, S., and Globus, M. Effect of some therapeutic agents on the developing rat fetus. Toxic. Appl. Pharmacol., 1967, 10:244–252.
49. Money, J. Sex reassignment as related to hermaphroditism and transsexualism. In: Green, R. and Money, J. (Eds.) Transsexualism and Sex Reassignment. Baltimore: Johns Hopkins Press, 1969.
50. Murai, N. Effect of maternal medication during pregnancy upon behavioral development of offspring. Tohoku J. Exp. Med., 1966, 89:265–272.
51. Nadler, R. Differentiation of the capacity for male sexual behavior in the rat. Hormones Behav., 1969, 1:53–63.
52. Nichols, N. Acute alcohol withdrawal syndrome in a newborn. Am. J. Dis. Child., 1967, 113:714–715.
53. Nora, J., Sommerville, R., and Fraser, F. Homologies for congenital heart diseases: murine models, influenced by dextroamphetamine. Teratology, 1968, 1:413–416.
54. Ordy, J., Samorajski, T., Collins, R., and Rolsten, C. Prenatal chlorpromazine effects on liver, survival and behavior of mice offspring. J. Pharmacol. Exp. Ther., 1966, 151:110–125.
55. Paget, G. Dexamphetamine sulphate in mice. Lancet, 1965, 2:1129.
56. Peeke, H., LeBoeuf, B., and Herz, M. The effect of strychnine administration during development on adult maze learning in the rat. II: Drug administration from day 51 to 70. Psychopharmacologia, 1971, 19:262–265.
57. Perlmutter, J. Drug addiction in pregnant women. Am. J. Obstet. Gynecol., 1967, 99:569–572.
58. Persaud, T., and Ellington, A. Cannabis in early pregnancy. Lancet, 1967, 2:1306.
59. Persaud, T., and Henderson, W. The teratogenicity of barbital sodium in mice. Arzneim. Forsch., 1969, 19:1309–1310.
60. Peterson, W., Morese, K., and Kaltreider, D. Smoking and prematurity. A preliminary report based on study of 7740 Caucasians. Obst. Gynecol., 1965, 26:775–779.
61. Phoenix, C., Goy, R., Gerall, A., and Young, W. Organizing action of prenatally administered testosterone propionate on the tissues mediating mating behavior in the female guinea pig. Endocrinol., 1959, 65:369–382.
62. Phoenix, C., Goy, R., and Resko, J. Psychosexual differentiation as a function of androgenic stimulation. In Diamond, M. (Ed.) Reproduction and Sexual Behavior. Bloomington: Indiana University Press, 1968.
63. Poulson, E., and Robson, J. The effect of amine oxidase inhibitors on pregnancy. J. Endocrinol., 1963, 27:147–152.
64. Poulson, E., and Robson, J. Effect of phenelzine and some related compounds on pregnancy and on sexual development. J. Endocrinol., 1964, 30:205–215.
65. Proceedings, Third National Conference on Methadone Treatment. U.S. PHS Pub. No. 2172, 1970.
66. Ravenholt, R., and Levinski, M. Smoking during pregnancy. Lancet, 1965, 1:961.
67. Rolsten, C. Effects of chlorpromazine and psilocin on pregnancy of C57BL/10 mice and their offspring at birth. Anat. Rec., 1967, 157:311.
68. Roux, C. Action teratogene de la prochlorpemazine. Arch. Fr. Pediat., 1959, 16:968–971.
69. Salas, M., and Schapiro, S. Hormonal influences upon the maturation of the rat brain's responsiveness to sensory stimuli. Physiol. Behav., 1970, 5:7–11.
70. Schaefer, O. Alcohol withdrawal syndrome in a newborn infant of a Yukon Indian mother. Canad. Med. Ass. J., 1962, 87:1333–1334.
71. Schapiro, S. Some physiological, biochemical, and behavioral consequences of neonatal hormone administration: cortisol and thyroxine. Gen. Comp. Endocr., 1968, 10:214–228.
72. Schapiro, S., and Norman, R. Thyroxine: effects of neonatal administration on maturation, development and behavior. Science, 1967, 155:1279–1281.
73. Setala, K., and Nyyssonen, O. Hypnotic sodium pentobarbital as a teratogen for mice. Naturwissenschaften, 1965, 51:413.
74. Shimada, H., and Gorbman, A. Long lasting changes in RNA synthesis in the forebrains of female rats treated with testosterone soon after birth. Biochem. Biophys. Res. Comm., 1970, 38:423–430.
75. Speirs, A. Thalidomide and congenital abnormalities. Lancet, 1962, 1:303–305.

76. Stechler, G. Newborn attention as affected by medication during labor. Science, 1964, 144:315–317.
77. Steele, R., and Langworth, J. The relationship of antenatal and postnatal factors to sudden unexpected death in infancy. Can. Med. Ass. J., 1966, 94:1165–1171.
78. Stern, R. The pregnant addict. A study of 66 case histories. Am. J. Obstet. Gynecol., 1966, 94:253–257.
79. Swanson, H. Alteration of sex-typical behaviour of hamsters in open field and emergence tests by neo-natal administration of androgen or estrogen. Anim. Behav., 1967, 15:209–216.
80. Swanson, H., and McKeag, A. Effects of neonatal administration of cortisol to hamsters on their adult behavior in the open field. Hormones Behav., 1969, 1:1–5.
81. Swanson, H., and van der Werff ten Bosch, J. Sex differences in growth of rats, and their modification by a single injection of testosterone propionate shortly after birth. J. Endocrinol., 1963 26:197–207.
82. Takano, K., Tanimura, T., and Nishimura, H. Effects of psychoactive drugs on the fetus. Proc. Cong. Anom. Res. Ass. Jap., 1963, 3:2.
83. Thompson, W., and Olian, S. Some effects on offspring behavior of maternal adrenalin injection during pregnancy in three inbred mouse strains. Psychol. Rep., 1961, 8:87–90.
84. Tobach, E., Aronson, L., and Shaw, E. (Eds.) The Biopsychology of Development. New York: Academic Press, 1971.
85. Tuchmann-Duplessis, H., and Mercier-Parot, L. Répercussion d'un somnifère, le glutethimide, sur la gestation et le développement foetal du rat, de la souris et du lapin. C.R. Acad. Sci., 1963, 256:1841–1843.
86. Vincent, N. The effects of prenatal alcoholism upon motivation, emotionality, and learning in the white rat. Am. Psychol., 1958, 13:401.
87. Wade, G., and Zucker, I. Taste preferences of female rats: modification by neonatal hormones, food deprivation and prior experience. Physiol. Behav., 1969, 4:935–943.
88. Werboff, J., Gottlieb, J., Dembicki, E., and Havlena, J. Postnatal effect of antidepressant drugs administered during gestation. Exp. Neurol., 1961, 3:542–555.
89. Werboff, J., and Havlena, J. Postnatal behavioral effects of tranquilizers administered to the gravid rat. Exp. Neurol., 1962, 6:263–269.
90. Whalen, R., and Nadler, R. Suppression of the development of female mating behaviour by estrogen administered in infancy. Science, 1963, 141:272–275.
91. Wolstenholme, G., and Porter, R. (Eds.) Drug Responses in Man. Boston: Little, Brown and Co., 1967.
92. Woolley, D. The Biochemical Basis of Psychoses. New York: John Wiley and Sons, 1962.
93. Woolley, D., and van der Hoeven, T. Alteration in learning ability caused by changes in cerebral serotonin and catecholamines. Science, 1963, 139:610–611.
94. Yerushalmy, J. Mother's cigarette smoking and survival of infant. Am. J. Obstet. Gynecol., 1964, 88:505–518.
95. Young, R. Developmental psychopharmacology: a beginning. Psychol. Bull., 1967, 67:73–86.
96. Young, R. Drug administration to neonatal rats: effects on later emotionality and learning. Science, 1964, 143:1055–1057.
97. Young, R. Effect of prenatal drugs and neonatal stimulation on later behavior. J. Comp. Physiol. Psychol., 1964, 58:309–311.
98. Young, R. Effect of tranquilization of neonatal rats on later behavior. Psychol. Rec., 1965, 15:401–407.
99. Young, R. Effects of differential early experiences and neonatal tranquilization on later behavior. Psychol. Rep., 1965, 17:675–680.
100. Young, R., and Klepinger, B. Effect of neonatal catecholamine administration on later behavior in rats. Psychopharmacologia, 1966, 8:445–453.
101. Zbinden, G., Bagdon, R., Keith, E., Phillips, R., and Randall, L. Experimental and clinical toxicology of chlordiazepoxide (Librium). Toxic. Appl. Pharmacol., 1961, 3:619–637.

CHAPTER 9

METHODOLOGICAL ISSUES

Methodological issues are discussed throughout this book. Most of them are not unique to psychopharmacology. The reader who wishes to pursue a career in psychopharmacology, or even to be able to interpret meaningfully the literature, would be wise to read a good textbook of experimental psychology (for example, Underwood's *Experimental Psychology* [78]).

CHOICE OF SUBJECTS

Rats and mice are convenient subjects with which to work. They are inexpensive to buy and maintain, are easily handled, and are well adapted to laboratory conditions. They have short-lived generations, which makes them valuable in teratological work. Mice are especially convenient because many inbred strains have been developed, which can be selected for particular qualities. More than 125 mutant genes have been identified, and mice bearing specific mutants can be purchased. Rats are valuable because their behavior, anatomy, and physiology have been so well studied. As for other species, Irwin (28) feels that cats are very reliable indicators of human responses to drugs; they require an oral dose (in mg/kg) approximately three times that of man. Monkeys have many advantages, but they are expensive. In addition, according to Irwin, they are relatively insensitive to drug-induced neurologic impairment. Another problem, when the dependent variable is behavior, is related to their intelligence: monkeys and apes probably suffer greater abnormalities than do other animals as a result of confinement in cages. Still another species was suggested by Modell (82, p. 248). He asserted that if the goal of pharmacological research is to apply results to man, then man is the ideal animal for testing.

Animal Research

Animal Models

A popular research strategy has been to attempt to produce in animals an analogue to some behavioral state in man. The problem may seem absurd on the face of it, e.g., what is a schizophrenic rat? In some cases it may incorrectly appear simple; for example, as will be seen in Chapter 14, it is easy to make laboratory animals aggressive, but the aggression may have little relevance to the study of aggression in man. One of the first behavioral researchers to use animal models in drug research was Masserman (47). He created conflicts in hungry cats and monkeys by shocking them or giving them an aversive blast of air whenever they pressed a lever to secure food. The animals developed signs of strong emotion: their hearts beat rapidly, their behaviors became stereotyped, they developed phobias, and they chewed imaginary food while refusing real food. These and several other symptoms seemed to justify Masserman's labeling of the rats as "neurotic." Then he studied the effects of drugs on the behaviors. Alcohol, morphine, and barbiturates had similar effects: all impaired the performance of complex behaviors in both normal and neurotic animals, but all also offered some protection against the development of neurotic symptoms. For example, only three of nine cats subjected to the conflict experience while intoxicated developed abnormal behavior, while all of the untreated controls became neurotic. More than half of the cats which received alcohol during the conflict experience became addicted to it, i.e., they preferred alcoholic drinks to water. All of the above-mentioned drugs also relieved the symptoms of neurosis. On the other hand, mephenesin, a muscle relaxant closely related to meprobamate, had no significant effects on either normal or neurotic behaviors.

It is an empirical question as to whether or not Masserman's animal models are useful in explaining the etiology of neurosis or alcoholism, or in suggesting any methods of treatment. Observations made in the laboratory are not always applicable to other situations; benactyzine, for instance, is effective against neurosis created in the laboratory, but is not effective clinically (75, p. 28). Still, models offer an interesting strategy for conducting experiments. Even if a successful laboratory cure is not directly applicable to man, it may point the way to more effective curative techniques. The relevant differences between the animal model and the actual disease as manifested in man can be sought out. Then, appropriate modifications in the technique for cure can be tried.

Screening Techniques

Screening techniques are used for the purpose of identifying, among the enormous number of new drugs developed each year, those which have useful or potentially useful pharmacological activity. One important point to note is that a test, to be useful, need not bear any known relationship to the manner in which the drug is to be used in man. For example, drugs which counteract self-stimulation in rats (see Chap. 16) may accurately predict antipsychotic activity in man. The information is valuable, even if the mechanism is obscure. Certain types of information which can be derived from screening tests are almost always generalizable to man. Steinberg (75) has listed, among them, factors which influence sensitivity to a drug; these include age of subjects and their initial level of reactivity, and ambient temperature. In addition, latencies and durations of action, chronic effects, dose-response curves, and interactions can be studied.

DOSE-RESPONSE RELATIONSHIPS. Turner (77) suggested establishing dose-response relationships by using logarithmic dosing series. He recommended one series — 10, 30, 100, 1000 mg/kg — as being particularly informative. Other authors favor starting with a very low dose and doubling it with successive groups of animals.

When responses to a drug are plotted graphically against doses, it is an easy matter to calculate the ED_{50}. Occasionally, more accurate measurements are desired, and arithmetic methods are used. Of those given by Turner, the easiest method is one attributed to G. Karber. Consider the data in Table 9.1 which was collected from seven groups of eight animals, and in which the response is death. Column 3 is calculated from the information in column 2, and column 5 from column 4. When there is 100 percent mortality (or 100 percent of whatever response is being measured) in two or more successive groups, data from the groups given the higher doses are discarded; similarly, when there is 0 percent mortality in two or more successive groups, data from those given the lower doses are not used.

The sum of the products listed in column 6 is obtained and is divided by the number of animals per group. The result is subtracted from the smallest dose which was lethal to all of the animals. The result is the LD_{50}. In the example given,

$$LD_{50} = 10.0 - (32.3/8) = 6.0 \text{ mg/kg}$$

BEHAVIORAL TESTS.   Below are brief descriptions of a few behavioral tests which require minimal apparatus. For detailed information on particular tests, see Turner's thorough review of screening and testing in *Screening Methods in Pharmacology* (77).
1. Tests for CNS Depression
    a. The runway test: thirsty animals are trained to run down a run-
    way for water reward. The runway has three components: a
    starting box, an alley, and a goal box. When times to exit from
    the box have stabilized, the animals are injected with the test
    substance. The measure used is the percent of animals with
    exit latencies greater than 10 seconds.
    b. The loss of righting reflex: animals are injected with the test
    substance, then placed on their backs; if they do not right them-
    selves within 30 seconds, they are said to have lost their righting
    reflex.
    c. The loss of corneal reflex: the cornea and conjuctiva of both
    eyes are touched with a fine hair; if there is no response for one
    second, the reflex is said to be lost.
2. Tests for Tranquilization
    a. Prolongation of sleeping time of animals given a barbiturate
    after the test drug.
    b. Decrease in spontaneous motor activity.
    c. Reduction of body temperature.
    d. Ratio of ED_{50} for loss of corneal reflex to ED_{50} for loss of pinna
    reflex (the pinna reflex is said to be lost when the animal does
    not respond after its ear is touched with a fine hair): tranquil-
    izers block the pinna reflex at low doses, but leave the corneal
    reflex intact even at lethal doses; mephenesin and alcohol have

TABLE 9.1 LD_{50} Computed by Karber's Method*

Group	Dose	Difference Between Successive Doses	Number Dead	Mean Dead, Successive Groups	Product, Columns 3 × 5
1	12.5		8		result discarded
2	10.0	2.5	8		
3	8.0	2.0	7	7.5	15
4	6.4	1.6	7	7	11.2
5	5.0	1.4	1	4	5.6
6	4.0	1.0	0	0.5	0.5
7	3.2	0.8	0	0	result discarded
					Total 32.3

*Adapted from G. Karber, in *Screening Methods in Pharmacology*, ed. R. Turner
(New York: Academic Press, 1965).

ratios greater than 1, and barbiturates and meprobamate have ratios less than 1.

3. Tests for Central Stimulation

a. The LD_{99} for groups of mice is determined, using pentobarbital; with a new group, at the same time of day and same room temperature as the earlier tests, a dose equivalent to twice the LD_{50} of the test drug is injected subcutaneously simultaneously with the pentobarbital. Many stimulants protect against the pentobarbital.

b. Rats are trained to obtain their nutritional requirements by drinking from a rich broth; then, after the test substance is injected, the amount of broth ingested per body weight of animal is measured. The test is meaningful because of the known relationship between stimulants and anorexia: not all stimulants decrease appetite, but almost all anorexic substances are stimulants.

Turner suggested that general observation of test animals can yield valuable information. He urged attention to these signs: alertness or stupor; stereotypy; excessive grooming, which may indicate stimulation; vocalizations, which suggest pain; startle response to a loud noise; motor incoordination; pupil size; urination or salivation, which indicates muscarinic activity; and heart rate. Several other screening tests not listed by Turner are given below:

4. Tests for Addiction Liability

a. Woods and Schuster (83) have found that all drugs which act as positive reinforcers for rhesus monkeys are abused by man. A drug is a "positive reinforcer" for monkeys when the animals will learn to make the responses which lead to injection of the drug. Woods and Schuster have been active in identifying positively reinforcing drugs. They found that patterns of self-administration vary with different drug classes. Central stimulants such as cocaine and methamphetamine are administered by the monkeys to the point of convulsions and exhaustion; then, after a self-imposed rest their responding begins anew. Narcotics intake increases daily until a stable asymptote is reached. The patterns of responding to alcohol and barbiturates are similar to each other: maximum intake is reached rapidly, is maintained for a period, and is followed by abstinence; after long exposure, the monkeys become debilitated. Table 9.2 lists some drugs which are reinforcers for rhesus monkeys and others which are not.

b. The D'Amour-Smith rat-tail-flick test indicates both analgesic activity and addiction liability. The test is simply a measure of the latency with which an animal moves its tail out of the path of an intense, painful beam of light.

TABLE 9.2   Drugs Acting as Reinforcers in the Rhesus Monkey*

Central Stimulants	Narcotics	Barbiturates
Cocaine	Morphine	Pentobarbital
D-Amphetamine	Methadone	Amobarbital
Pipradrol	Meperidine	
Phenmetrazine	Codeine	
SPA†	Pentazocine	
Methylphenidate		

Drugs not serving as reinforcers:

Pemoline	Nalorphine	
Chlorpromazine	Levallorphan	

*From Woods, J., and Schuster, C. Regulation of drug self-administration. *In* Harris, R., McIsaac, W., and Schuster, C. (Eds.) *Drug Dependence* (Austin; University of Texas Press, 1970), p. 159.
†L-1,2-Diphenyl-1-dimethylaminoethane-HCl.

c. Pellets containing a morphine base are subcutaneously implanted in mice so that they become addicted; the narcotic antagonist naloxone is then injected to precipitate the abstinence syndrome. One feature of the syndrome is that the animals jump quite a bit. The mice are placed on a platform, and their latency to jump is measured; drugs which can substitute for morphine suppress withdrawal, and hence prolong the jump latency (20).

5. Tests in Animals Which Predict Hallucinogenic Activity in Man

a. Gessner (19) reviewed several tests. When mice are used, many drugs which produce hallucinations in man elevate body temperature and also produce a fine tremor. Corne and Pickering (9) reported that head-twitching in mice is very sensitive to drugs which have hallucinogenic activity in man.

6. Tests of Emotionality

a. Estes and Skinner (12) and Brady (8) developed a powerful procedure for measuring emotionality. They reasoned that one effect of a fear-inducing stimulus would be the suppression of ongoing behavior. They trained rats to bar press for food, then presented a clicking sound for three minutes; at its termination, the rats received electric shock. After several pairings of the click and shock, the rats stopped responding when the click sounded. Rats injected with amphetamine increased overall responding, but showed a greater suppression effect to the click than they did without the drug. By contrast, reserpine reduced responding, but also reduced the suppressive effects of the click (8).

b. A very simple procedure for measuring emotionality is to place the animal in an arena and count the number of times it defecates.

Toxicity Testing

Koppanyi and Avery (33) listed several useful drugs, including penicillin, digitalis, ipecac, cinchona bark, ether, and chloroform, which were introduced into therapeutics prior to the development of elaborate screening procedures. This is most fortunate, because otherwise they might have been discarded; all are toxic, in one way or other, to at least one commonly used laboratory species.

Litchfield (43) tabulated the results of several studies with six different drugs which he did not name, but for which he said considerable information was available. He described 39 toxic physical signs which are potentially observable in man, dogs, and rats, and then tabulated the number of signs actually reported with each species for each drug. Since each species was tested with six drugs, there were $39 \times 6 = 234$ possible responses. Litchfield reported the numbers of toxic responses as follows: man: 53; man only: 23; rats and man: 18; rats but not man: 19; dogs and man: 29; dogs but not man: 24. Thus, positive responses in rats correctly forecast positive responses in man 18 times, while incorrectly forecasting 19 times. On 35 $(53 - 18)$ occasions, absence of a sign in rats was not predictive of such an absence in man. Similarly, toxic signs in dogs predicted toxic signs in man on 29 occasions and incorrectly predicted toxicity in man 24 times. On 24 occasions, absence of a sign in dogs was not predictive of absence in man.

Although the results expose weaknesses in the program of testing animals to determine drug toxicity, they should be viewed in perspective. For one thing, in $197 - 35 = 162$ instances, a negative response in rats correctly predicted a negative response in man; for dogs, the figure was $181 - 24 = 157$ times. Secondly, there were dosage differences: humans received the therapeutic dose while animals received the maximum tolerated dose. A third consideration is that the studies were spread out over time and involved many experimenters who undoubtedly differed somewhat in their criteria for scoring a sign positive. Some of the signs may have existed even before the drug was administered. Another factor is that the first-time administration of a drug has different nonpharmacological effects for man and animals; in man, the placebo effect is likely to be operative, while in animals the stress of handling and injection is likely to be maximal on the first trial. Finally, it is not essential that a particular sign correspond in animals and man. What is important is that the animal screen should enable scientists to make accurate predictions about the likelihood of toxicity in man. Suppose, for example, that the sole effect of a drug on rats was to make them permanently comatose. Suppose further that its sole effect on man was to cause a severe rash. Does this hypothetical example illustrate a failure of the animal screen? No, because the purpose of the screen is to identify toxic substances, which would have been accomplished.

Zbinden (85) pointed up other shortcomings of the animal screen. He listed the 41 most frequently recorded untoward physical effects observed in more than 11,000 patients treated with 77 different drugs or drug combinations. Twenty-one of the effects are unlikely to be observed in an animal experiment. In addition, a variety of psychic effects such as hallucinations and euphoria cannot be observed (see Table 9.3). Moreover, certain unfavorable reactions require special preconditions such as stress, pregnancy, vitamin deficiencies, or the like; this should be a point of some concern, since subjects for toxicity testing are typically healthy, normal animals.

There are several reasons for differential responsiveness to drugs. Koppanyi and Avery (33) stated that the effective dose of a drug is the effective concentration which is maintained at the site of action. This is influenced by several factors, including weight, sur-

TABLE 9.3 The Most Frequent Untoward Reactions to Drugs Observed in 11,115 Patients Treated with 77 Different Drugs or Drug Combinations*

SIDE EFFECT†	No.	SIDE EFFECT	No.
Drowsiness	426	Skin rash	29
Nausea	211	Anorexia	23
Dizziness	198	Depression	23
Sedation	176	Increased appetite	21
Dry mouth	133	Tremor	21
Nervousness	98	Perspiration	21
Epigastric distress	98	Dermatitis	19
Headache	91	Increased energy	18
Vomiting	83	Vertigo	16
Weakness	61	Palpitations	16
Nasal stuffiness	57	Blurred vision	16
Hypertension	57	Lethargy	15
Insomnia	56	Nocturia	15
Fatigue	55	Excitation	14
Constipation	54	Abdominal distention	14
Tinnitus	49	Frequent bowel movement	14
Weight gain	39	Flatulence	14
Hypotension	38	Stiffness	13
Dryness of nasopharynx	38	Urticaria	13
Heartburn	38	Tachycardia	13
Diarrhea	30		

*From Zbinden, G. The significance of pharmacological screening tests in the preclinical safety evaluation of new drugs. J. New Drugs, 1966, 6: p. 6. The data used in the table is summarized from 86 recent drug evaluation papers.
†Side effects for the detection of which there is no satisfactory animal model available are printed in italics.

face area, absorption from site of administration, metabolism by enzymes, distribution and storage in tissues, and excretion. The major sources of differences are enzymatic.

Welch (80) described many substantial differences between species, in response to drugs. For example, azauracil does not produce toxic effects in monkeys even when given in massive doses, yet it is sufficiently toxic to man that its many clinical features cannot be used to advantage. The related drug azauridine is nontoxic to man, but is fatal to dogs even when given in small doses. The reason for the differences in the pharmacology of the two substances is incompletely understood. Welch continued with the example of the two drugs in order to take issue with prevailing standards for the evaluation of toxicity. He pointed out that orally administered azauridine is not readily absorbed in man, and that the unabsorbed portion is converted in the lower bowel to the more toxic azauracil. As a result, the clinical utility of azauridine—a drug with many therapeutic applications—is greatly limited. However, a synthetic compound, 2', 3', 5'-triacetyl-6-azauridine, can be administered as a source of azauridine without producing azauracil. Yet, since it was a new drug (when Welch was writing), it had to be subjected to costly and time-consuming tests before it could be used, even though its pharmacology was thoroughly understood. Welch noted that toxicity results with 2', 3', 5'-triacetyl-6-azauridine would be highly dependent on the choice of animal species: dog or monkey. He affirmed, rightly, that the exercise of caution in releasing potentially hazardous drugs on the market must be weighed against the possibility of harm done by withholding a drug of proved effectiveness against certain diseases.

A good reason for not withholding clinically useful drugs is the inaccuracy of extrapolations from animal to man, some of which have already been cited. The record of the Food and Drug Administration reflects the difficulty. Of the thousands of new drugs developed from 1958 to 1964, the commission approved 251 for clinical use. Of these, eight—about three percent—ultimately proved to be so hazardous that they were withdrawn from the market (48).

More emphasis should be placed on testing drugs directly on man. Sadusk (65) defined three phases in such tests. First, the maximum tolerated dose is determined, along with side effects. Then, there is an actual clinical trial with hundreds of patients tested in accordance with dosage schedules as determined in the first phase. Finally, the drug is distributed to selected physicians, where it is hoped that all benefits and dangers will manifest themselves. Unfortunately, Zbinden (85) has shown that many adverse drug actions are unlikely to be noticed until the drugs are introduced on the market.

Human Research

The Problem of Volunteers

Most studies on man require volunteer subjects, a practice which has generated a great deal of controversy (see the discussion of ethical issues at the end of this chapter). A considerable body of recent research has indicated that volunteers for any type of experiment are not representative of the general population. For example, volunteers for hypnosis research have more favorable attitudes toward hypnosis, and volunteers for interviews about sexual attitudes have more sexually permissive attitudes than nonvolunteers (73, 84). Rosenthal and Rosnow (62) evaluated the literature comparing volunteers and nonvolunteers, and they concluded the following:

1. It is highly likely that volunteers, as a group, have greater educational attainments, higher occupational status, higher need for approval, and higher intelligence, and are less authoritarian.

2. The evidence is less adequate, but suggestive, that volunteers are younger, more sociable, more unconventional, more seeking of arousal, and more frequently firstborn.

Several of these differences have important implications for psychopharmacological research. The various factors almost surely contribute to differential drug use between volunteers and nonvolunteers (70). The difference in need for approval is of special importance. If volunteers perceive that an experimenter has a strong preference for a particular outcome, they may attempt to influence the results toward that outcome. Such a possibility underscores the need for double blind experiments.

Several differences between volunteers for drug studies and nonvolunteers have been reported (11, 37, 55). Lasagna and von Felsinger (37) noted that problems of emotional adjustment were likely to be greater with volunteers. Esecover et al. (11) found that 46 percent of volunteers for studies with hallucinogenic drugs had some form of psychiatric disorder.

EXPERIMENTAL DESIGN

The Placebo Effect

Orne (49) has argued emphatically that a subject's perceptions about what is expected of him contribute greatly to his experimental performance. For example, two groups of college students were asked to try to deceive a lie detector (62, p. 149). Members of one

group were told that the apparatus was virtually infallible except
in the case of psychopathic personalities or habitual liars. Members
of the second group were told that only highly intelligent, emotionally stable, mature individuals were capable of successful deception.
After a single trial, one-half of the members of each group were
randomly chosen to be told that they had fooled the machine, and
the other half that they had been detected. They were then given
a second trial. Large, detectable responses were given both by those
who had wanted to be detected and were told that they had not
been, and by those who had wanted to deceive and were told that
they had not deceived. The other two groups did not give such large
responses.

Orne noted that psychopharmacologists are in the enviable
position of being able to control against the effects of expectations
by using placebos. Even here, the subjects are typically aware that
they are receiving medication of some sort, so that the data generated
by such experiments only provide comparisons between the effects of
a placebo and the effects of placebo plus drug. Rarely is the action
of the drug alone, without the placebo effect, obtained. Lyerly et al.
(45) devised a solution for parceling out the drug effect. They used
middle-aged to elderly men and randomly assigned them to receive
either amphetamine, chloral hydrate, or placebo. One third of the
men in each group, regardless of what they actually received, were
told that they were getting amphetamine; they were given a brief
description of what amphetamine might be expected to do. Another third were told that they were receiving chloral hydrate, and
that it would make them relaxed or drowsy. The remainder were
given drug or placebo in disguised form, and were told that they
were being used as non-drug controls. Then, after waiting at least
an hour for the drugs to take effect, the experimenters measured
mood and motor performance of the men. There were large differences between subjects who were aware they had received a drug
and those who had unknowingly been given the same drug. Among
those men who were aware, drug action was influenced to a great
extent by whether subjects were told they were receiving amphetamine or chloral hydrate.

Extent of Placebo Effect

Beecher (5) compiled a list of patient complaints which have
been successfully treated with placebo (reproduced on p. 238). He
claimed that placebos were relatively ineffective against experimentally induced pain. However, Gelfand et al. (18) used placebos to
modify both perception of and tolerance to pain produced by ultra-
sound. Frankenhaeuser et al. (17) observed greater effects on sub-

jective measures such as mood than on objective measures like reaction time. Nevertheless, physiological systems are responsive.
Cleghorn et al. (cited in 5) found that injection of isotonic saline into
severely anxious patients produced several reliable changes in the
composition of the blood. Keats and Beecher (cited in 5) found that
7 of 15 subjects given a placebo which they thought was a narcotic
responded with constricted pupils. Still, the most dramatic effects
are psychic. Reed and Witt (56) reported a full-blown LSD reaction
in a man who had received placebo, while a second, who thought
he had received placebo but who had actually ingested a usually
effective dose of LSD, was unaffected by the drug. They invoked
cognitive factors to explain both events. Several participants at the
Josiah Macy conference on LSD described similar findings (74, pp.
72–73).

Beecher (6, p. 70) cited evidence that placebos frequently produce side effects. These include dry mouth, nausea, headache, drowsiness, and fatigue. The side effects are dose-dependent (25, 54). One
side effect is dependence; Vinar (79) described a case of a schizophrenic woman who was given placebo; she began increasing the
dosage, was unable to stop taking it without help, and had an abstinence syndrome when it was taken away from her.

Effects of Varying the Physical Nature of the Placebo

Leslie (39) suggested that red, yellow, and brown pills are more
effective than blue or green; that unusual sizes (very small or very
large) and dosages (9 or 11, but not 10, drops) yield best results;
and that strange and bitter tastes are more effective than common
tastes. Four placebos per day are more effective than one per day (58).
Although placebo effects generally become attenuated over time,
changes in color, size, or shape often lead to dramatic new improvements (57). The effect varies with the situation in which the placebo
is administered; it is much more powerful when given on the battle-
field than in civilian hospitals. In general, placebo effects are potentiated by stressful situations (6).

The Role of Conditioning

If, as suggested above, the placebo effect depends on conditioning, it should be obtainable in animals. Several studies have shown
that the effect is indeed obtainable. Studies have been conducted
in which rats were injected repeatedly (or even just once) with an
active drug and then were injected with saline; the saline produced
behavioral changes in the same direction as those produced by the
drug (26, 63, 65). One popular paradigm has been called conditioned

hypoglycemia. To produce it, a neutral stimulus is paired with large doses of insulin. Insulin by itself normally leads to a fall in the level of blood glucose. Eventually (after several pairings), the previously neutral stimulus is by itself sufficient to cause the drop in blood glucose. See Reference 41 for a review of studies on conditioned hypoglycemia in man.

Park and Covi (52) tried a novel approach which further demonstrates the role of conditioning. They suggested to a group of anxious neurotic patients that they take placebos. All were informed that the pills contained no active drug but had nevertheless been useful in treating others with the same symptomatology. All but one of fifteen patients who were asked to participate agreed to do so, and all but one of these showed significant improvement. The results indicate that placebo responsiveness does not depend solely on belief in the efficacy of a drug; rather, it is a function of all of the factors which constitute the therapeutic situation. The results are not completely convincing because no control groups were used. Perhaps the mere act of visiting a therapist reduces anxiety? Perhaps anxious neurotics have a high rate of spontaneous recovery?

Placebo Reactors

What type of person responds best to placebos? This important question has engendered controversy ever since Jellinek (30) observed that most headache sufferers respond consistently to placebo, whether with relief or with continuation of pain. By 1956 Tibbetts and Hawkings (76) had listed age, duration of illness, and degree of anxiety as important determinants of placebo responsiveness, while eliminating such factors as sex, intelligence, work record, and severity of illness. Liberman (40), however, denied the existence of an identifiable class of placebo reactors. He administered placebos to 51 women in three situations, each involving pain from a different source. He found that relief in one situation was not predictive of relief in either of the others, and concluded that there are no personality correlates for placebo responsiveness. It might appear that suggestible individuals, or those who are readily hypnotizable, would respond most strongly to inactive medication. Evans (13) tested the notion and found that it was not supported by the evidence.

Fisher (15) has emphasized the inadequacy of most research on this problem, as expressed in these comments:

Most investigators ... have relied upon essentially a single placebo situation from which a subject's placebo reactivity score is inferred. From a psychometric point of view, the use of one response in one situation as the basis for a score purporting to measure "placebo reactivity" is near indefensible. This is virtually the equivalent of using only one item from the Taylor Manifest Anxiety Scale to measure anxiety, using one item from the Wechsler-Bellevue scale of intelligence to measure I.Q., or using one item from any acceptable scale to measure anything. One simply cannot expect a score based upon a single behavioral sample to have sufficient reliability to significantly relate necessarily to anything else (be it another personality trait or another situational score).

Fisher's criticisms are reasonable and important. Yet they lead to the prediction that responses to two different placebo situations, just as to two different items on the Taylor or Wechsler-Bellevue scales, should be highly correlated. As we have just seen, Liberman showed this not to be the case. Probably the safest conclusion is that placebo responsiveness in a given situation is determined in large part by personality factors, but the evidence as to whether high and low responsiveness are trans-situational is inconclusive.

The attempts to identify placebo reactors have given rise to two related questions: (1) Does the magnitude of response to a particular drug indicate probable responsiveness to other drugs? (2) Can strong and weak drug reactors be differentiated in advance? With respect to the first question, Lasagna et al. (36) reported that morphine alleviates pain best in strong placebo reactors. Kornetsky et al. (35) found low but significant correlations between pentobarbital-induced depression and amphetamine-induced potentiation of lever pressing for food reward in rats. Kornetsky (34) also cited data on humans which showed that the degree of responsiveness to one drug is predictive of responsiveness to others.

Rickels and his co-workers believe that strong and weak drug reactors *can* be identified in advance. They advocate personality diagnoses as tools for selecting appropriate drugs for patients. Rickels et al. (60) and Overall et al. (50) showed that the antidepressive action of imipramine is strongest in patients with low anxiety, while high anxiety patients react most strongly to benactyzine. Different populations of patients respond differentially to diazepam (59) and to phenothiazines (22). In rats, modification of activity level by stimulant and depressant drugs is greatest in those which are initially most active (29).

The Double Blind

The pervasiveness of the placebo effect, together with the well-documented observations that outcomes of experiments are influenced by the expectations and hopes of the experimenters (61), underscores the need for conducting research in such a manner that neither experimenter nor subject knows the condition to which the subject has been assigned. The double blind is mandatory in clinical studies. In double blind experiments there are at least two groups, one given a drug and the other placebo; both groups are otherwise treated identically, with neither attending physician nor patients knowing the assignment of patients to groups. It is not enough to keep the patients alone unaware, for if a physician is knowledgeable about the composition of the drug and placebo groups, he is likely to show great solicitude toward recipients of the drug. This is especially true if the drug is relatively untried or known to be powerful. At the same time, complaints and queries of patients who receive placebos may be sloughed off.

Objections to the Double Blind

Several prominent scientists dispute the need for double blind studies. Hoffer and Osmond (27, p. 202) have been particularly vocal critics. They argue that clinicians do not use double blind techniques when they are required to make important decisions, such as when they determined that thalidomide is toxic; that many currently used clinical techniques, such as electroconvulsive shock therapy, tranquilizers, antidepressants, and open wards, were introduced without resorting to the double blind; that it is both costly and cumbersome; that it is impossible to use the double blind with drugs such as LSD because its effects are too easily recognizable; and that the experimental situation is antithetical to good therapeutic practice because experimenters are trained to be cold and aloof. In support of this last point, Fisher et al. (16) asked physicians to maintain an attitude of either scientific skepticism or enthusiasm toward meprobamate. The improvement rates of their patients were compared with those who received placebo. Patients treated with meprobamate in a scientific atmosphere did not differ from those treated with placebo under similar conditions. Yet, meprobamate was superior to placebo when both were administered by enthusiastic physicians. This demonstration of interaction between drug and condition of testing helps explain why many enthusiastic claims of clinicians fail to receive substantiation within the sterile confines of the laboratory. Before attempting to defend the use of the double blind, three additional criticisms shall be mentioned for the sake of completeness. These were given by Plutchik et al. (53), who nevertheless feel that double blind studies are useful except in selected instances:

1. Double blind studies are not always applicable, such as when the effects of electroconvulsive shock therapy are compared with those of a drug.

2. They lead too readily to the use of fixed dose preparations, with the result that none of the patients may receive the optimal dose.

3. When, as is commonly the case, two drugs have different time courses of effect, and their efficacy is compared at a single fixed time, one drug may inappropriately seem better.

Answers to Objections

In answer to the preceding objections, the following points are offered for consideration:

1. The fact that some important decisions have not required the use of double blind studies does not refute their general usefulness. When effects are of a very large order of magnitude, as was the case with thalidomide, the double blind is probably not needed. Even then, there are precedents where extremely powerful effects which were attributed to a particular treatment were actually the result of something else. For example, Barber (2) has questioned the role of hypnotic induction procedures in eliciting hypnotic phenomena. He showed that simply asking people to simulate hypnosis is just as effective in producing analgesia, age regression, unique body experiences, and psychophysiological changes. In any event, very large effects are rare, and cannot be fully understood unless confounding variables such as experimenter bias are eliminated.

2. While many successful clinical methods were introduced without recourse to the double blind, many other apparently successful procedures were used until double blind methodology showed that they should be discarded. For example, see pages 153 to 155 concerning the efficacy of many antidepressant drugs. The therapeutic value of many forms of psychotherapy has recently been questioned (81). Rest cures and frontal lobotomies were once very popular, but are no longer used.

3. There is no need for the experimental situation to be cold and impersonal. Researchers should profit by the experiment of Fisher; they should treat all patients, whether given a placebo or an active drug, with the same enthusiasm and optimism that would be given in the clinic.

4. There is an acceptable strategy for surmounting the problems of fixed dose and single time for testing. All that need be done is to assign the administration of drugs to a competent observer who is not involved in making the final determinations about the value of the drugs. Dosage can then be adjusted as deemed necessary. Patients should be maintained on the drugs until their responsiveness reaches peak values, if that is the measure of interest, or until their behavior stabilizes; in this way, different time courses can cause only inconvenience, but not misinterpretation of results.

5. Although it may be impossible to disguise the acute effects of certain drugs or treatments, the purpose of therapy is to promote

long range beneficial changes. It is quite easy to conduct an experiment with LSD or electroconvulsive shock. All that is needed is to have an experimenter wait to analyze the results until after the acute effects have dissipated. Residual effects are the only relevant ones.

6. The cost and difficulty of the double blind are excessive only if they exceed the benefits to be derived. The inadequacy of many popular forms of treatment suggests that the cost of not using double blind techniques may, in fact, be enormous.

Alternatives to the Double Blind

Plutchik et al. offered three alternatives to double blind experiments. The first is to measure the bias introduced by experimenters of a particular persuasion by having them indicate their strength of belief in a drug. Their answers would then be correlated with their judgments of efficacy. Alternatively, a second observer could rate the first. Plutchik et al. cited a study by Shapiro (71) in which drops in blood pressure produced by hypotensive agents were greater when physician attitudes were rated as enthusiastic than when they were rated as unenthusiastic.

A second approach is to distribute bias by using either experimenters who have opposite beliefs in the efficacy of the drug or groups of patients who differ in their optimism about the outcome.

The third possibility is to exaggerate the bias by selecting experimenters who are very favorable to the drug and comparing the results with those obtained normally. Presumably, a big difference between the two conditions would be indicative of a large experimenter bias effect. Of course, the study by Fisher (cited previously) suggests that an enthusiastic physician attitude may substantially increase the difference in effects of active drugs and placebos independently of experimenter bias.

In sum, the goal of clinical psychopharmacology is to develop drugs which yield maximum clinical utility. Hence, they should be tested under conditions which promote maximal effectiveness. These generally include an enthusiastic attitude, adjustable dosage regimens, and careful attendance to the complaints of patients, along with other appropriate measures. None of these conditions precludes the use of the double blind.

Importance of Cognitive Factors

Schachter (67) recognized that there are many conflicting reports of drug effects, such as those which attribute to LSD either stimulant, depressant, euphoriant, or dysphoriant effects. Even a drug like epinephrine produces varied effects. Maranon (46) reported that some of his subjects were unaffected by epinephrine, while others reported intense emotional responses which ranged from euphoria to violent anger. Others reported feeling "as if" they were angry, fearful, or happy. Schachter and Singer (68) tried to reconcile the disparate findings. They noted that epinephrine produces the same physiological effects as do strong emotions. However, although emotionality is marked by certain physiological changes, many emotions have similar patterns of change. Thus, the meaning given to the physiological changes may depend on the individual's cognition. If a person is aware of the cause of the changes, as when he is told that he is receiving a drug which will increase heart rate and blood pressure, he is unlikely to report emotionality. On the other hand, if the drug is administered without his knowledge, the particular emotion evoked will depend on the situation.

Schachter and Singer tested the correctness of their analysis. They injected subjects with epinephrine or a placebo. They told one-half of the members of each group to expect that their hearts would begin pounding and their hands shaking; the other half of each group was told to expect no side effects. The four groups thus formed were further divided by placing one-half of each in a situation designed to evoke anger reactions, while the rest were encouraged by the circumstances in which they were placed to become euphoric.

The results bore out what had been expected. Those subjects who had been told to expect side effects were relatively uninfluenced by the context in which they were observed; moreover, epinephrine and placebo subjects did not greatly differ. The uninformed drugged subjects, however, caught the mood of the situation. They became appropriately angry or euphoric. These results are not limited to the emotions of anger and euphoria, or to the drug epinephrine (69). With regard to how a response to a drug may be shaped, Schachter quoted Becker's observations (4) on the reactions of novice marijuana smokers: "Being high consists of two elements: the presence of symptoms caused by marijuana use and the recognition of these symptoms and their connection by the user with his use of the drug. It is not enough, that is, that the effects be present; they alone do not automatically provide the experience of being high. The user must be able to point them out to himself and consciously connect them with his smoked marijuana before he can have this experience. Otherwise, regardless of the actual effects produced, he considers that the drug has had no effect on him."

The physiological changes produced by marijuana are thus shown to be intrinsically neither good nor bad. Users must learn to recognize the state and be taught that it is pleasant. Schachter offered one final example of a physiological condition which can be viewed subjectively: vomiting. Twentieth century Americans find vomiting disagreeable, but Romans at banquets probably regarded it as pleasant.

SOME OTHER METHODOLOGICAL PROBLEMS

Determining Mechanism and Site of Action

Just because two drugs produce the same overt behavioral effects is no assurance that they act either by the same mechanism or at the same site. For example, activity may be increased because of a direct stimulant action or because of increased pain, fear, hunger, or hypothermia. A partial solution toward identifying primary drug effects is to test congeners which share some but not all of the actions. Thus, if two related drugs both lower body temperature to about the same extent, but only one produces hyperactivity, it is unlikely that the lowered temperature is the cause of the hyperactivity.

The technique of autoradiography is a powerful means of localizing the sites of drug action. It consists of labeling a suitable drug with a radioactive isotope; by then examining the tissues of injected subjects, the distribution of the drug can be determined. In general, small molecules enter the brain more easily. The methylated analogues of many drugs (such as atropine and scopolamine) do not enter readily. Their actions can be compared with those of the unmethylated drugs. If there are differences in effect, they are attributed to the central activity of the unmethylated drugs. Domino's work with selective blocking agents (described on pp. 355–356) indicates still another strategy for determining site of action.

There are several techniques for administering drugs locally. Grossman (24) developed a technique using cannulas, which enables researchers to administer minute amounts (one to five μg) of a drug directly into specific parts of the brain. However, Routtenberg (64) has questioned the specificity of the technique. Feldberg (14) injects drugs directly into the ventricles of the brain and then perfuses dyes over specific ventricular regions in order to localize site of action. A relatively simple technique is to implant recording electrodes within parts of the brain suspected of being affected by a drug. Through the use of this procedure, it can be shown that both stimulant and hypnotic drugs modify activity within the reticular formation (32). However, even with sophisticated techniques, it is not possible to tell whether a response is due to the structure stimulated or to secondary activation of other structures.

Behavior-behavior Correlations

There are two popular approaches toward understanding the mechanisms of drug action. First, as described before, researchers try to determine the site of action. Secondly, they focus on the identification of the neurotransmitters which underlie specific behaviors. (This latter strategy is discussed in appropriate places throughout the remainder of the book.) Both approaches are currently being pursued with great vigor in many laboratories throughout the world. There is a third paradigm, which has been largely neglected, that may be called the search for behavior-behavior correlations. The idea is to distinguish between the primary and secondary behavioral effects of drugs, and to determine relationships among behaviors. The scientist who studies behavior-behavior correlations might compare the effects of 10 different drugs on two behaviors, e.g., sex and aggression. He would see if changes of one behavior paralleled changes of the other. Perhaps both changes would be seen to be secondary to changes in activity or sensitivity to stimuli. These could then be tested by both pharmacological and non-pharmacological means. Perhaps some behavior could be shown to be primary, and then knowledge of a drug's action on that behavior might enable predictions of its effects on a much wider range of behaviors.

Special Problems of the Clinician

Clinical psychopharmacologists encounter several difficulties which are unique to their profession. Of necessity, their experimental designs generally deviate greatly from the ideal. In the ideal experiment, a fairly homogeneous group of subjects is randomly divided into two or more treatment and control groups. The size of the experimental sample is chosen before the start of testing; the aim is to maximize the likelihood of uncovering important differences, without testing so many subjects that even very slight differences among groups will attain statistical significance. The problem of subject attrition, or dropouts, is rarely a serious one.

In the clinic, the patient population is rarely homogeneous. As a consequence, the variability of responsiveness to drugs is large, and statistical analyses are less likely to yield positive results. A partial solution would be to use factorial designs, as they enable experimenters to test two or more variables simultaneously (see Reference 31 for a simple exposition of the use of such designs in research).

The problem of sample size is a difficult one. It may be impossible to conduct a meaningful test of a drug believed to be efficacious against schizophrenia if the test is done in a small mental hospital where only a few patients are schizophrenic. Perhaps joint programs would help, although the investigators would have to recognize that responsiveness to drugs varies among different clinics (42). The alternative may be to restrict government funding of such research to only those scientists with access to a large patient population.

The problem of subject attrition, which is often quite large in drug studies, can be reduced to some extent by the preselection of patients and by devoting considerable attention to all participants. An additional possibility which reduces the impact of dropouts is to test each subject one or more times under each drug condition. This within-subject design is efficient and reduces variability. However, it cannot be used when the effects of a treatment are irreversible, or when the dependent variable is permanent mental functioning. One additional problem is that the difference between treatment and control conditions is generally magnified when subjects serve as their own controls (23); thus, results would not be completely comparable to those reported in other studies.

ETHICAL ISSUES

In 1966, Henry Beecher of the Harvard Medical School published a very important paper on ethics in scientific research (7). Beecher examined 100 consecutive reports of medical studies involving man which were published in a reputable, unnamed journal. At least 12 of the studies were of questionable ethical standards. Procedures reported in the studies included the removal of the thymus glands of young children—not out of medical need but merely to determine function—and the withholding of drugs which were known to be effective in treating certain diseases, with the result that some patients died. The experiments were conducted without patient consent in charity wards, VA hospitals, private hospitals, and some of the finest medical centers in the world. It is clear that one need not be a practicing or prospective scientist to be concerned with the question of ethics in medical research.

Kline (10, p. 345) believes that it is often inadvisable to seek patient consent. He cited several reasons: emotionally disturbed patients may be incapable of acting in their own best interests; labeling a drug "investigational" might cause refusal by many patients, especially those already suffering from overwhelming anxiety or paranoia, even though the drug may have already demonstrated effectiveness in many similar cases; lastly, the delays involved in obtaining consent may have unfortunate consequences. In rebuttal, Curran (10, p. 346) observed that patient consent is the first commandment in both the Decalogue of Nuremberg and the code of the World Medical Association. He also remarked that, where the same individual is both therapist and investigator, he may be tempted to rationalize a patient's refusal to take a particular drug as unwise and something to be disregarded.

Many scientists believe that consent, by itself, is an insufficient criterion for inclusion of a patient in an experiment. Pappworth (51) argued that certain types of individuals should not be allowed to volunteer under any circumstances. These include "minors, the very elderly, the very poor, prisoners, patients suffering from fatal, incurable, or seriously debilitating diseases, the insane or seriously emotionally disturbed, personnel in the Armed Forces, medical students, laboratory workers and conscientious objectors." Lehmann (38) ridiculed the list, noting that it excludes all but those who would have no desire to participate in such experiments.

Baumrind (3) attacked prevailing standards in psychological research, where the same types of problems arise. She began by quoting from the Introduction of a draft of the report of the Committee on Ethical Standards in Psychological Research:

> Almost any psychological research on human subjects entails some compromise among ethical ideals, some choice of one particular ethical standard over others. For this reason, there are those who would call a halt to the whole endeavor, or who would erect barriers that would exclude research on many central psychological questions as out of bounds. But for a psychologist, the decision not to do research is an ethically questionable solution, since it is one of his obligations to use his research skills to extend knowledge for the sake of ultimate human betterment.

Baumrind disagrees emphatically with the above viewpoint of the Ethics Committee. She expressed the opinion that because researchers enjoy special status in the eyes of their subjects, they have a special responsibility to behave morally and to ensure that no harm befalls the subjects. She did approve of the section of the ethics code devoted to potential outcomes of experiments, which states that "the subject must be fully informed of these benefits and costs, competent to judge them, and must accept the arrangement free of duress"; she deplores sections elsewhere which are worded so as to permit evasion of the principle. She stated that "scientific ends, however laudable these may be, do not by themselves justify the use of means that in ordinary transactions would be regarded as reprehensible." She does not accept that part of the draft which states, "The general ethical question always is whether the subject runs a risk of being harmed that the importance of the research does not warrant." Baumrind feels that the individual must be the sole judge of risk which he is willing to accept for the sake of others.

Beecher's exposure of research which seriously endangered

human life has raised profound ethical questions. He, Curran, Papp-worth, and Baumrind believe that the rights of the individual are pre-eminent. On the other side, some scientists stress that many medical advances which have relieved suffering and prolonged the lives of millions of people originated from experiments which sacri-ficed the lives of human subjects. Walter Reed's isolation of the *Aedes* mosquito as the carrier of yellow fever is a prominent example. Medical researchers would be seriously handicapped if there were a ban on experiments which endangered human lives. Tests for possible toxicity of drugs and chemical additives would be dis-allowed because their nature entails risks but no direct gain for the participants. People who give consent would be adjudged to be emotionally disturbed; or perhaps to have been intimidated into participation, as is often the case within prisons; or to have been misled about the possible consequences of the experiment. No treat-ment, once it gained popular acceptance, would ever be withheld to further test its value. As a consequence, even totally useless treat-ments (which might also be painful, dangerous, time consuming, and costly) would persist even longer than they now do.

The problem is a weighty one. Philosophers such as Kant, J. S. Mill, and G. E. Moore have argued for centuries about proper ethical conduct. Many modern philosophers deny the existence of ethical absolutes. Whether the rights of the individual are inviolable or may occasionally be sacrificed for the good of society is nowhere carved in stone for all to see.

There is no doubt that many scientists and physicians have abused their privileged positions by conducting research where the primary motive has been to enhance personal status, even at the expense of human suffering or lives. In addition, animals have also been exposed to needless suffering. Ethical codes, such as the newly revised Americal Psychological Association code, contain provisions detailing the proper treatment of research animals. The author chooses to cast his vote on the side of those who believe in protecting the integrity of the individual even at the cost of hamper-ing research.

A BRIEF NOTE ON MEASUREMENT TECHNIQUES

The administration of a drug is no different in principle from the manipulation of any other independent variable, and therefore requires no special techniques for measurement of induced behavioral changes. This book may be considered to be a compilation of certain approaches to the measurement of behavior. Descriptions of many other types of independent variables may be found in any good textbook of experimental psychology. Techniques of operant conditioning, which can be used to generate very stable behavioral baselines, have been described in many books; one of the best is by Sidman (72). For a review of many useful questionnaires and rating scales (up to 1960), see Lorr (44). An updated version is provided by Gleser (21). For evaluating the efficacy of drugs in psychotherapy, skill in clinical assessment is needed. A helpful text in this area is Reference 1.

REFERENCES

1. Anastasi, A. *Psychological Testing*. New York: Macmillan, 1961.
2. Barber, T. *Hypnosis: A Scientific Approach*. New York: Van Nostrand Reinhold, 1969.
3. Baumrind, D. Principles of ethical conduct in the treatment of subjects: reaction to the draft report of the Committee on Ethical Standards in Psychological Research. Am. Psychol., 1971, 26:887–896.
4. Becker, H. Becoming a marihuana user. Am. J. Sociol., 1953, 59:235–242.
5. Beecher, H. Ethics and clinical research. New Eng. J. Med., 1966, 24:1354–1360.
6. Beecher, H. *Measurement of the Subjective Response*. New York: Oxford University Press, 1959.
7. Beecher, H. The powerful placebo. J.A.M.A., 1955, 159:1602–1606.
8. Brady, J. A comparative approach to the evaluation of drug effects upon affective behavior. Ann. N.Y. Acad. Sci., 1956, 64:632–643.
9. Corne, S., and Pickering, R. A possible correlation between drug-induced hallucinations in man and a behavioural response in mice. Psychopharmacologia, 1967, 11:65–78.
10. Efron, D. (Ed.) *Psychopharmacology: A Review of Progress*. U.S. PHS Pub. No. 1836, 1968.
11. Esecover, H., Malitz, S., and Wilkens, B. Clinical profiles of paid normal subjects volunteering for hallucinogenic drug studies. Am. J. Psychiat., 1961, 117: 910–915.
12. Estes, W., and Skinner, B. Some quantitative properties of anxiety. J. Exp. Psychol., 1941, 29:390–400.
13. Evans, F. The placebo response: relationship to suggestibility and hypnotizability. Paper read at Am. Psychol. Assoc. Convention, 1969.
14. Feldberg, W. *A Pharmacological Approach to the Brain From Its Inner and Outer Surfaces*. Baltimore: Williams & Wilkins, 1963.
15. Fisher, S. The placebo reactor: thesis, antithesis, synthesis, and hypothesis. Dis. Nerv. Syst., 1967, 28:510–515.
16. Fisher, S., Cole, J., Rickels, K., and Uhlenhuth, E. Drug-set interaction: the effect of expectations on drug response in outpatients. Neuropsychopharmacol., 1964, 3:149–156.
17. Frankenhaeuser, M., Post, B., Hagdahl, R., and Wrangsjoe, B. Effects of a depressant drug as modified by experimentally-induced expectation. Percept. Motor Skills, 1964, 18:513–522.
18. Gelfand, S., Ullman, L., and Krasner, L. The placebo response: an experimental approach. J. Nerv. Ment. Dis., 1963, 136:379–387.
19. Gessner, P. Pharmacological studies of 5-methoxy-N,N-dimethyltryptamine, LSD and other hallucinogens. *In* Efron, D. (Ed.) *Psychotomimetic Drugs*. New York: Raven Press, 1970.
20. Gibson, R., and Tingstad, J. Formulation of a morphine implantation pellet suitable for tolerance—physical dependence studies in mice. J. Pharm. Sci., 1970, 59:426–427.
21. Gleser, G. Psychometric contributions to the assessment of patients. *In* Efron, D. (Ed.) *Psychopharmacology: A Review of Progress*. U.S. PHS Pub. No. 1836, 1968.
22. Goldberg, S., and Mattsson, N. Schizophrenic subtypes defined by response to drugs and placebo. Dis. Nerv. Syst., 1968, 29:153–158.

23. Grice, G. Dependence of empirical laws upon the source of experimental variation. Psychol. Bull., 1966, 66:488–498.
24. Grossman, S. Eating or drinking elicited by direct adrenergic or cholinergic stimulation of hypothalamus. Science, 1960, 132:301–302.
25. Gruber, C. Interpreting medical data. Arch. Int. Med., 1956, 98:767–773.
26. Herrnstein, R. Placebo effect in the rat. Science, 1962, 138:677–678.
27. Hoffer, A., and Osmond, H. The Hallucinogens. New York: Academic Press, 1967.
28. Irwin, S. Considerations for the pre-clinical evaluation of new psychiatric drugs: a case study with phenothiazine-like tranquilizers. Psychopharmacologia, 1966, 9:259–287.
29. Irwin, S., Slabok, M., and Thomas, G. Individual differences: I. Correlation between control locomotor activity and sensitivity to stimulant and depressant drugs. J. Pharmacol. Exp. Ther., 1958, 123:206–211.
30. Jellinek, E. Clinical tests on comparative effectiveness of analgesic drugs. Biometrics, 1946, 2:87–91.
31. Keppel, G. Design and Analysis: A Researcher's Handbook. Englewood Cliffs, N.J.: Prentice-Hall, 1973.
32. Killam, E. Drug action on the brain stem reticular formation. Pharmacol. Rev., 1962, 14:175–223.
33. Koppanyi, T., and Avery, M. Species differences and the clinical trial of new drugs: a review. Clin. Pharmacol. Ther., 1966, 7:250–270.
34. Kornetsky, C. Alterations in psychomotor functions and individual differences in responses produced by psychoactive drugs. In Uhr, L. and Miller, J. (Eds.) Drugs and Behavior. New York: Wiley, 1960.
35. Kornetsky, C., Dawson, J., and Pelikan, E. In Rinkel, M. (Ed.) Specific and Non-Specific Factors in Psychopharmacology. New York: Philosophical Library, 1963.
36. Lasagna, L., Mosteller, F., von Felsinger, J., and Beecher, H. A study of the placebo response. Am. J. Med., 1954, 16:770–779.
37. Lasagna, L., and von Felsinger, J. The volunteer subject in research. Science, 1954, 120:359–361.
38. Lehmann, H. Problems in controlled clinical evaluations. In Efron, D. (Ed.) Psychopharmacology: A Review of Progress. U.S. PHS Pub. No. 1836, 1968.
39. Leslie, A. Ethics and practice of placebo therapy. Am. J. Med., 1954, 16:854–862.
40. Liberman, R. The elusive placebo reactor. Proc. Fifth Int. Cong. Neuropsychopharmacol., 1966, 557–566.
41. Lichko, A. Conditioned reflex hypoglycemia in man. Pavlov J. Higher Nerv. Act., 1959, 9:731–737.
42. Lipman, R., Park, L., and Rickels, K. Paradoxical influence of a therapeutic side effect interpretation. Arch. Gen. Psychiat., 1966, 15:462–474.
43. Litchfield, J. Evaluation of the safety of new drugs by means of tests in animals. Clin. Pharmacol. Ther., 1962, 3:665–672.
44. Lorr, M. Rating scales, behavior inventories, and drugs. In Uhr, L. and Miller, J. (Eds.) Drugs and Behavior. New York: Wiley, 1960.
45. Lyerly, S., Ross, S., Krugman, A., and Clyde, D. Drugs and placebos: the effects of instructions upon performance and mood under amphetamine sulphate and chloral hydrate. J. Ab. Soc. Psychol., 1964, 68:321–327.
46. Maronon, G. Contribution à l'étude de l'action émotive de l'adrénaline. Revue Française d'Endocrinologie, 1924, 2:301–325.
47. Masserman, J. Drugs, brain and behavior: an experimental approach to experiential psychoses. J. Neuropsychiat., 1962, 3:S104–S113.
48. Modell, W. Chairman's opening remarks. In Wolstenholme, G. and Porter, R. (Eds.) Drug Responses in Man. Boston: Little, Brown, 1967.
49. Orne, M. Demand characteristics and the concept of quasi-controls. In Rosenthal, R., and Rosnow, R. (Eds.) Artifact in Behavioral Research. New York: Academic Press, 1969.
50. Overall, J., Hollister, L., Meyer, F., Kimbell, I., and Shelton, J. Imipramine and thioridazine in depressed and schizophrenic patients: Are there specific antidepressant drugs? J.A.M.A., 1964, 189:605–608.
51. Pappworth, M. Human Guinea Pigs: Experimentation on Man. London: Routledge, 1967.

52. Park, L., and Covi, L. Nonblind placebo trial. Arch. Gen. Psychiat., 1965, 12:336–345.
53. Plutchik, R., Platman, S., and Fieve, R. Three alternatives to the double-blind. Arch. Gen. Psychiat., 1969, 20:428–432.
54. Pogge, R., and Coats, E. The placebo as a source of side effects in normal people: influence of gradually increasing doses. Neb. St. Med. J., 1962, 47:337–339.
55. Pollin, W., and Perlin, S. Psychiatric evaluation of "normal control" volunteers. Am. J. Psychiat., 1958, 115:129–133.
56. Reed, C., and Witt, P. Factors contributing to unexpected reactions in two human drug-placebo experiments. Confin. Psychiat., 1965, 8:57–68.
57. Rickels, K., Baumm, C., and Fales, K. Evaluation of placebo responses in psychiatric outpatients under two experimental conditions. Neuropsychopharmacology, 1964, 3:80–84.
58. Rickels, K., Hesbacher, P., Weise, C., Gray, B., and Feldman, H. Pills and improvement: a study of placebo response in psychoneurotic outpatients. Psychopharmacologia, 1970, 16:318–328.
59. Rickels, K., Raab, E., and Hesbacher, P. Diazepam, phenobarbital sodium, and placebo in three neurotic populations. Cited in Rickels, K. Antineurotic agents: specific and non-specific effects. In Efron, D. (Ed.) Psychopharmacology: A Review of Progress. U. S. PHS Pub. No. 1836, 1968.
60. Rickels, K., Ward, C., and Schut, L. Different populations, different drug responses. Am. J. Med. Sci., 1964, 247:328–335.
61. Rosenthal, R. On the social psychology of the psychological experiment. The experimenter's hypothesis as unintended determinant of experimental results. Am. Sci., 1963, 51:268–283.
62. Rosenthal, R., and Rosnow, R. The volunteer subject. In Rosenthal, R., and Rosnow, R. (Eds.) Artifact in Behavioral Research. New York: Academic Press, 1969.
63. Ross, S., and Schnitzer, S. Further support for a placebo effect in the rat. Psychol. Rep., 1963, 13:461–462.
64. Routtenberg, A. Drinking induced by carbachol: thirst circuit or ventricular modification. Science, 1967, 157:838–839.
65. Rushton, R., Steinberg, H., and Tinson, C. Effects of a single experience on subsequent reactions to drugs. Brit. J. Pharmacol., 1963, 20:99–105.
66. Sadusk, J. Drugs and government: the role of government in the development and distribution of medicinal agents. Georgetown Med. Bull., 1965, 18:173–181.
67. Schachter, S. On the assumption of "identity" in psychopharmacology. Symp. Med. Aspects of Stress in Military Clim., 1964.
68. Schachter, S., and Singer, J. Cognitive, social and physiological determinants of emotional state. Psychol. Rev., 1962, 69:379–399.
69. Schachter, S., and Wheeler, L. Epinephrine, chlorpromazine, and amusement. J. Ab. Soc. Psychol., 1962, 65:121–128.
70. Schubert, D. Arousal seeking as a motivation for volunteering: MMPI scores and central-nervous-system-stimulant use as suggestive of a trait. J. Proj. Tech. Person. Assess., 1964, 28:337–340.
71. Shapiro, A. Influence of emotional variables in evaluation of hypotensive agents. Psychosom. Med., 1955, 17:291–305.
72. Sidman, M. Tactics of Scientific Research. New York: Basic Books, 1960.
73. Siegman, A. Responses to a personality questionnaire by volunteers and non-volunteers to a Kinsey interview. J. Ab. Soc. Psychol., 1956, 52:280–281.
74. Stafford, P., and Golightly, B. (Eds.) LSD: The Problem Solving Psychedelic. New York: Universal Publishing and Distributing Corp., 1967.
75. Steinberg, H. Methods of assessment of psychological effects of drugs in animals. In Marks, J., and Pare, C. (Eds.) Symposium on the Scientific Basis of Drug Treatment in Psychiatry. London: Pergamon, 1965.
76. Tibbetts, R., and Hawkings, J. The placebo response. J. Ment. Sci., 1957, 102:60–66.
77. Turner, R. Screening Methods in Pharmacology. New York: Academic Press, 1965.
78. Underwood, B. Experimental Psychology. New York: Appleton-Century Crofts, 1966.
79. Vinar, O. Dependence on a placebo: a case report. Brit. J. Psychiat., 1969, 115:1189–1190.

80. Welch, A. Pharmacological differences, qualitative and quantitative, between man and other species. *In* Wolstenholme, G., and Porter, R. (Eds.) *Drug Responses in Man.* Boston: Little, Brown, 1967.
81. Wolpe, J., Salter, A., and Reyan, L. (Eds.) *The Conditioning Therapies: The Challenge in Psychotherapy.* New York: Holt, Rinehart, and Winston, 1964.
82. Wolstenholme, G., and Porter, R. (Eds.) *Drug Responses in Man.* Boston: Little, Brown, 1967.
83. Woods, J., and Schuster, C. Regulation of drug self-administration. *In* Harris, R., McIsaac, W., and Schuster, C. (Eds.) *Drug Dependence.* Austin: U. Texas, 1970.
84. Zamansky, H., and Brightbill, R. Attitude differences of volunteers and nonvolunteers and of susceptible and nonsusceptible hypnotic subjects. Int. J. Clin. Exper. Hypnosis, 1965, *13*:279–290.
85. Zbinden, G. The significance of pharmacological screening tests in the preclinical safety evaluation of new drugs. J. New Drugs, 1966, *6*:1–7.

CHAPTER 10

SENSORY PHENOMENA

Several commonly used drugs must be administered with great caution because of the possibility that they will produce irreversible damage to sensory systems. Others have transient side effects, which may be toxic or facilitatory; still other drugs are used in large part because of their profound influences on sensory and perceptual processes.

If there is reason to suspect that a drug has damaged tissue, a pathologist may be called in for consultation. Pathologists have relatively direct procedures for determining the extent of injury, if any. However, more complex techniques of assessment are necessary for the detection of temporary impairment, facilitation, or modification of sensory functioning. An approach favored by neurophysiologists utilizes evoked responses (ER's). This involves the stimulation of a sensory receptor and the simultaneous recording of responses of individual neurons or populations of neurons along the sensory pathway. For example, an electrode implanted in the retina or the visual cortex may be used to investigate differential sensitivity to various wavelengths of light. The technique has the advantage of not requiring cooperation on the part of the subject; ER's can even be recorded from anesthetized animals. Unfortunately, it is often easier to obtain drug-induced modifications of ER's than it is to interpret their behavioral significance. Thus, although it is known that LSD reduces the amplitude of the response evoked in several brain sites by median nerve stimulation (116), the finding does little to clarify the behavioral actions of LSD.

The work of Granit (53) puts the problem into clearer perspective.

He found that retinal cells of cats respond differently to different wavelengths of light, even though there is little evidence for color discrimination in the cat (58). Because of our limited understanding of the behavioral significance of ER's, they will be mentioned only occasionally in this chapter; the interested reader is referred to Reference 37 for several informative articles.

Problems of interpretation also plague psychologists. They must infer changes in the capacity of sensory systems from altered responsiveness to stimuli; however, altered responsiveness may be caused by changes in motor capacity, vigilance, learning ability, memory, or motivation. The experiments of Terrace and of Dews, described in Chapter 2, are relevant; they showed that discrimination performance after the administration of various drugs is determined to a great extent by the prior history of the subjects, and by the particular schedule of reinforcement.

The picture is not all bleak. Several powerful techniques have been developed which enable scientists to estimate drug effects on sensory processes with considerable accuracy. These are described below as they have been used to study olfaction, taste, vision, audition, time estimation, and the perception of pain.

OLFACTION

In order for a substance to be odorous, it must be volatile. That is, it must evaporate quickly, thereby losing molecules to the air which can be breathed into the nose. It is also necessary that the molecules be of the right size and shape for collecting on the tissue lining of the nose. Most highly volatile substances are odorous.

The sensation of taste is partially determined by odor. With smell eliminated as a cue, e.g., when the nostrils are held shut, it is very difficult to distinguish by taste between such otherwise easily discriminable substances as Coca-Cola and 7-Up, or slices of potato and apple. Schutz and Pilgram (115) reported that when subjects were stimulated by a pleasant odor, their sensitivity to the taste of sour substances was modified. The direction of change depended upon the initial level of sensitivity; thresholds were raised in sensitive subjects and lowered in insensitive ones. Because of the interactions between olfaction and taste, it is not surprising that most drugs which modify the one sense also modify the other.

It is a relatively straightforward matter to determine an absolute threshold: it is simply that intensity of a stimulus to which a subject responds 50 percent of the time. A differential threshold is the intensity of the difference between two stimuli which is correctly reported as a difference 75 percent of the time. The procedures for obtaining threshold values are described in most experimental psychology books. Most of the studies on drug-induced changes in olfaction have used absolute thresholds as the measure of acuity. Problems with the threshold concept are discussed in the section on audition.

Increased Acuity

Hormones

There is a sex difference in olfactory acuity; women have a more highly developed sense of smell than men (103), and the difference is hormonally dependent.* It varies with the menstrual cycle, reaching a peak at mid-cycle when estrogen levels are highest.

Olfactory acuity is deficient in those women whose ovaries are less active than normal. The condition can be remedied with estrogen, whereas androgen makes it even worse (114). The hormones probably act by changing the size of the vessels in the mucous membrane (104).

There are sex differences in odor preferences; as Kenneth (84) reported, women enjoyed the smell of xylol more than did men. There are also hormonally dependent preferences of males for odors associated with sexual receptivity in females; for example, whereas normal male rats readily discriminate between the odors of sexually receptive and unreceptive females, castrated males make the discrimination only if some other reward is contingent upon it (such as water when they are thirsty) (92).

Amphetamines

Amphetamine is well known as an appetite suppressant. The mechanism by which it exerts its effects is not fully understood, and one early suggestion was that it affected the senses of olfaction or taste. Turner and Patterson (130) tested the hypothesis by determining olfactory thresholds both prior to amphetamine administration and hourly for three hours afterward. The subjects were men and women, and the test substance was xylol. In addition to amphetamine, each subject also was tested with a placebo and with a preparation containing the appetite depressants phenmetrazine and phen-

---

*Differential acuity can be quite specific. For instance, women are more capable of detecting by odor the presence of 17-keteosteroid compounds, which are urinary metabolites of the adrenal glands. The ability is lost upon the removal of the ovaries, and can be restored by treatment with estrogen (LeMagnen, reported in 54).

butrazate. The subjects fasted during the period when thresholds were being measured.

The results did not confirm the hypothesis that amphetamine impairs the sense of smell. In fact, there were no changes in threshold during the three hours after administration for which data were obtained; by contrast, when the subjects were given the placebo, thresholds to detect xylol rose over time, which means that acuity declined. The authors suggested that the rise in threshold was caused by the cumulative effects of fatigue and fasting. If anything, then, amphetamine enhanced acuity. A more clear-cut enhancement was seen after administration of the phenmetrazine preparation, when thresholds actually fell over time.

Caffeine

Turner (129) cited Mysnikov, who studied olfactory thresholds in dogs. He found that several stimulant agents, including caffeine, improved the sense of smell. The results are consistent with the amphetamine findings.

Niacin

Green (55) has treated many patients who came to him with serious impairment of several sense modalities, but most prominently that of smell. He believes that the problem is caused by niacin deficiency, and hence prescribes large doses of the vitamin. He reported many cases of dramatic relief of symptoms following this simple treatment.

Decreased Acuity

Local Anesthetics

Several authors (listed in Reference 129) have reported that the local anesthetics, of which cocaine has been best studied, temporarily depress olfactory acuity. For some odors, such as that of rubber, the deficit often persists for several months. If only one nostril is treated, the other often becomes hypersensitive to odors.

Alcohol

Marguiles et al. (97) reported that small amounts of ethyl alcohol caused elevations of olfactory thresholds. However, Pangborn (106) offered several methodological objections to the study, the most serious of which were that the environment was contaminated with odors, temperature and humidity were not controlled, and the subject may have responded to fluctuations in air pressure as well as to odor.

Miscellaneous Effects

Neoarsphenamine, a drug once used to treat syphilis, induced ether-like sensations in some patients, with the disturbances often lasting for several hours. Several hallucinogenic drugs give rise to strange olfactory sensations. No threshold testing has been done, but some people who take LSD, mescaline, psilocybin, or marijuana report subjective changes in acuity (21, 31). They become aware of smells which nonusers cannot sense. Until more refined testing is conducted, the possibility that they are hallucinating the smells cannot be excluded. A substantial percentage of users of psychedelic drugs report that smells become richer and take on new qualities when they are high (127).

TASTE

There are four primary taste sensations: sweet, salt, acid, and bitter. Drugs often act differentially on the four.

Hormones

The adrenal glands secrete several hormones. One type, exemplified by desoxycorticosterone, acts primarily to promote retention of sodium; prednisolone is representative of a second class which helps to regulate sugar balance. People who suffer from untreated adrenal cortical insufficiency, a disease characterized by easy fatigability and inability to cope with environmental change, are able to detect sodium chloride (and a great many other substances as well) at about 1/100th the concentration required by people with normal adrenal functioning. Surprisingly, injections of desoxycorticosterone correct the defects associated with the hypoadrenal state, but do not affect salt thresholds. Prednisolone, on the other hand, returns the threshold to normal (68). Olfaction is affected in the same way by both the disease and the hormone treatment.

Sex hormones affect taste acuity. Allara (2) reported that castrated animals show a change in the number of taste buds, but in the animals he studied, the change did not modify taste preferences (81, p. 148). However, gonadal hormones affect the composition of saliva, which is very important for taste perception (48). Female mice were found to be more sensitive to the taste of 6-n-propyl-thiouracil than were males, and castration decreased the sensitivity of both sexes. The taste thresholds of the castrates were increased by testosterone and decreased by estrogen (74).

In contrast to the work with mice, Henkin's measurements of taste thresholds in postmenopausal and ovariectomized women, and in patients receiving estrogen or testosterone therapy, showed no significant alterations from the norm (81, p. 148). Patients with the symptom of underdeveloped gonads (found in certain disease states) did show changes: they had both poor olfactory acuity and reduced taste sensitivity to sour and bitter. Estrogen helps to return taste thresholds toward normality in hypogonadal women.

Pangborn (81, p. 149) did not find consistent variation with the menstrual cycle in taste sensitivity. There were large individual differences in the effects of the normal hormonal variations.

There is a sex difference in preferences for sweets in humans and rats. Females of both species have a stronger preference than do males. In an elegant series of studies (9, 131, 139, 140), Zucker and his colleagues have determined the hormonal basis for the difference. Removal of the ovaries of female rats reduced their preferences for saccharin, and the preferences were restored by replacement therapy with estrogen and progesterone. Preferences were also diminished during pregnancy, at which time the secretion of progesterone is increased and estrogen secretion decreased. The authors suggested that an optimal balance of estrogen and progesterone may act directly on the brain to control the reactivity of taste stimuli. (Zucker's work on the effectiveness of very small doses of gonadal hormones during the neonatal period in influencing adult responsiveness to sweet solutions is described in Chapter 8.)

Zucker's group described several parallels between saccharin preferences and aversion toward quinine. When their water supply is adulterated with quinine, intact female rats reduce intake to a greater extent than do ovariectomized ones. Pregnancy also reduces the aversion toward quinine.

Increased Acuity

Vitamins

Taste receptors are modified epithelial cells, and epithelial cells are sensitive to the actions of certain vitamins. Therefore, it is not surprising that the sensation of taste is impaired by vitamin deficiency. In particular, deficiencies of vitamin A result in histological changes in the tongue and virtual elimination of preferential taste behavior. Administration of vitamin A restores normal preferences (11). Deficiencies of several other nutrients also modify taste preferences (128).

Sympathetic Stimulation

A useful measure of sensory acuity is the just noticeable difference (jnd). If a stimulus has an intensity S, and if the intensity of the smallest increment in the stimulus which can be detected by a perceiver is given by ΔS, then the jnd is defined by the ratio of $\Delta S/S$. For example, if a 10-decibel tone can just barely be distinguished from one of 11 decibels, the jnd is $1/10 = 0.1$. The smaller the jnd, the greater the sensitivity. Fischer and Kaelbling (45) measured the jnd's detected by humans when they tasted saccharin and sucrose. When the experimenters administered psilocybin or amphetamine, both drugs reduced the size of the jnd's. The authors argued that the drugs increased sensitivity by activating the sympathetic nervous system. As further evidence, they contrasted the sensitivity of mental patients who were or were not on phenothiazine or imipramine medication. These drugs are antiadrenergics — that is, they reduce sympathetic activity. Patients treated with the drugs had larger jnd's than did untreated patients. However, Herxheimer (69) found no effect of amphetamine on taste thresholds.

Dinitrophenol used to be a popular appetite-suppressant. Chronic use of dinitrophenol induces several alterations of taste perception. Bitter tastes are accentuated, while tastes for salt — and occasionally for sweet and sour as well — are lost (Bogaert, reported in 57).

Decreased Acuity

Smoking

Although many of the effects of smoking are due to nicotine, other substances, such as carbon monoxide, also contribute. In an early study, Sinnot and Rauth (120) found that absolute taste thresholds are greater for smokers than for non-smokers. Smokers are especially insensitive to bitter tastes; their thresholds for quinine and the odorless compound 6-n-propylthiouracil, for instance, are elevated (80).

Arfmann and Chapanis (4) asked female smokers and non-smokers to compare the intensity of a solution of vanilla extract which was sprayed into their nostrils with the intensity of a similar solution which was placed on their tongues. Smokers consistently rated the smell as stronger. Although the experiment shows that the sense of smell relative to the sense of taste is greater in non-smokers, it does not indicate whether smoking improves olfactory acuity or reduces taste sensitivity. In light of the evidence previously cited, the results of Arfmann and Chapanis can most easily be accounted for by assuming that smoking impairs taste while not affecting smell. The fact that smoking dulls taste sensitivity may account in part for the problem of weight gain which often plagues people who quit smoking. The food tastes so good that they are unable to stop eating.

Alcohol

The chorda tympani nerve conveys taste sensations from most of the tongue. Alcohol reduced the activity of the chorda tympani nerve in rats, cats, and dogs (66). Like other nerves, the chorda tympani is composed of many individual fibers, and those in the cat are readily distinguishable into two types. They react differently to alcohol. About one-half of the fibers show a reduction in activity following application of alcohol, and increased activity after a water rinse (67). The rest of the fibers are increased in activity by alcohol, and water restores them to their resting level; these latter fibers are very sensitive to salt.

The response of the entire nerve was studied prior to and after administration of alcohol. Several different tastes were used, representing each of the primary tastes. Alcohol reduced responsiveness to sweet (sucrose), acid (acetic acid), salt (sodium chloride), and, most strongly, to bitter (quinine).

Methylpentynol

When rats are given the sedative methylpentynol, they drink solutions of alcohol which they otherwise do not accept (29). The most probable reason for the change is that the drug increases the taste threshold for alcohol.

Local Anesthetics

Skramlik (121) reported that most of 15 local anesthetics which he tested were effective taste suppressants. Bitter was most strongly affected, and salt was also affected to a considerable extent. Sweet and sour were hardly affected. The local anesthetics often produced transient phases of hyperacuity.

Miscellaneous Effects

Hallucinogenic drugs affect taste much as they do smell. Taste sensation takes on new qualities, and eating becomes very pleasant (127). After marijuana use, sweet substances are particularly enjoyed.

Two plants have greatly intrigued workers in the field of taste research. The first, Synsepalum dulcificum, has been dubbed miracle fruit. When a person takes a leaf of it, the tastes of sweet, bitter, and salty substances remain unchanged, but sour tastes are converted to sweet tastes. Lemons taste quite sweet (76).

The second plant is Gymnema sylvestre, which virtually eliminates sweet tastes in man, but leaves other tastes unaffected (138). Combinations of the two plants yield interesting results. When miracle fruit is taken prior to the ingestion of citric acid, it greatly reduces the sourness of the taste and embellishes it with sweetness. Ingestion of Gymnema sylvestre abolishes the sweetness and returns the sourness to its original intensity (5). It seems only a matter of time before manufacturers will begin converting vitamin C–rich lemon or grapefruit juice into delectable sweet juices capable of competing with carbonated soft drinks.

Taste Thresholds as Indicators of Drug Activity

Fischer et al. (43) have made some intriguing discoveries in regard to stereoisomeric drugs. Stereoisomers are compounds which differ from each other only in the way their atoms are joined in space; otherwise, they have the same molecular formula and are like one another with respect to which atoms are joined with which. Fischer and his colleagues found that taste thresholds were lower for the stereoisomer which was biologically most active on the entire organism. Thus D-amphetamine, which is several times more active than L-amphetamine, is tasted at much lower concentrations. It was further found that individuals who were most sensitive to the taste of a drug were also most reactive to its pharmacological effects. People who taste psilocybin at low thresholds, for instance, react strongly to it, while non-tasters barely react to the same dose.

Fischer has classified tastes into three partially independent types on the basis of the reactions of subjects to them. The first type is represented by 6-n-propylthiouracil; the threshold for 6-n-propylthiouracil is bimodally distributed, which means that the distribution has two peaks, just as height is bimodally distributed with one peak for men and a different peak for women. In this case, there is one peak for tasters and another for non-tasters. Tasters of 6-n-propylthiouracil also taste compounds which are structurally

similar to it. All are bitter. Thresholds for the other two tastes, quinine and hydrochloric acid, are normally distributed, as are most biological and physiological traits. Sensitivity to the taste of quinine is a
good predictor of sensitivity to the taste of other compounds with
normally distributed taste. This includes most compounds. The
significance of these findings is that they offer an excellent assay for
predicting drug activity. Dosage given to an individual can be adjusted in accord with his taste sensitivity, and new compounds can
be rapidly screened for biological activity.

VISION

Many drugs affect visual functioning by modifying the pupillary
response to light. The pupils become dilated or constricted, and as

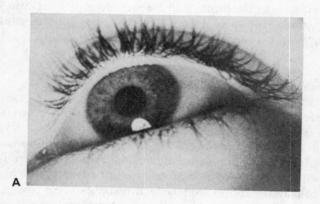

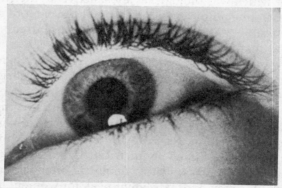

Figure 10–1 A normal pupil is shown in *A*, a dilated pupil is shown in *B*. (From
"Attitude and pupil size," by Eckhard H. Hess. Copyright © 1965 by Scientific
American, Inc. All rights reserved.)

a result the individual is more or less sensitive to light. (See Figure 10–1 for examples of normal and dilated pupils.) Ophthalmologists use the mydriatic (pupillary dilating) effects of atropine and related drugs to advantage; they apply the agent topically to the retina so that it may be thoroughly examined. The effects often persist for days, during which time photophobia (abnormal sensitivity to light) and blurry vision for near objects may occur. Other drugs, such as the antidepressant imipramine and the antianxiety agents benactyzine and diazepam, must be used with care because they have some atropine-like actions. All mydriatics are contraindicated when there is evidence of glaucoma, because when intraocular pressure is initially high, mydriatic agents produce further increases.

Ocular side effects during drug use are common. They are especially prevalent with the phenothiazine derivatives. DeLong (26) reviewed the literature on phenothiazine toxicity and noted that there were many reports of changes in the lens, cornea, and retina; these changes were most frequently observed during long-term therapy. A small sample of other drugs which often impair vision includes the following: chloroquinine, an antimalarial drug which is also effective against rheumatoid arthritis and several other ailments, but which may cause generalized retinal damage (51, p. 1094); quinine, which often produces serious visual deficits (51, p. 1110); the antiepileptic drug trimethadione, which reduces acuity and leads to color blindness (122); and aspirin, which may cause dimness of vision (51, p. 327).

Increased Acuity

Visual acuity can be measured in several different ways. Visual threshold measurements have the same significance as thresholds in other modalities. A very popular technique is to measure critical flicker fusion (CFF), which is a sensitive test for drug effects. CFF is measured by flashing a light at moderate intervals from a stationary source, so that an observer would report a series of flashes. The interval between flashes is then gradually reduced until, at some point, the observer reports seeing a steady, continuous light. That interval is the CFF. The higher the frequency at which successive stimuli merge, the better is the receptor system functioning.

Simonson and Brozek reviewed studies of drug effects on CFF through 1952 (119). A problem with many of the older studies is that they lacked placebo controls. The importance of the deficiency can be appreciated by considering the findings of Misiak and Rizy (101), who reported that CFF generally decreases over long periods of testing, probably because the subjects become fatigued; if this factor is ignored, a decline in CFF during pre- and postdrug tests might be falsely attributed to the drug. Nevertheless, the review by Simonson and Brozek included many instances of improvements in acuity as measured by CFF. Amphetamine, desoxyephedrine (methamphetamine), and large doses of caffeine all enhanced performance, as did smoking and vitamins B and C. Subsequent studies with the amphetamines reveal either no effect or a small positive one (73, 101). Warwick and Eysenck (133) confirmed the small positive effect of nicotine. Other drugs which improve CFF performance are LSD and psilocybin (88).

Several of the drugs which improved CFF performance had negative effects on other measures of visual acuity. For example, Blough (16) developed a very precise technique for measuring visual thresholds in animals and found that LSD increased the threshold in pigeons. Carlson (19) reported similar results in man. LSD is often accompanied by blurred vision (72, p. 111), slower adaptation to darkness (105), and greater than normal Mueller-Lyer illusion (35).*
On the other hand, Bennett (10), using himself as a subject with many different drugs, found that low doses of LSD improved acuity. Bennett also took amphetamine, which raises the CFF. Vision was impaired, as it was with the MAOI iproniazid. MAOI's often cause blurred vision (51, p. 197).

Although smoking elevates CFF, it reduces the ability of subjects to make brightness intensity discrimination, probably because of the carbon monoxide which is absorbed from inhaled smoke. Smoking also impairs nighttime visual discrimination (60, 111).

A well-known drug-induced improvement of visual functioning is that provided by vitamin A. People with a vitamin A deficiency suffer from night blindness, but the condition can rapidly be remedied by administration of large doses of the the vitamin (65). Several other drugs which have been tested, including strychnine, caffeine, morphine, phenobarbital, and amphetamine, have little effect on the time course of dark adaptation (96).

There is some evidence that visual acuity in women varies with the menstrual cycle, being poorest just prior to and during menstruation (24, p. 95). The hormone progesterone is often prescribed for those women who suffer from severe anxiety and tension during menstruation. It relieves all symptoms, presumably including the visual ones, in most patients (24, p. 51).

---

*Muller-Lyer illusion: both lines are the same length. The line on the right is normally perceived as longer.

Decreased Acuity

There is a fairly good consensus that stimulant drugs improve CFF performance. By contrast, most depressant drugs consistently lower CFF. Among those tested have been phenobarbital (89), reserpine (10), chlorpromazine (70), and other phenothiazines (94). In the case of chlorpromazine, tolerance develops to its effects during chronic usage (70), and over time, the effects disappear. Meprobamate has had variable effects, decreasing CFF in some but not all studies (10, 73, 102).

In adddtion to lowering CFF, alcohol has several other effects on vision. The appearance of blurred and double vision in the severely intoxicated is well known, and excessive intake is also associated with defects in red-green color vision (15, p. 144; 62).

Miscellaneous Effects

Hallucinogens

Among the best known effects of various hallucinogenic drugs are those on vision. LSD becomes concentrated in the visual system (125). LSD-like drugs produce mydriasis. When a person who has taken LSD rubs his eyeballs while in the dark, there is a great increase in the number of phosphenes (phosphorescent-like glows of light) that are perceived (87). In describing visual experiences with mescaline, Aldous Huxley wrote:

First and most important is the experience of light. . . . All colors are intensified to a ptich far beyond anything seen in the normal state, and at the same time the mind's capacity for recognizing fine distinctions of tone and hue is notably heightened.
The typical mescalin or lysergic-acid experience begins with perceptions of colored, moving, living geometrical forms. In time, pure geometry becomes concrete, and the visionary perceives, not patterns, but patterned things, such as carpets, carvings, mosaics. . . . Fabulous animals move across the scene. Everything is novel and amazing (75, pp. 89–96).

Hartman and Hollister (63) carefully analyzed the effects of hallucinogenic drugs on color vision. They tested psilocybin, LSD, and mescaline on volunteer subjects. All three drugs reduced accuracy of color discriminations, although only psilocybin did so significantly. Several other tests were administered in which subjects were asked to describe their experiences of color after exposure to various stimuli. The types of stimuli used included some which normally induce the experience of color and others which normally do not. The stimuli were as follows:

1. Incandescent bulb: subjects looked at an incandescent bulb

for five seconds and were then asked to match the colors of any afterimages which they saw with colors on a color chart. The procedure normally induces the experience of color. Drugs facilitated the experience; all three increased the number of colors reported, and psilocybin also increased the duration of the afterimage.

2. Rotating disk: subjects fixated on a rotating black and white disk which was spun at each of four different frequencies. The disk is normally a marginally adequate stimulus for inducing color. All three drugs increased the perception of color; the particular colors reported were very similar for LSD and mescaline (those reported for psilocybin were different).

3. Tone plus disk: when a tone was sounded while subjects observed the rotating disk, the number of color reports increased in the case of LSD and was unchanged for the other two drugs. The additional stimulation normally has no effect on the perception of color.

4. Tone alone: pure tones, which normally do not affect visual experience, did so after the subjects received LSD or mescaline. Although colors were perceived only infrequently, the drugs did evoke changes in the brightness and patterning of the visual field.

In sum, all three drugs increased color experiences. An additional finding was that subjects who were initially unable to discriminate accurately between two hues reported the perception of those hues less frequently during trials with drugs than they reported hues which they were easily able to discriminate prior to drug administration.

The study by Hartman and Hollister, especially points two to four, confirms the commonly reported finding that hallucinogenic drugs increase the likelihood of synesthesia (a sensation in one sensory modality which is elicited by stimulation of a different modality). Another example of synesthesia is that people who take mescaline and then listen to music with their eyes closed report the experience of moving patterns which change colors and match the tempo of the music (59). Marijuana-induced synesthesia has also been reported (21).

Fischer et al. (44) had volunteers take psilocybin and then asked them to adjust the levels of illumination of three slide projections of abstract paintings. Their task was to select the levels of illumination at which the artist would have wanted them to view the painting. Twelve of the fifteen subjects preferred lower levels of illumination than they did without psilocybin. The remaining three preferred higher levels, and also reacted least to the drug as measured by changes in performance on the Minnesota Multiphasic Personality Inventory. They also had the greatest pre-drug variability on perceptual tasks, i.e., before drug administration their scores on two successive administrations of the same test were most different.

Fischer's work with drugs and taste sensitivity has already been described. His experiments on drug-induced visual effects are complementary. In both sets of experiments he has been able to identify characteristics of individuals which predict reactivity to drugs.

Marijuana evokes several visual phenomena: colors appear brighter and more luminous (132, p. 104); there are changes in depth perception (3); people and objects often appear distorted in size (127). Hallucinations are rare, but visual imagery, especially while reading, is quite common.

Pigeons trained to peck a key whenever the color of a standard visual display changed showed striking increases in the number of changes reported after they had been injected with LSD, a marijuana extract, or bufotenine, a hallucinogenic drug first isolated from the skin of toads (118). When marijuana was inhaled rather than injected, their performance was impaired.

The extent to which changes in learned performance involving vision reflect alterations of visual functioning is not clear. Low doses of LSD improve visual discrimination in pigeons (6), while higher doses lead to performance decrements in both pigeons and monkeys (6, 49). Several drugs, including LSD (85), flatten gradients of generalization.* In a study by Hearst (64), monkeys were trained to bar press to avoid shock whenever light of a particular intensity was turned on. Seven other intensities were interspersed with the critical one. Animals typically respond most to the critical stimulus and show decreasing rates of response to stimuli far removed from the critical one. After receiving caffeine, amphetamine, or scopolamine — and independent of the drug's effects on their total number of responses — the animals emitted a higher percentage of responses to stimuli which were far different from the stimulus paired with shock. The effects of LSD on auditory generalization gradients are similar. However, a recent study by Dykstra and Appel (33) calls into question the interpretation that LSD affects acuity of discrimination. They found that auditory generalization gradients were changed only after doses which greatly reduced rates of responding. They argued that the changes were caused by an artifact, because at very low rates of responding slight shifts in response patterns yield big differences in percent of responses to each stimulus.

---

*Subjects who learn to respond to a particular stimulus also emit responses to other, related stimuli. The strength of response is greatest to stimuli which are most like the original one, and diminishes with increasing dissimilarity between stimuli. The relationship between the distance of a stimulus from the original and the strength of response is the generalization gradient. The steeper the generalization gradient, the finer the discriminations that are being made between stimuli.

Motivation for Visual Stimuli

Fox (47) studied response rates of light-deprived monkeys under conditions where they could bar press for brief flashes of light. Each animal was tested under three conditions involving: (1) no drug, with each bar press rewarded with light; (2) amphetamine, with each press rewarded; and (3) amphetamine, with no reward light. The third condition was used to control for the possibility that amphetamine might have activating effects on behavior irrespective of any light reward. There was a small activating effect, but it was insufficient to account for the very substantial increase in responding in the second condition as compared with the first; in other words, amphetamine increased the reward value of light. The important aspect of the stimulus may have been its novelty or unfamiliarity; as further evidence, Day and Thomas (25) reported that amphetamine increases the proportion of time spent looking at more complex (as opposed to simpler) visual patterns.

AUDITION (HEARING)

Many popular prescription and nonprescription drugs impair hearing. Chronic users of aspirin, antihistamines, and sulfonamides often experience tinnitus, or ringing in the ears. Many antibiotics damage both the auditory and the vestibular systems; the latter is essential for maintenance of equilibrium, and drugs like streptomycin may therefore result in loss of balance (137). The antibiotic kanamycin causes both hearing loss and morphological degeneration of the auditory apparatus (126). Although small doses of quinine sometimes increase acuity of hearing (51, p. 1107), large doses produce serious deficits (51, p. 1110).

Increased Acuity

The auditory flutter fusion (AFF) is analogous to CFF. It is defined as the interval at which a listener first reports successive tones as a continuous tone. There have been very few studies of drug effects on AFF. Eysenck and Easterbrooke (41) reported that amphetamine did not alter AFF, but Besser, using a more sensitive technique, reported elevated thresholds (13).

The hallucinogens are noted for increasing the subjective awareness of sounds, especially enhancing one's enjoyment of music. There is some evidence that they improve acuity. Eddy et al. (34) said that marijuana lowers the threshold for acoustical stimuli, but the LaGuardia Report (98) stated that marijuana does not alter auditory acuity. Marijuana helps make music sound more beautiful to many users (17). Bennett (10) claimed that LSD improved his own hearing. LSD does not normally elicit auditory hallucinations in sighted individuals; however, there is some indication that when given to blind people, LSD both improves auditory acuity and causes powerful distortions in the realm of hearing (72, p. 115). The blind do not report vivid visual effects (1, 113), nor do blindfolded people (71, p. 77).

Along the same lines, Edwards and Cohen (36) and Cohen and Edwards (23) have demonstrated that the effects of LSD are dependent to a great extent on external stimulation. They administered LSD or a placebo to men who had never before taken the drug. The men were placed under conditions of sensory deprivation or sensory normalcy. In the deprivation condition, they were instructed to sit quietly in a darkened, soundproof, temperature-controlled room; without any drug, the procedure is sufficient to induce hallucinations in a high proportion of subjects. In the normal condition the men were placed in the same room, but the lights were on, the door was open, and magazines and a radio were available. Each subject was tested under each combination of drug and environment.

The actions of LSD on the cardiovascular system—measured by changes in heart rate and finger pulse volume—were largely independent of environment. However, the drug did not exert its usual effects on measures of activation such as respiration rate, EEG, and palmar skin resistance. The critical determinant of changes in the activation variables was environmental condition. The authors suggested that many conflicting reports concerning the actions of LSD could be attributed to unspecified differences in the environment which greatly altered the course of action of the drug.

A second intriguing aspect of the aforementioned studies is that, under the combined conditions of LSD and sensory deprivation, the subjects believed that they had received either a placebo or a very weak dose of LSD. Visual changes did not appear until they were let out of the darkened room, at which time all of the men became aware of the LSD effects.

Decreased Acuity

The results of a very old study (61) suggest that alcohol interferes with the perception of tone. Other CNS depressants—amobarbital, diazepam, and chlorpromazine—produce AFF decrements (12). The latter finding plus the data on amphetamine parallel the results for the visual system: depressant drugs impair ability to distinguish successive pulses from continuous stimulation, while stimulants facilitate performance.

Rappaport et al. (109) utilized signal detection procedures for determining auditory thresholds in normal subjects and paranoid and non-paranoid schizophrenics. Signal detection was developed by Peterson et al. (107) to overcome some of the inadequacies of traditional threshold measures. It is applicable to all sensory modalities and is potentially of great value in drug research; accordingly the rationale of signal detection will be briefly elaborated before further discussion of Rappaport's findings.

The CNS is spontaneously active, and there is always some activity in sensory systems. Thus, the response which a stimulus elicits is the summated effect of the stimulus and the random "noise" within the system. When a subject is asked whether or not he has detected a stimulus, his report is based on the criterion which he adopts for deciding whether his perception is of noise alone or of signal plus noise. The criterion is influenced by several factors, including his expectations, the actual probability of a signal on a given trial, and the rewards for correct and incorrect responses. If the subject is given $1.00 for each correct detection and loses $.05 for each false alarm, his criterion and hence his threshold are likely to be different than if correct responses are rewarded by a nod from the experimenter and incorrect ones by a look of stern disapproval.

Signal detection theorists avoid many of the problems of traditional threshold measurement by calculating the difference between the frequency of "Yes" responses when the signal is presented, and the frequency to noise alone, divided by a measure of the variability (standard deviation) of responses to noise alone. The obtained result is practically uncontaminated by changes in criterion and is taken as a measure of sensitivity. Signal detection theorists have also developed measures for calculating the criterion used and the probability of a correct detection on a given trial.

Rappaport et al. found that chlorpromazine medication interacted with diagnostic subtype in influencing auditory thresholds. Performance of non-paranoid schizophrenics and of many normal subjects deteriorated; performance of other normal individuals was unimpaired, while paranoid schizophrenics showed improvement.

TIME ESTIMATION

Time perception is altered by LSD, mescaline, psilocybin, and marijuana in both human subjects and rats (46, 95, 134). All four usually lead to overestimation of elapsed time, so that 10 clock minutes might feel like 20. LSD, but not marijuana, elevates body temperature (77), and time is generally experienced as passing more slowly when body temperature is high (42). Subjects underestimate time when given alcohol (79), and alcohol is hypothermic.

Under the schedule known as Differential Reinforcement of Low Rates of Responding (DRL), a response is rewarded only if it is emitted after a minimal interval of time has elapsed since the last response. Premature responding resets the timer to zero. Many factors influence performance on DRL schedules, including the length of the intervals; one factor is the acuity of temporal discrimination. In evaluating performance under DRL schedules, the rate of responding conveys less information than the percent of successive responses which occur at different time intervals, i.e., the relative frequency distribution of inter-response times (IRT's). Weiss and Laties (135) found that salicylate increased IRT's, but aspirin left them unchanged. Alcohol greatly suppressed responding, but did not change IRT's (117). Amphetamine, a stimulant, and chlordiazepoxide, a depressant, both decreased IRT's (117, 112).

Goldstone et al. (50) devised an ingenious technique for studying ability to estimate elapsed time. They sounded tones which varied in duration between 0.1 and 2.0 seconds, and asked their subjects to estimate whether the duration was more or less than one second. Each subject was tested with many durations, and that duration which was reported as more than one second on exactly 50 percent of the trials was calculated. It was called the Second Estimation Point (SEP). The effects of drugs on the SEP were evaluated.

Medical students and interns were tested prior to drug administration and then 30 and 60 minutes post-drug. Prior to administration, there was a slight tendency to overestimate clock time. Secobarbital increased the SEP, and D-amphetamine reduced it. A group given placebo changed in the same direction as the secobarbital group, but to a lesser extent.

The authors reported that rises in the value of SEP are associated with subjective reports of time "flying," while decreases occur when time seems to drag. The authors postulated that clock time is estimated by making unconscious reference to certain unspecified internal recurring events. Heart rate can be taken as an example. People become aware through experience of the frequency with which their hearts beat while they are at rest; then they are able to estimate an elapsed time of one minute by counting, say, 70 heart beats. Stimulant drugs speed up these internal events, so that an external clock would appear to slow down by contrast. Hence, time would drag.

Estimation of the SEP by humans is a much different task from DRL performance of rats and pigeons. As such, seeming incompatibilities between the two measures — the findings that the depressant chlordiazepoxide decreased IRT's (slowed subjective time?), while the depressant secobarbital increased the SEP (made time fly?) — should not cause great concern. Because the estimation of SEP is less contaminated by factors such as motivational variables, it is probably better than DRL schedules for measuring ability to make temporal discriminations. In fact, Reynolds (110) has shown that the emission of frequent short and hence unrewarded IRT's does not result from inability to discriminate between short and long intervals. He devised a procedure whereby pigeons were required to peck twice at a key lit by a red light in order to change the light to blue. Pecks at the blue key were rewarded only when the two responses on red had been separated from each other by at least 18 seconds. The response rate of the pigeons to the blue key was found to vary according to the interval between their responses to red; that is, even though they emitted many responses on the red key which eliminated the possibility that they would be rewarded on the next trial with the blue key, they were able to discriminate when they had made such inappropriate responses.

PAIN

Agents for relieving pain are indispensable to physicians. Hippocrates made use of opium, and Osler called morphine God's own medicine. Meperidine, a synthetic opiate, is routinely used in many hospitals to relieve the pains of childbirth. Of the several classes of drugs which have analgesic action, the narcotic analgesics are best known.

Narcotic Analgesics

Morphine is the standard against which all other analgesics are measured. Its action is rapid in onset, reliable, and long-lasting. It is inexpensive. Morphine is selective, relieving pain at doses which have little effect on other sensory modalities or on intellectual or emotional processes. It has a direct action on cells within the pain pathway, reducing their responsiveness to painful stimuli (99). Painful stimuli take longer to reach the frontal lobes of the brain (20).* Morphine is effective in the laboratory; monkeys exposed to increasing intensities of shock, which could be reduced by pressing a bar, tolerated higher levels of shock with morphine than under control conditions (136).

---

*Pethidine, a synthetic analgesic, also reduces pain responses, but acts on a somewhat different population of cells than does morphine (99).

Certain side effects make morphine a less than ideal analgesic. It often produces dizziness, nausea, headache, and lethargy (78). Respiratory depression occurs at doses below the narcotic threshold, constituting a serious drawback for use in obstetrics. Tolerance develops to many of the effects of morphine, and with it the possibility of addiction. Some people, although relatively few, become dependent upon opiates as a means of relieving pain. Physicians are therefore acutely aware of the addiction liability of morphine, and as a consequence, it is often administered in insufficient doses to properly obtund pain (90).

Jaffe (78) listed 20 potent narcotic analgesics, but noted that differences between them are not great. Although some synthetic analgesics are extremely powerful — much more so than morphine — they also have a greater potential for producing physical dependence. As a rule there is a strong parallelism between analgesic activity and the likelihood of producing dependency (27). Some exceptions to the generalization lend hope that a better analgesic will someday be found. For example, nalorphine, which under certain circumstances relieves pain, is a narcotic antagonist. Nalorphine not only reverses the respiratory depressant effects of morphine, but actually precipitates withdrawal symptoms in physically dependent individuals. It is not a drug which has clinical utility as an analgesic because it produces many unpleasant side effects. However, its discovery has provided an impetus to the search for related compounds in which there is a separation of analgesic activity and dependence liability. Pentazocine, naloxone, and cyclazocine are three of the many drugs which have been developed as a result and which may have some value as analgesics.

A second promising separation of analgesia and dependence liability was found in compounds structurally similar to morphine, the N-methyl substituted 6,7-benzomorphans. Each of the six compounds which have been studied in this series can be synthesized in two forms: the levo and dextro stereoisomers. In each case, the levo form has the more powerful analgesic action of the pair, yet precipitates withdrawal symptoms in physically dependent subjects; the dextro forms are weak analgesics and suppress withdrawal symptoms, i.e., they have morphine-like actions and are likely to produce physical dependence (28).

Salicylates

The salicylates, the best known of which is aspirin, are widely used for relieving minor pains. They reduce pain both by a direct action on the central nervous system and by eliminating inflammation as a source of pain. The salicylates act best against low intensity pain such as that caused by headache, dysmenorrhea, and arthritis. In a laboratory situation, they increased the level of shock which rats tolerated before the animals began working to reduce the shock (135). By contrast, pentobarbital, when given in any dose up to that which produced severe ataxia, did not affect responding to reduce shock. The ability of animals to escape high intensity shock was not impaired by salicylates.

Salicylates increase pain thresholds, but to a lesser extent than does codeine. Phenylbutazone, an ingredient in many nonprescription preparations, is a less effective analgesic than aspirin.

Hallucinogens

Two components of marijuana have pronounced analgesic activity (14), and marijuana was at one time commonly prescribed for the relief of pain (124). In fact, Reynolds, physician to Queen Victoria, ranked it foremost among all drugs for relieving pain.

Kast and Collins (82) compared the effectiveness of LSD with that of meperidine and dihydromorphinone, both commonly used analgesics, in several terminally ill cancer patients. LSD gave more prolonged and complete relief.

Benzimidazoles

A group of substances with very similar structures, collectively called benzimidazoles, are central depressants and muscle relaxants. Several of them are powerful analgesics as well, and one, 4'-ethoxybenzyl, is over 1000 times more powerful than morphine (56). Their extreme toxicity greatly limits their usefulness. However, they have been used with some success in surgery (reported in 18).

Miscellaneous Drugs

Many drugs have some analgesic actions under some circumstances. Chlorpromazine and reserpine relieve pain directly and also potentiate the effects of morphine (93). The method of producing pain is important; chlorpromazine has much more powerful actions on pain induced by thermal stimulation than it has on pain induced by electrical or mechanical stimuli (52, p. 62). The antianxiety agents diazepam, chlordiazepoxide, and aminopyrine, the stimulant methamphetamine, some MAOI's, and the local anesthetic procaine all relieve pain under some conditions (38, 108).

Theories of the Mechanism of Pain Relief

Beecher (7) has emphasized the power of placebos to relieve pain. His table indicating the wide variety of complaints which are assuaged by placebos is reproduced as Table 10.1. The power of the placebo effect encouraged Beecher to resuscitate a theory first formulated by Strong in 1895: pain has two components — the original sensation, and the emotional reaction to it. He believes that morphine and other analgesics act only on the latter. His supporting evidence comes from a variety of sources, foremost of which is the finding that the effectiveness of both morphine and placebos in relieving laboratory-induced pain in humans differs greatly from the effectiveness of the two in relieving pain resulting from illness or injury. In one comparison of the two, placebos relieved only 3.2 percent of 173 volunteers in laboratory studies, as opposed to 34.6 percent of 831 clinical patients (8). Beecher also stated that about 15 different groups of investigators have failed to demonstrate a dependable effect of even large doses of narcotics on experimental pain threshold in man. The reason for the difference between experimental and pathological pain, according to Beecher, is that vastly more stress accompanies the latter. Morphine, he believes, acts only on the stress component. He tested his assumption by adding stress to the experimental situation, and then found dependable responses to morphine (123). Still another type of support comes from his work with Lasagna et al. (91); they found that surgical patients treated for postoperative pain who reacted favorably to placebos were more likely than nonreactors to obtain relief from morphine. Also, both morphine and placebos were less effective in patients whose pain was of long duration.

As surprising as Beecher's theory is, it has received confirmation from other sources. Clark (22) used a signal detection paradigm to measure the sensitivity of volunteers to thermal pain. They were given a placebo described as a potent analgesic, and it reduced their responsiveness to pain. However, analysis by the methods of signal detection showed that the change was mediated not by reductions in thermal sensitivity, but rather by altering motivational factors.

Along other lines, Evans (39) used a procedure developed by Kimble (86) in which the intensity of shock delivered to a rat determined the form of response which was elicited; the animals crouched or flinched after receiving low intensity shocks, but jumped off the floor at higher intensities. Evans reported that the flinch response was rarely accompanied by signs of agitation, while animals which jumped usually vocalized and showed other signs of distress. He therefore suggested that animals might flinch at the first perception of pain, and jump as an emotional reaction to severe

TABLE 10.1 Therapeutic Effectiveness of Placebos in Several Conditions*

Condition	Study	Placebo Agent	Route†		Patients, No.	% Satisfactorily Relieved by a Placebo
Severe post-operative wound pain	Keats, A. S., and Beecher, H. K.: J. Pharmacol. & Exper. Therap. 100:1–13, 1950	Saline	I. V.		118	21
	Beecher, H. K., and others: U. S. Armed Forces M. J. 2:1269–1276, 1951	Saline	S. C.		29	31
	Keats, A. S., and others: J. A. M. A. 147:1761–1763 (Dec. 29) 1951	Saline	I. V.		34	26
	Beecher and others (1953)	Lactose	P. O.		52 / 36 / 44 / 40	40 / 26 / 34 / 32 } 33
	Lasagna and others (1954)	Saline	S. C.		14 / 20 / 15 / 21 / 15 / 15	50 / 37 / 53 / 40 / 40 / 15 } 39
Cough	Gravenstein, J. S., and others: J. Appl. Physiol. 7:119–139, 1954	Lactose	P. O.		22 / 23	36 / 43 } 40
Drug-induced mood changes	Lasagna, L., and others: J. A. M. A. 157:1006–1020 (March 19) 1955	Isotonic sodium chloride	S. C.	Normal / "Post-addicts"	20 / 30	30 / 30

Condition	Reference	Placebo agent	Route	Total patients	% relieved
Pain from angina pectoris	Evans, W., and Hoyle, C.: Quart. J. Med. 2: 311–338, 1933	Sodium bicarbonate "Placebo"	P. O.	66	38
	Travell, J., and others: Ann. New York Acad. Sc. 52:345–353, 1949		P. O.	19	26
	Greiner, T., and others: Am. J. Med. 9:143–155, 1950	Lactose	P. O.	27	38
Headache	Jellinek (1946)	Lactose	P. O.	199	52
Seasickness	Gay and Carliner (1949)	Lactose	P. O.	33	58
Anxiety and tension	Wolf and Pinsky (1954)	Lactose	P. O.	31	30
Experimental cough	Hillis (1952)	Isotonic sodium chloride	S. C.	Many experiments 1	37
Common cold	Diehl, H.S.: J. A. M. A. 101:2042–2049 (Dec. 23) 1933	Lactose	P. O.	Cold acute 110, Subacute chronic 48	35, 35
				Total patients 1,082	Average 35.2 ± 2.2% relieved

*From Beecher, H. The powerful placebo. J. A. M. A., 1955, *159*: p. 1604.

†I. V., intravenous; S. C., subcutaneous; P. O., oral.

pain. Drugs which were known to have some analgesic action—chlor-promazine, perphenazine, morphine, codeine, nalorphine, and acetylsalicylate—raised the jump threshold, but had no effect on the flinch response. Other drugs had no effect on either response. Evans concluded that the results support Beecher's hypothesis that drugs relieve pain by diminishing the emotional components of the reaction to it. A plausible alternative explanation, which also accounts for some although not all of Beecher's findings, is that analgesics limit the total possible amount of pain input, while not altering thresholds. The alternative could be tested by seeing if drugs modify jnd's to increments in experimentally produced pain.

Dinnerstein et al. (30) proposed a somewhat different mechanism of action for analgesics, while sharing with Beecher the belief that they do not act directly on pain pathways. It should be noted that the latter point ignores a great body of data; pain pathways are known, and analgesics do influence transmission through them (see preceding discussions and Ref. 100). Nevertheless, Dinnerstein et al. postulated that the action of drugs on pain or anxiety can be explained solely in terms of amplification or inhibition of placebo effects. The general line of reasoning for their provocative hypothesis is given as follows (see bibliography in Ref. 30).

1. Although the presentation of a strong sound by itself has no effect on tolerance to pain, the coupling of a strong sound with instructions that it will be analgesic does produce analgesia. Weak sound accompanied by the same instructions is not effective. Thus, in order to obtain analgesia, it is necessary to have both a strong stimulus and appropriate expectations. Effective drugs may provide strong internal stimuli.

2. The internal stimuli interact with expectations. Thus, when chloral hydrate and amphetamine were described as energizers and administered to aged patients, amphetamine produced more comfort; it also produced more comfort when both were described as sedatives; however, when both were administered in concealed form, they produced the same effect. Both were better than lactose. Dinnerstein et al. interpreted the results as follows:

a. The general effectiveness of drugs increases with increasing ability to produce distinctive internal stimuli.

b. Effectiveness in a particular situation depends on both the distinctiveness and the pattern of the internal stimuli. In the study on sound analgesia, a strong sound was more effective than a weak one. If the intent had been to induce sleep, a weak sound probably would have been better.

3. Procedures which focus attention away from pain are analgesic. The same procedures, if they focus attention on the pain, in-

crease its perceived intensity. One of the actions of methamphetamine is to narrow the focus of attention. Accordingly, the effects of methamphetamine on perceived pain should depend on the extent to which the pain is at the center of attention. When administered in the laboratory, under conditions where the perception of pain is salient, amphetamine increased the painfulness of shocks. When used in a clinical setting with morphine, where attention was focused on relief from pain, amphetamine potentiated the effects of morphine. The authors predicted that amphetamine, if described as an analgesic, would be effective with weak pain (attention could be focused elsewhere), but not with strong.

4. The initial state of a subject may determine the direction of change induced by a drug. For instance, nicotine has differential actions on high and low activity rats. Similarly, tranquilizers reduce anxiety in high anxiety patients but increase anxiety in low anxiety patients. (Could these findings serve as a basis for a diagnostic test of level of anxiety?) The analgesic effects of aspirin may be restricted to people with low levels of anxiety; in one study, aspirin actually increased sensitivity to pain in high anxiety subjects.

5. As already discussed, morphine is effective against pain only when anxiety is a major component.

The authors concluded that a drug, in order to justify being labeled an analgesic, should have two properties. First, it should produce a physiological effect independent of the initial physiological state of the individual. Second, it should produce an unambiguous pattern of internal stimuli, so that all recipients would "interpret" it in the same way. They believe that no such drug now exists, and question the possibility that one could exist even in theory. They urged physicians to prescribe analgesics and to adjust the contexts in which they are administered according to the characteristics and needs of their patients. Whether or not all analgesic drugs are essentially placebos, a point made by Beecher should be well noted. He said that placebos have powerful effects; they should not be discarded, because in most cases it is much better to administer a placebo than to give no treatment at all.

CONCLUSIONS

The British psychologist H.J. Eysenck has constructed an elaborate theory about biological determinants of behavior (40). A major tenet is that drugs have different effects on introverts and extroverts. An introvert, by his definition, is a quiet, reserved person who does not crave excitement and who keeps his feelings under control.

Extroverts are sociable, easygoing, eager for excitement, and emotional. Stimulant drugs, by raising the level of cortical arousal, reduce the need for additional stimulation, i.e., they shift the personality to make it more introverted. Depressants have the opposite effect. In general, according to Eysenck, stimulant drugs lower sensory thresholds while depressants raise them; and, in general, stimulants have the biggest effects on extroverts, depressants on introverts.

The theory is appealing. It is simple and is supported by a large body of data (see Ref. 40 for a review). It has been useful to Eysenck and other scientists in suggesting many interesting experiments. Nevertheless, the sensory systems are too complex to fit into any such simple schema. Even within a single modality, the direction of change in sensitivity following drug administration varies with the type of measurement. Mydriatic drugs increase sensitivity to light, but often blur vision; the effects of amphetamine on pain depend on the context in which it is administered; LSD may improve or impair ability to make visual or temporal discriminations. A final point, as noted in Chapter 2, is that environmental variables determine to a great extent whether a drug has stimulant or depressant properties.

REFERENCES

1. Alema, G. Allucinazioni da acido lisergico in cieco senza balbi oculari. Riv. Neurol., 1952, 22:720–733.
2. Allara, E. Sull'influenza esercitata dagli ormoni sessuali sulla struttura delle formazioni gustative di Mus rattus albinus. Riv. Biol., 1952, 44:209–299.
3. Allentuck, S., and Bowman, K. The psychiatric aspects of marihuana intoxication. Am. J. Psychiatry, 99:248–251.
4. Arfmann, B., and Chapanis, N. The relative sensitivities of taste and smell in smokers and non-smokers. J. Gen. Psychol., 1962, 66:315–320.
5. Bartoshuk, L., Dateo, G., Vandenbelt, D., Buttrick, R., and Long, L. Effects of Gymnema sylvestre and Synsepalum dulcificum on taste in man. In Pfaffman, C. (Ed.) Olfaction and Taste, III. New York: Rockefeller University Press, 1969.
6. Becker, D., Appel, J., and Freedman, D. Some effects of LSD on visual discrimination in pigeons. Psychopharmacologia, 1967, 11:354–364.
7. Beecher, H. Increased stress and effectiveness of placebos and "active" drugs. Science, 1960, 132:91–92.
8. Beecher, H. The powerful placebo. J.A.M.A., 1955, 159:1602–1606.
9. Bell, D., and Zucker, I. Sex differences in body weight and eating: organization and activation by gonadal hormones in the rat. Physiol. Behav., 1971, 7: 27–34.
10. Bennett, C. The drugs and I. In Uhr, L., and Miller, J. (Eds.) Drugs and Behavior. New York: John Wiley and Sons, 1960.
11. Bernard, R., Halpern, B., and Kare, M. The reversible effect of vitamin A deficiency on taste. Fed. Proc., 1962, 21:362.
12. Besser, G. Centrally acting drugs and auditory flutter. In Proc. Symposium on Drugs and Sensory Functions, Royal Coll. Physicians, 1966.
13. Besser, G. Some physiological characteristics of auditory flutter fusion in man. Nature, 1967, 214:17–19.

14. Bicher, H., and Mechoulam, R. Pharmacological effects of two active constituents of marihuana. Arch. Int. Pharmacodyn., 1968, 172:24–31.
15. Bjerver, K., and Goldberg, L. Alcohol and Road Traffic. Stockholm: Kugelbergs Boktrykeri, 1951.
16. Blough, D. Effect of lysergic acid diethylamide on absolute visual threshold of the pigeon. Science, 1957, 126:304–305.
17. Bouquet, R. Cannabis. Bull. Narcot. Drugs, 1950, 2:14–30.
18. Cain, C., and Roszkowski, A. Benzoxazoles, benzothiazoles, and benzimidazoles. In Gordon, M. (Ed.) Psychopharmacological Agents, Vol. 1. New York: Academic Press, 1964.
19. Carlson, V. Effect of lysergic acid diethylamide (LSD-25) on the absolute visual threshold. J. Comp. Physiol. Psychol., 1958, 51:528–531.
20. Chin, J., and Domino, E. Effects of morphine on brain potentials evoked by stimulation of the tooth pulp of the dog. J. Pharmacol. Exp. Ther., 1961, 132:74–86.
21. Chopra, I., and Chopra, R. The use of cannabis drugs in India. Bull. Narcot. Drugs, 1957, 9:4–29.
22. Clark, W. Sensory-decision theory analysis of the placebo effect on the criterion for pain and thermal sensitivity. J. Abnorm. Psychol., 1969, 74:363–371.
23. Cohen, S., and Edwards, A. The interaction of LSD and sensory deprivation: physiological considerations. In Wortis, J. (Ed.) Recent Advances in Biological Psychiatry, 6. New York: Plenum Publishing Corp., 1964.
24. Dalton, K. The Premenstrual Syndrome. Springfield, Ill.: Charles C Thomas, 1964.
25. Day, H., and Thomas, E. Effects of amphetamine on selective attention. Percept. Mot. Skills, 1967, 24:1119–1125.
26. DeLong, S. Ocular reactions to psychopharmacologic drugs. In Efron, D. (Ed.) Psychopharmacology: A Review of Progress. U.S. PHS Pub. No. 1836, 1968.
27. Deneau, G., and Seevers, M. In Lawrence, D., and Bacharach, A. (Eds.) Evaluation of Drug Activities: Pharmacometrics. London: Academic Press, 1964.
28. Deneau, G., Villareal, J., and Seevers, M. Addendum, Minutes of the 28th Meeting of the Committee on Problems of Drug Dependence, NAS-NRC, 1966.
29. Dicker, S. The effects of methylpentynol on ethanol drinking and on water metabolism in rats. J. Physiol., 1958, 144:138–147.
30. Dinnerstein, A., Lowenthal, M., and Blitz, B. The interaction of drugs with placebos in the control of pain and anxiety. Perspect. Biol. Med., 1966, 10:103–117.
31. Ditman, K., Moss, T., Forgy, E., Zunin, L., Lynch, R., and Funk, W. Dimensions of the LSD, methylphenidate, and chlordiazepoxide experiences. Psychopharmacologia, 1969, 14:1–11.
32. Dove, W. A study of individuality in the nutritive instincts and of the causes and effects of variations in the selection of food. Am. Natur., 1935, 69:469–544.
33. Dykstra, L., and Appel, J. Lysergic acid diethylamide and stimulus generalization: rate-dependent effects. Science, 1972, 177:720–722.
34. Eddy, N., Halbach, H., Isbell, H., and Seevers, M. Drug dependence: its significance and characteristics. Bull. WHO, 1965, 32:721–733.
35. Edwards, A., and Cohen, S. Persistence of an evaluative response conditioned under LSD and sensory deprivation. In Wortis, J. (Ed.) Recent Advances in Biological Psychiatry, 7. New York: Plenum Publishing Corp., 1965.
36. Edwards, A., and Cohen, S. Visual illusion, tactile sensibility and reaction time under LSD-25. Psychopharmacologia, 1961, 2:297–303.
37. Efron, D. (Ed.) Psychopharmacology: A Review of Progress. U.S. PHS Pub. No. 1836, 1968.
38. Emele, J., Shanaman, J., and Warren, M. The analgesic activity of phenelzine and other compounds. J. Pharmacol. Exp. Ther., 1961, 134:206–209.
39. Evans, W. A new technique for investigation of some analgesic drugs on a reflexive behavior in the rat. Psychopharmacologia, 1961, 2:318–325.
40. Eysenck, H. The Biological Basis of Personality. Springfield, Ill.: Charles C Thomas, 1967.
41. Eysenck, H., and Easterbrook, J. Drugs and personality. XI. The effects of stimulant and depressant drugs upon auditory flutter fusion. J. Ment. Sci., 1960, 106:855–857.

42. Fischer, R., Griffin, E., and Liss, L. Biological aspects of time in relation to (model) psychoses. Ann. N.Y. Acad. Sci., 1962, 96:44–65.
43. Fischer, R., Griffin, F., and Pasamanick, B. The perception of taste: some pathophysiological, pharmacological and clinical aspects. In Hoch, P., and Zubin, J. (Eds.) Psychopathology of Perception. New York: Grune and Stratton, 1965.
44. Fischer, R., Hill, R., and Warshay, D. Effects of the psychodysleptic drug psilocybin on visual perception. Changes in brightness preference. Experientia, 1969, 25:166–168.
45. Fischer, R., and Kaelbling, R. Increase in taste acuity with sympathetic stimulation: the relationship of a just noticeable difference to systemic psychotropic drug dose. In Wortis, J. (Ed.) Recent Advances in Biological Psychiatry, 9. New York: Plenum Publishing Corp. 1967.
46. Fischer, R., and Mead, E. Time contraction and psychomotor performance produced by "Psilocybin." Nature, 1966, 209:433–434.
47. Fox, S. Self-maintained sensory input and sensory deprivation in monkeys. J. Comp. Physiol. Psychol., 1962, 55:438–444.
48. Fregly, M., and Waters, I. Effect of desoxycorticosterone acetate on NaCl appetite of propylthiouracil treated rats. Physiol. Behav., 1966, 1:65–74.
49. Fuster, J. Lysergic acid and its effects on visual discrimination in monkeys. J. Nerv. Ment. Dis., 1959, 129:252–256.
50. Goldstone, S., Boardman, W., and Lhamon, W. Effect of quinal barbitone, dextroamphetamine, and placebo on apparent time. Brit. J. Psychol., 1958, 49: 324–328.
51. Goodman, L., and Gilman, A. (Eds.) The Pharmacological Basis of Therapeutics. New York: Macmillan, 1965.
52. Gordon, M. (Ed.) Psychopharmacological Agents, Vol. 1. New York: Academic Press, 1964.
53. Granit, R. Sensory Mechanisms of the Retina. London: Oxford University Press, 1955.
54. Green, J. The function of the hippocampus. Endeavour, 1963, 22:80–84.
55. Green, R. Subclinical pellegra and idiopathic hypogeusia. J.A.M.A., 1971, 218: 1303.
56. Gross, F., and Turrian, H. On benzimidazole derivatives with strong analgesic activity. Experientia, 1957, 13:401–403.
57. Grossman, S. Drug effects on taste, olfaction, and food intake. In Herxheimer, A. (Ed.) Drugs and Sensory Functions. Boston: Little Brown and Co., 1968.
58. Gunter, R. The discrimination between lights of different wave lengths in the cat. J. Comp. Physiol. Psychol., 1954, 47:169–172.
59. Guttmann, E. Artificial psychoses produced by mescaline. J. Ment. Sci., 1936, 82: 203–221.
60. Halperin, M., McFarland, R., Niven, J., and Roughton, F. The time course of the effects of carbon monoxide on visual thresholds. J. Physiol., 1959, 146:583–593.
61. Hansen, K. Untersuchungen uber den Einfluss des Alkohols auf die Sinnestatigkeit bei bestimmten Alkoholkonzentrationen im Organismus. Heidelberg, 1924.
62. Harrington, D. The Visual Fields. London: Henry Kimpton, 1956.
63. Hartman, A., and Hollister, L. Effect of mescaline, lysergic acid diethylamide and psilocybin on color perception. Psychopharmacologia, 1963, 4:441–451.
64. Hearst, E. Drug effects on stimulus generalization gradients in the monkey. Psychopharmacologia, 1964, 6:57–70.
65. Hecht, S., and Mandelbaum, J. The relation between vitamin A and dark adaptation. J.A.M.A., 1939, 112:1910–1916.
66. Hellekant, G. Electrophysiological investigation of the gustatory effect of ethyl alcohol. I: The summated response of the chorda tympani in the cat, dog and rat. Acta Physiol. Scand., 1965, 64:392–397.
67. Hellekant, G. Electrophysiological investigation of the gustatory effect of ethyl alcohol. II: A single fibres analysis in the cat. Acta Physiol. Scand., 1965, 64:398–404.
68. Henkin, R. Abnormalities of taste and olfaction in various disease states. In

Kare, M., and Maller, O. (Eds.) *The Chemical Senses and Nutrition.* Baltimore: Johns Hopkins Press, 1967.

69. Herxheimer, A. Amphetamine and taste in man. *In* Herxheimer, A. (Ed.) *Drugs and Sensory Functions.* Boston: Little, Brown, 1968.

70. Hoehn-Saric, R., Bacon, E., and Gross, M. Effects of chlorpromazine on flicker fusion. J. Nerv. Ment. Dis., 1964, *138*:287–292.

71. Hoffer, A. *In* Cholden, L. (Ed.) *Lysergic Acid Diethylamide and Mescaline in Experimental Psychiatry.* New York: Grune and Stratton, 1956.

72. Hoffer, A., and Osmond, H. *The Hallucinogens.* New York: Academic Press, 1967.

73. Holland, H. Drugs and personality. XII. A comparison of several drugs by the flicker-fusion method. J. Ment. Sci., 1960, *106*:858–861.

74. Hoshishima, K. Endocrines and taste. *In* Kare, M., and Maller, O. (Eds.) *The Chemical Senses and Nutrition.* Baltimore: Johns Hopkins Press, 1967.

75. Huxley, A. *The Doors of Perception* and *Heaven and Hell.* New York: Harper and Row, 1963.

76. Inglett, G., Dowling, B., Albrecht, J., and Hoglan, F. Taste-modifying properties of miracle fruit (*Synsepalum dulcificum*). J. Agr. Food Chem., 1965, *13*:284–287.

77. Isbell, H., and Jasinski, D. A comparison of LSD-25 with (-)-Δ^9-trans-tetrahydrocannabinol (THC) and attempted cross tolerance between LSD and THC. Psychopharmacologia, 1969, *14*:115–123.

78. Jaffe, J. Narcotic analgesics. *In* Goodman, L., and Gilman, A. *The Pharmacological Basis of Therapeutics.* New York: Macmillan, 1965.

79. Jones, R., and Stone, G. Psychological studies of marijuana and alcohol in man. Psychopharmacologia, 1970, *18*:108–117.

80. Kaplan, A., and Glanville, E. Taste thresholds for bitterness and cigarette smoking. Nature, 1964, *202*:1366.

81. Kare, M., and Maller, O. (Eds.) *The Chemical Senses and Nutrition.* Baltimore: Johns Hopkins Press, 1967.

82. Kast, E., and Collins, V. Lysergic acid diethylamide as an analgesic agent. Anesth. Analges., 1964, *43*:285–289.

83. Keeler, M. Interrelations of the effects of psilocybin on subjective sensation, photopic critical frequency of fusion and circulating non-esterified fatty acids. Experientia, 1963, *19*:37–38.

84. Kenneth, J. A few odor preferences and their constancy. J. Exp. Psychol., 1928, *11*: 56–61.

85. Key, B. Alterations in the generalization of visual stimuli induced by LSD in cats. Psychopharmacologia, 1964, *6*:327–337.

86. Kimble, G. Shock intensity and avoidance learning. J. Comp. Physiol. Psychol., 1955, *48*:281–284.

87. Knoll, M., Kugler, J., Hofer, O., and Lawder, S. Effects of chemical stimulation of electrically-induced phosphenes on their bandwidth, shape, number and intensity. Confin. Neurol., 1963, *23*:201–226.

88. Landis, C., and Clausen, J. Certain effects of mescaline and lysergic acid on psychological functions. J. Psychol., 1954, *38*:211–221.

89. Landis, C., and Zubin, J. The effects of thonzylamine hydrochloride and phenobarbital sodium on certain psychological functions. J. Psychol., 1951, *31*: 181–200.

90. Lasagna, L. Addicting drugs and medical practice: toward the elaboration of realistic goals and the eradication of myths, mirages, and half-truths. *In* Wilner, D., and Kassebaum, G. (Eds.) *Narcotics.* New York: McGraw-Hill, 1965.

91. Lasagna, L., Mosteller, F., von Felsinger, J., and Beecher, H. A study of the placebo response. Am. J. Med., 1954, *16*:770–779.

92. LeMagnen, J. Les phénomènes olfacto-sexuels chez le rat blanc. Arch. Sci. Physiol., 1952, *6*:295–331.

93. Leme, J., and Rocha e Silva, M. Analgesic action of chlorpromazine and reserpine in relation to that of morphine. J. Pharm. Pharmacol., 1961, *13*:734–742.

94. Lloyd, D., and Newbrough, J. Sensory changes with phenothiazine medication in schizophrenic patients. J. Nerv. Ment. Dis., 1964, *139*:169–175.

95. Maffii, G., and Constantini, D. Effects of drugs on timing behavior. Biochem. Pharmacol., 1961, *8*:61–62.

96. Mandelbaum, J. Dark adaptation: some physiologic and clinical considerations. Arch. Ophthal., 1941, 26:203–239.
97. Marguiles, N., Irvin, D., and Goetzl, F. The effect of alcohol upon olfactory acuity and the sensation complex of appetite and satiety. Permanente Found. Med. Bull., 1950, 8:1–8.
98. Mayor's Committee on Marihuana. The Marihuana Problem in the City of New York. Lancaster, Penna.: Jaques Cattell, 1944.
99. McKenzie, J., and Beechey, N. The effects of morphine and pethidine on somatic evoked responses in the midbrain of the cat, and their relevance to analgesia. EEG, 1962, 14:501–519.
100. Melzack, R. The perception of pain. Sci. Am., 1961, 204:41–49.
101. Misiak, H., and Rizy, E. The effects of dextroamphetamine and phenobarbital on a simplified standardized CFF measure. Psychopharmacologia, 1968, 13: 346–353.
102. Misiak, H., Zenhausern, R., and Salafia, W. Continuous temporal evaluation of the effects of meprobamate on critical flicker frequency in normal subjects. Psychopharmacologia, 1966, 9:457–461.
103. Money, J. Psychosexual differentiation. In Money, J. (Ed.) Sex Research: New Developments. New York: Holt, Rinehart and Winston, 1965.
104. Mortimer, H., Wright, R., and Collip, J. The effect of the administration of oestrogenic hormones on the nasal mucosa of the monkey (Macaca mulatta). Canad. Med. Assoc. J., 1936, 35:503–513.
105. Ostfeld, A. Effects of LSD-25 and JB318 on tests of visual and perceptual functions in man. Fed. Proc., 1961, 20:876–883.
106. Pangborn, R. Some aspects of chemoreception in human nutrition. In Kare, M., and Maller, O. (Eds.) The Chemical Senses and Nutrition. Baltimore: Johns Hopkins Press, 1967.
107. Peterson, W., Birdsall, T., and Fox, W. The theory of signal detectability. Inst. Radio Engrs., 1954, PGIT-4:171–212.
108. Randall, L., Schallek, W., Heise, G., Keith, E., and Bagdon, R. The psychosedative properties of methaminodiazepoxide. J. Pharmacol. Exp. Ther., 1960, 129: 163–171.
109. Rappaport, M., Hopkins, H., Silverman, J., and Hall, K. Auditory signal detection in schizophrenics. Psychopharmacologia, 1972, 24:6–28.
110. Reynolds, G. Discrimination and emission of temporal intervals by pigeons. J. Exp. Anal. Behav., 1966, 9:65–68.
111. Rhee, K., Kim, D., and Kim, Y. The effects of smoking on night vision. In: Tokyo, 14th Pacific Med. Conf. (Professional papers), 1965.
112. Richelle, M., Xhenseval, B., Fontaine, O., and Thone, L. Action of chlordiazepoxide on two types of temporal conditioning in rats. Int. J. Neuropharm., 1962, 1:381–391.
113. Rinkel, M. Neuropharmacol. Trans. 2nd Conf., New York: Josiah Macy, 1956.
114. Schneider, R., Costiloe, J., Howard, R., and Wolf, S. Olfactory perception thresholds in hypogonadal women: changes accompanying administration of androgen and estrogen. J. Clin. Endocr., 1958, 18:379–390.
115. Schutz, H., and Pilgrim, F. Psychophysiology in food acceptance research. J. Am. Diet. Assoc., 1953, 29:1127–1128.
116. Shagass, C. Effects of LSD on somatosensory and visual evoked responses and on the EEG in man. In Wortis, J. (Ed.) Recent Advances in Biological Psychiatry, 9. New York: Plenum Publishing Corp., 1967.
117. Sidman, M. Technique for assessing the effects of drugs on timing behavior. Science, 1955, 122:925.
118. Siegel, R. Hallucinogenic-induced effects on a visual discrimination task in pigeons. Paper presented at Fourth International Congress on Pharmacology. Basel, Switzerland, 1969.
119. Simonson, E., and Brozek, J. Flicker fusion frequency. Physiol. Rev., 1952, 32: 349–378.
120. Sinnot, J., and Rauth, J. Effect of smoking on taste thresholds. J. Gen. Psychol., 1937, 17:155–161.
121. Skramlik, E. The fundamental substrates of taste. In Zotterman, Y. (Ed.) Olfaction and Taste. Oxford: Pergamon, 1963.

122. Sloan, L., and Gilger, A. Visual effects of Tridione. Am. J. Ophthal., 1947, *30*: 1387–1405.
123. Smith, G., Lowenstein, E., and Beecher, H. Experimental pain produced by the submaximum effort tourniquet technique: further evidence of validity. J. Pharmacol. Exp. Ther., 1968, *163*:468–474.
124. Snyder, S. *Uses of Marijuana.* New York: Oxford University Press, 1971.
125. Snyder, S., and Reivich, M. Regional localization of lysergic acid diethylamide in monkey brain. Nature, 1966, *209*:1093–1095.
126. Stebbins, W., Miller, J., Johnsson, L., and Hawkins, J. Behavioral measurement and histopathology of drug-induced hearing loss in subhuman primates. *In* Vagtborg, H. (Ed.) *Use of Nonhuman Primates in Drug Evaluation.* Austin: University of Texas Press, 1968.
127. Tart, C. *On Being Stoned.* Palo Alto: Science and Behavior Books, 1971.
128. Tribe, D., and Gordon, J. Choice of diet by rats deficient in members of the vitamin B complex. Brit. J. Nutr., 1953, *7*:197–201.
129. Turner, P. Amphetamines and smell threshold in man. *In* Herxheimer, A. (Ed.) *Drugs and Sensory Functions.* Boston: Little, Brown and Co., 1968.
130. Turner, P., and Patterson, D. Smell threshold as a test of central nervous function. Acta Oto-Laryngol., 1966, *62*:149–156.
131. Wade, G., and Zucker, I. Hormonal modulation of responsiveness to an aversive taste stimulus in rats. Physiol. Behav., 1970, *5*:269–273.
132. Walton, R. *Marihuana, America's New Drug Problem.* Phila.: Lippincott, 1938.
133. Warwick, K., and Eysenck, H. Experimental studies of the behavioural effects of nicotine. Pharmakopsychiat., 1968, *1*:145–169.
134. Weil, A., Zinberg, N., and Nelsen, J. Clinical and psychological effects of marihuana in man. Science, 1968, *162*:1234–1242.
135. Weiss, B., and Laties, V. Changes in pain tolerance and other behavior produced by salicylates. J. Pharmacol. Exp. Ther., 1961, *131*:120–129.
136. Weitzman, E., and Ross, G. A behavioral method for the study of pain perception in the monkey. Neurol., 1962, *12*:264–272.
137. Wersall, J., and Lundquist, P. Ototoxic drugs. *In* Herxheimer, A. (Ed.) *Drugs and Sensory Functions.* Boston: Little, Brown and Co., 1968.
138. Yackzan, K. Biological effects of *Gymnema sylvestre* fractions. Ala. J. Med. Sci., 1966, *3*:1–9.
139. Zucker, I. Body weight and age as factors determining estrogen responsiveness in the rat feeding system. Behav. Biol., 1972, *7*:527–542.
140. Zucker, I., Wade, G., and Ziegler, R. Sexual and hormonal influences on eating, taste preferences, and body weight of hamsters. Physiol. Behav., 1972, *8*: 101–111.

CHAPTER 11

LEARNING AND MEMORY

The processes of learning and memory are generally conceptualized as involving three broad phases. The first is registration: information is selected from all the incoming sensory data and registered in the CNS. It is not the case that all suprathreshold stimuli are equally well registered. A study by Hernandez-Peon et al. (72) offers a classic example of the influence of attention on registration. They recorded ER's to clicking sounds within the cochlear nucleus of unanesthetized cats. The responses were greatly attenuated when the experimenters presented mice in a jar or fish odors to the cats during the sounding of the clicks. Removal of the distracting stimuli was followed by return of the ER's to their previous levels. Other influences on registration include learning capacity, motivational state, and perceptual abilities.

The second phase is storage. Once registered, material to be remembered must be stored. There appear to be at least two types of storage, called short- and long-term memory. Short-term memory is probably maintained by a transient activation of a population of neurons. An example of short-term memory is that of the person who remembers a telephone number he has looked up only long enough to dial it. More permanent storage probably involves both anatomical and biochemical changes within the CNS. The process whereby short-term memories are converted into long-term memories is called memory consolidation. Memories which have been recently consolidated are very fragile and are easily disrupted by various natural and experimental procedures. For example, Russell and

248

Nathan (115) reported that more than 70 percent of people who had suffered serious head injury were amnesic for events which occurred within one half-hour of the injury.

The third phase is retrieval. Retrieval refers to the capacity to call up stored memory as needed. Knowledge of something does not assure that it will be recalled on demand. The tip of the tongue phenomenon, in which retrieval of a familiar name or place is temporarily blocked, is well known. Interference with the retrieval mechanism also takes place when material learned in one physiological state is not readily accessible in another. (State dependent learning will be discussed in detail later in this chapter.)

All active drugs affect registration. The processes of registration, storage, and retrieval are not generally analyzed separately; accordingly, the many studies of drug effects on "learning" are grouped under the general heading "acquisition." Following the discussion of acquisition are sections on consolidation of short-term memory, long-term storage, and retrieval. Several laboratories have conducted research programs which focus on the role of cholinergic mechanisms in all aspects of learning and memory. These programs are best considered together and are covered in the latter part of the chapter.

It is impossible in a book of this size to review even a fairly substantial proportion of the studies on drug effects on learning. Therefore, only highlights are discussed. However, it must be realized that the actions of drugs on acquisition depend on the conditions of testing. The particular task used in a testing situation is of considerable importance. Perhaps the clearest example of a drug-task interaction can be seen in the work of Cook and Davidson, which will be discussed later. In any experiment, the nature of the task is always a relevant consideration.

DRUGS WHICH AFFECT ACQUISITION

Miscellaneous Stimulants

Karl Lashley noted in 1917 (80) that low doses of strychnine improve maze learning in rats. His findings were largely ignored until the relatively recent work of McGaugh and his colleagues (88–90). They reported facilitation of learning with subconvulsive doses of several different stimulant drugs which were administered immediately prior to testing. They were aware of the possibility that the drugs were not acting directly on learning, but were instead improving it secondarily by increasing vigilance, motivation, or motor skills. Accordingly, they used diverse tasks, such as mazes and avoidance boxes, and diverse rewards, such as food and escape from shock. In these and other situations, and in several species of animals, stimulants improved performance.

Strychnine has been the most widely used drug, but many other stimulants have been tried with success. These include picrotoxin, diazadamantanol, pentylenetetrazol, bemegride, amphetamine, and caffeine. These drugs do not share a common mechanism of action. For example, picrotoxin blocks the release of neurotransmitters by inhibitory fibers; strychnine permits the release of inhibitory neurotransmitters, but competes with them at postsynaptic sites; and pentylenetetrazol stimulates by reducing neuronal recovery time.

Caffeine improves some types of learning (98), as does nicotine. Domino (45) found that small doses of nicotine enhanced learning of an avoidance response in rats, while larger doses led to slower learning. Erickson (51) reported similar findings, and in addition used nicotine bismethiodide, which does not cross the blood-brain barrier, to test the possibility that the effect is a peripheral one. The latter drug did not facilitate learning, which suggests that the nicotine effect is central. The results of several other studies confirm the facilitating effects of nicotine on some types of learning (20, 62).

Miscellaneous Depressants

The minor tranquilizer chlordiazepoxide generally impairs acquisition (32, 33), as does alcohol (130). The long-acting barbiturate sodium barbital likewise slows acquisition (92). Amobarbital has been shown to slow the process of classical conditioning (59).

Pentobarbital (a short-acting barbiturate) leads to reduced memory span in man (107). Meprobromate, on the other hand, may facilitate learning, especially in situations where anxiety depresses performance (43).

Marijuana

A variety of studies point to a marijuana-induced impairment of acquisition. Abel (1) read lists of words aloud to volunteers, immediately after which they were asked to write down as many words as they could recall. They were again asked to recall the words after an interval of 25 minutes. Both types of recall were impaired after the subjects were given marijuana.

Scheckel et al. (116) tested the effects of two chemical components of marijuana on delayed matching in monkeys. The monkeys were required to press a lever under one of two lights. The correct response was determined by the color of a light which was presented at some time prior to their response. Behavior was seriously disrupted for a period of up to nine days.

Melges et al. (91) were unable to demonstrate any serious effects of marijuana on memory until they devised a very complex task. Subjects were required to alternate between subtracting 7 from, and adding 1, 2, or 3 to, a starting number between 106 and 114. They were required to stop calculating when they reached a specified number between 46 and 54. Errors increased as the subjects who had been injected with a constituent of marijuana came closer to the target number; apparently, they were unable to calculate while keeping track of the goal.

Drugs Which Affect the Adrenergic System

The amphetamines enhance the learning of many types of tasks. Many (but not all) investigators have found that amphetamine improves avoidance conditioning in rats (47, 78). Classical conditioning is likewise affected by amphetamine; Franks and Trouton (59) demonstrated an increase in the rate of conditioning of an eye-blink response to a puff of air. Nash (99) employed a battery of intellectual tasks and reported general improvements. Laties and Weiss (82) pointed out that the improvement in learning under some conditions may be an artifact attributable to the use of electric shock. Rats tend to become immobile when shocked, as this reduces current density; however, because the immobility interferes with their capacity to make responses, their learning is slowed. Amphetamine thus "enhances" learning because it reduces the immobility. However, Weitzner has shown that in humans amphetamine improves both verbal learning and the ability to learn a series of numbers (138).

Latane and Schachter (81) claimed that low doses of epinephrine improved avoidance conditioning in rats. A role for epinephrine in avoidance responding seemed even more evident when Wenzel and Jeffrey (139) showed that mice in which activity in the sympathetic nervous system was eliminated learned more slowly than did controls. However, Moran et al. (97) were unable to replicate the Latane and Schachter findings. Conner and Levine (36) argued that the normal level of circulating epinephrine is optimal for avoidance learning in intact rats; both adrenalectomy and treatment of intact rats with epinephrine impaired performance.

Rech et al. (109), Moore (96), and Hanson (69) administered α-methyltyrosine, which inhibits the formation of dopamine and norepinephrine, to rats and guinea pigs. There were decrements in avoidance conditioning. Hanson found a strong correlation between the deficits and brain levels of catecholamines.

Serotonin

Essman (53) has argued for a central role of serotonergic mechanisms in learning and memory. Stevens et al. (122) and Essman (54) have modified levels of brain serotonin through the use of precursors and depletors. The results of both studies were similar: elevation of brain serotonin level impaired learning, while reduced levels improved it. These results should be contrasted with those of Woolley and van der Hoeven (see p. 174), who suggested that serotonin deficiency may lead to impaired learning ability.

Glutamic Acid

One of the products of amino acid metabolism is ammonia, which is highly toxic and must therefore be rapidly excreted or changed into some other form. One pathway is via reaction with glutamic acid to form glutamine. The reaction not only rids the body of ammonia but also provides, in the form of glutamine, a readily available store of nitrogen. Thus, glutamic acid serves a vital physiological function. It is also one of the amino acids which occur most frequently in proteins, and is found in especially high concentration in the brain. Glutamic acid is metabolized, in part, to gamma aminobutyric acid (GABA), which is a neurotransmitter in some crustaceans and has been proposed as a possible neurotransmitter in mammals. Glutamic acid may itself be a neurotransmitter.

In 1944 Zimmerman and Ross (141) reported that glutamic acid (GA) facilitated maze learning in rats. Their study precipitated a wave of others, which culminated in a 1960 review by Astin and Ross (7); they commented on the methodological inadequacy of most of the positive studies and noted that there was a strong association between positive results and absence of control groups. Their critique dimmed the enthusiasm for GA. However, in 1966, Vogel et al. (132) argued that the role of GA in intellectual functioning is still an open issue. They observed that Astin and Ross had failed to cite all the relevant literature, and had incorrectly classified some of their cited studies. Correcting their work, Vogel et al. tabulated the results of the studies as follows: 14 positive, with control groups; 17 positive, lacking controls; 16 negative, with controls; and 6 negative, without. They argued against summary dismissal of the studies lacking control groups because of the 30 in which they were used, only 4 reported that control group subjects changed significantly during the course of the experiment. The changes, although statistically significant, were small, and were in sharp contrast to the often substantial increases in subjects given GA in studies without controls. The problem of disposition of positive uncontrolled studies is a knotty one; it would seem that the best solution would be to conduct additional experiments which are methodologically sound.

Most of the early GA research used different types of retardates as subjects. Authors who reported positive results often indicated that some subjects were much more affected by treatment than were others. Perhaps GA is effective only on certain types of people, and the failure of experimenters to discriminate among their subjects obscured positive effects on some of them.

Vogel et al. discussed a problem which has continued to plague methodologically oriented psychopharmacologists. Individuals differ in responsiveness to drugs. Therefore, subjects in a study should not all receive the same dose; rather, the optimal dose for each should be determined. When experimenters use blind procedures, it is difficult for them to adjust dosage to individuals (the problem is more fully discussed on p. 202). While most of the positive studies used individualized drug administration, few of the negative studies did so. In at least some of the negative studies, the authors chose to administer large doses to all subjects, with the likely consequence that many suffered toxic side effects.

Another variable which distinguishes among positive and negative studies is the actual drug used. Some investigators assumed that the common household product monosodium glutamate (MSG) was equivalent to GA in its effects, so both drugs have been employed, seemingly interchangeably. However, there are important differences between them. In direct comparison, GA resulted in IQ rises of retardates, but MSG did not. GA reduced epileptic activity, while MSG increased it. Four of the negative studies with controls used MSG; in no MSG study were positive effects observed.

GA has been studied with normal subjects as well as with retardates. There have been 10 positive reports, most with control groups, and only three negative ones. The most frequent interpretation applied to GA is that it increases drive and other components of personality which are related to intelligence.

Drugs Which Affect RNA Synthesis

Pemoline and Magnesium Hydroxide

Considerable attention has been focused on the possibility that ribonucleic acid (RNA) is a "memory molecule." The pros and cons of this proposition will be discussed later; for now, suffice it to say that many studies of memory function have been prompted by the report (disputed by Stein and Yellin [120]) that the combination of pemoline and magnesium hydroxide (PMH) stimulates brain RNA polymerases (64). In 1966, Plotnikoff (104) described a shock avoidance task for rats in which a buzzer signaled the imminent onset of shock; learning was enhanced by injections of PMH. However, Beach and Kimble (17) showed that PMH sensitized rats to the *sound* of a buzzer, independent of the role of the buzzer in signaling shock onset. Other experimenters either failed to obtain a facilitation of memory or attributed positive results to hyperactivity or to heightened sensitivity to shock (60).

Not all of the work has been with avoidance conditioning. There is some evidence that hungry rats given PMH learn mazes more rapidly for food reward (39). Plotnikoff and Evans (106) tried to overcome some of the objections to the studies involving shock by using an entirely different procedure. Rabbits with recording electrodes implanted in the visual cortex were the subjects. A light was flashed every two seconds, and the ER was measured; its amplitude declined over time, and then, after about three hours, stabilized. (See Chapter 10 for a discussion of ER's.) The light flash was then paired with electric shocks to the hind legs until the ER to the light flash alone increased in amplitude; this indicated that conditioning had occurred. The amplitude of the ER was markedly increased by PMH, but not by several other stimulants which were tried; the results were interpreted by the authors to mean that PMH has a distinct central activity which facilitates learning. In a subsequent study (105) the powerful stimulant picrotoxin was used, and it too had positive effects.

Burns et al. (23), Smith (118), and Talland and McGuire (127) all tested the effects of PMH on conditioning in humans. The results on several different learning tasks were essentially negative. In those situations in which PMH did facilitate learning, the most plausible explanation seems to be that it did so via a general alerting effect, especially in subjects who were performing poorly because of fatigue.

Vitamin B$_{12}$*

Enesco (49) noted that vitamin B$_{12}$ stimulates both RNA and protein synthesis in mammalian tissues, and that deficiencies of vitamin B$_{12}$ are associated with neurological and psychiatric disorders. She further tested its role in affecting brain RNA by injecting it into laboratory rats maintained on a standard diet which was not

---

*The reader should be reminded that "drug" has been defined as any chemical agent which affects living protoplasm. Hence vitamins are drugs.

deficient in the vitamin; neuronal RNA concentration increased. Enesco then tested the effects of vitamin B_{12} on the acquisition of a bar pressing response, with water as the reward. The animals first merely observed for 15 minutes while trained rats bar pressed; then they were given access to the bar.

Although there were no differences among experimental and control animals in response acquisition, the vitamin-treated rats emitted more responses than did controls during the course of several days of training. When they were placed on a variable interval schedule (reward being given following the first response after a specified time interval, which varied from trial to trial), the experimentals again emitted more responses.

The results are difficult to interpret. The experimental and control animals did not differ significantly in basal metabolism rate, body weight, or open field activity; nevertheless, some factor other than a difference in learning ability may have accounted for the results. B_{12} may have increased thirst or activity under the specific conditions of the experiment. In any event, the clearest test of learning ability is acquisition, which was not affected in Enesco's experiment.

Yeast RNA

Yeast is a good source of RNA. Cameron and Solyom (27) tested the effects of yeast extracts of RNA on the intellectual functioning of senile patients. The patients, selected on the basis of established severe memory defects, were given three different tests of memory and learning ability; then they were given either oral RNA or a placebo. In later modifications of the procedure additional tests were used, and the RNA was injected rather than given orally.*

Cameron claimed substantial improvement in the drugged subjects, with the best results reported for those patients who had the smallest initial defects. He concluded that the results favor the interpretation that RNA provides the organic substrate for the memory trace. However, other interpretations are possible. Enesco (50) found that RNA leads to an increase in serum uric acid level, and uric acid may be a cortical stimulant. Uric acid improves acquisition of a water maze (52). Milner (95, p. 466) claimed that at least one of Cameron's experiments was not conducted as carefully as would appear from reading of the published reports.

Cook, Davidson, and their colleagues (37, 38) have published an

---

*Patients were pretreated with metaraminol (which is used to elevate blood pressure when it is dangerously low) and meperidine (an analgesic) to protect against toxicity from the RNA injections.

intriguing set of papers on the effects of yeast RNA on learning in rats. When the animals were required to climb a pole in order to avoid shock, yeast RNA facilitated acquisition of the response. The study has been replicated several times with similar results. Yeast RNA also improves maze learning in rats. However, the authors were not willing to assume generality for the effects of RNA on learning; they tested it in other situations, including discrimination learning and shock avoidance behavior, when the appropriate response was something other than pole climbing. Under these circumstances, there was no improvement in animals given RNA. The learning enhancement appears to be specific to a few situations, not all of them involving either shock or pole climbing.

CONSOLIDATION

Enhancement

Following his demonstration that stimulant drugs facilitate response acquisition, McGaugh tested the possibility that they do so by enhancing consolidation of the memory trace. (Nicotine has also been tested [51, 62].) The drugs were administered soon after learning had already occurred, and the animals were tested at a later time when the drugs were no longer active. Dosage was a crucial factor, with the optimum dosage being dependent on the particular strain of rats used (103). The performance of experimental animals was superior to that of controls. However, the assumption that the drugs had been excreted or metabolized by the time of testing may have been incorrect. Some drugs, e.g., amphetamine, have been shown (by Bauer and Duncan) to improve acquisition even when administered 24 hours prior to the start of training (16). Thus, if a drug is given immediately after learning but only 24 hours before retest, it may affect new learning rather than consolidation — that is, it may have proactive effects. Twenty-four hours may be close to the upper limit for proactive effects of drugs of the type used by McGaugh; Alpern and Crabbe (4) found no proactive effects in mice when discrimination training was begun 48 hours after injection of strychnine.

Although the findings of Bauer and Duncan require explanation, they do not substantially weaken McGaugh's interpretation that the drugs affect consolidation. He showed that effects are not only dose-dependent, but time-dependent as well. In general, the sooner after training the drug is administered, the stronger the facilitation of learning. Thus it is unlikely that the facilitation is the result of proactive effects; if that were the case, the strongest effects would be expected when the drug was administered just prior to retesting.

The time dependence of facilitatory effects is mirrored by studies of drugs which interfere with consolidation. In both cases, the time during which drug administration is effective varies with species, strain, task, and deprivation schedule. Rarely does the gradient extend beyond an hour.

Impairment

When animals receive an electric shock immediately after making a response, they inhibit the response on subsequent trials. When high intensity shock is used, it is easy to train the animals in only a single trial. Shock is used as a punishment in two popular procedures for obtaining one-trial learning; in one, rats or mice are placed on a small platform which rests on an electrified grid; in the other, they are placed in a box which has a hole in it. When they step off the platform, or through the hole, they receive the shock. As all the learning occurs in one trial, the procedure enables experimenters to specify with maximum precision the time involved between learning and experimental treatment.

Electroconvulsive Shock

Electroconvulsive shock (ECS) is used with humans to treat depression. ECS is a current passed through the head which causes brief convulsions. Attending psychiatrists had frequently noted that upon recovery from ECS, patients had amnesia for events immediately preceding the treatment. Careful experimentation with animals confirmed these early impressions. When animals are given electroconvulsive shock immediately after learning trials, they behave like naive animals. That is, when they are placed back in the original situation, they readily repeat the response that was followed by shock. The extent of their retrograde amnesia (RA) is highly dependent upon the interval between training and ECS. The sooner after training it is administered, the greater the RA; ECS has little effect on memory when the interval is greater than three hours. Several scientists reacted to the early ECS experiments with ingenious hypotheses which attempted to account for the results in ways which did not involve interference with memory consolidation. Their ideas stimulated some interesting experiments, but the original interpretation generally prevailed. One persistent difficulty with the hypothesis that ECS interferes with memory consolidation is that the forgotten material is often remembered at a much later date (142). Recently, Quatermain et al. (108) made a start toward identifying the critical variables which promote later recall. They used ECS to induce amnesia in rats, and the protein inhibitor cyclo-heximide to induce it in mice. They used one-trial passive avoidance conditioning in which animals received foot shock for making a response. The shock was immediately followed by the amnestic treatment. Twenty-four hours later, the subjects were returned to the test apparatus, but the shock mechanism was inoperative. Animals which had been treated with ECS or cycloheximide made the previously punished response as quickly as they had on the first trial, i.e., they behaved like naive animals. By contrast, the control animals took significantly longer to respond on the second trial. The results indicated, as expected, that the treatments were effective in producing amnesia. Yet the amnesia was reversible; when the animals were shocked outside the test apparatus within four hours of the test, they evidenced substantial recovery of the memory when retested 24 hours later. The results indicate that the amnestic treatments affect not consolidation, but rather the mechanism of retrieval.

The results of Quatermain et al. should be borne in mind when attempting to interpret the drug studies to be cited. However, even if the consolidation hypothesis is incorrect, the data are fascinating.

Drugs and RA

Although ECS is the most powerful technique known for producing RA, many drugs approach its effectiveness. Picrotoxin and pentylenetetrazol, which in subconvulsive doses improve consolidation, produce RA when given in doses large enough to produce convulsions. Yet convulsive doses of strychnine, which also facilitates consolidation at subconvulsive doses, do not impair consolidation (128). Moreover, the administration of anticonvulsant drugs such as diphenylhydantoin (DPH) and phenobarbital prior to ECS protects against the convulsions which normally accompany ECS, but not against RA (137).

The results of research on anesthetic and depressant drugs are equally confusing. The barbiturates thiopental and pentobarbital produce RA, but general anesthesia does not (70, 74, 102). The barbiturate amobarbital actually helps to restore memories forgotten after ECS (19). Anesthetic doses of halothane and carbon dioxide are effective in producing RA, but nitrogen is not (31, 126). Chlorpromazine also is effective (46). Consider the results with ether: there have been both positive and negative reports, and recently it was proposed that temperature may determine the outcome—that hot ether is much more effective than cold (5).

Weissman (137) tested 29 different drugs from more than 10 different classes for ability to produce RA. None was more effective than ECS, and only the stimulants picrotoxin and pentylenetetrazol yielded powerful effects. Among the ineffective drugs were ether, pentobarbital, and chlorpromazine. Reasons for the discrepancies between Weissman's and other studies are not known. Another puzzle is the vast differences in the time span during which the drugs are effective. Pentobarbital produces RA when injected 10 minutes after learning, but not at 20; pentylenetetrazol produces substantial effects when administered as late as four days after training.

One of the most striking effects of marijuana intoxication is memory lapse. Abel (1) has shown that the lapses do not result from failure to recall previously acquired material. Rather, acquisition of new material is impaired because of interference with consolidation. In Abel's study, adult volunteers were asked to learn lists of words prior to smoking marijuana cigarettes. Then they smoked and tried to recall the words; they also tried to recognize the previously learned words from larger lists. They performed as well as placebo controls on the recall task, but were poorer on the recognition task. When tested while intoxicated, their ability to learn new lists was greatly reduced. Abel analyzed the positions in the lists of items which were not recalled and, in accord with a recently proposed model of human memory, suggested that the items missed were those held in short-term store. He concluded that marijuana impairs acquisition by blocking the conversion of memories from short-term store to long-term storage, i.e., by blocking consolidation.

Weil and Zinberg (135) analyzed speech patterns of people high on marijuana. They reported two types of difficulties: forgetting the thing to be said next, and going off on irrelevant tangents. Their interpretation of the deficit is that marijuana interferes with retrieval of memory for events over the past few seconds, probably because users fail to rehearse. Their idea is compatible with the data of Abel, because his evidence indicated that the rehearsal of just learned material is important for consolidation.

Protection Against ECS

Weissman (136) has noted that memory consolidation is best defined as the development of resistance to disruption. He reasoned that since ECS is a means of disrupting consolidation, agents which protect against the effects of ECS may be said to facilitate consolidation. McGaugh reported that certain stimulants which facilitate consolidation also attenuated the amnesia following ECS, even though they potentiated the convulsant effects. Conversely, the anticonvulsant drugs phenobarbital, DPH, ether, and phenacemide blocked ECS convulsions without protecting against RA. DPH actually potentiated the effects of ECS. Meprobamate, on the other hand, blocked both convulsions and RA. Thus it seems that convulsions are irrelevant to the memory loss.

LONG-TERM MEMORY STORAGE

Effects of Strychnine on Long-Term Storage

Evidence has already been presented to show that strychnine improves the acquisition of new responses, presumably by enhancing the consolidation process. Alpern and Crabbe (4) have recently shown that strychnine also enhances long-term storage. Mice were trained in a complex maze, with access to saccharin solution as reward. Twenty-four hours after the last trial, they were assigned to one of six groups, each with a different dosage regimen of strychnine or tap water; the period of drug administration extended over 10 days. Twenty-four hours after the last injection, the mice were retested in the maze. The group whose members had received low daily doses of strychnine exceeded all the others in maze performance; high daily doses did not improve performance, nor did single high or low doses. The effect of strychnine was not the result of action on learning ability; naive mice which received low daily doses of strychnine for 10 days, and which were trained 48 hours after the last injection, did not learn the maze faster than controls. The facilitatory effect was only on animals that had received prior exposure to the maze. Thus, it must have influenced long-term memory.

Memory Molecules

Within the nucleus of every cell are chromosomes which contain deoxyribonucleic acid (DNA), the molecule in which is encoded the genetic information. Because of its large size, DNA is called a macromolecule. The DNA molecule is composed of large numbers of four nucleotides which can be combined in endless combinations, just as a four-letter alphabet could be arranged to construct an infinite number of words of unspecified length. DNA forms a template for the synthesis of a structurally similar macromolecule, RNA, which is also found in the cell nucleus. RNA plays a crucial role in the synthesis of proteins which, because they are composed of as many as 20 different amino acids, have the highest information content of all known molecules (129).

In 1950, Katz and Halstead (77) speculated that neuronal stimulation resulted in the ordering of originally random configurations of protein molecules. Their idea was seminal, and the search for a molecule in which memory is stored has led to the development of an exciting research frontier. Many investigators believe that long-term memory is chemically encoded; DNA, RNA, proteins, and lipids have all been proposed as meeting the criteria for being memory molecules. The criteria vary among experimenters, but those advanced by Dingman and Sporn (44) seem acceptable:

1. In order for a molecule to be considered a memory molecule, it must undergo a change of state in response to the experience to be remembered.

2. Its altered state must persist as long as the memory can be demonstrated.

3. Specific destruction of the altered state must result in permanent loss of the memory.

It is necessary to realize, in light of some of the evidence which has been cited in support of the different macromolecules as memory molecules, that satisfaction of the first criterion does not by itself constitute sufficient proof; neurons change as a result of stimulation, and constituents of neurons, which help to maintain their integrity, can be expected to change as well. However, failure to meet any of the criteria should eliminate a substance from consideration as a memory molecule. The structure of DNA is not changed by neuronal stimulation (79), and it need not be further discussed.

Dingman and Sporn stressed the inadvisability of considering the substrate of memory to be exclusively chemical or exclusively anatomical. There are almost surely interconnections — in order for axons to grow, proteins must by synthesized, and both RNA and proteins are essential for the maintenance of synaptic structure (133) — therefore, if memory molecules exist, their role is probably to modify the functioning of neurons. If such is the case, molecular theories would be compatible with theories of changes in neurotransmitter action (e.g., the work of Deutsch, which is discussed later).

Inhibitors of Protein Synthesis

Because of its complex structure and its involvement in so many aspects of cellular function, protein received early consideration as a memory molecule. Although the evidence is somewhat controversial, it appears that neuronal stimulation results in modification of protein structure, protein synthesis, and protein degradation (128, pp. 150–152). Neurons are very active protein synthesizers (85, p. 173). Flexner and his colleagues (reviewed in 57) initiated a research program utilizing the drug puromycin, which reduces the rate of protein synthesis by about 80 percent for several hours. They trained mice to run a maze to avoid shock, and stopped the training after the animals had chosen the correct side on 9 of 10 trials. Different groups of mice were injected with puromycin at varying times both prior and subsequent to training. They were also retested at varying intervals after the original training. The relationship between the number of trials necessary to achieve the criterion of 9 correct responses in 10 trials, during original learning and relearning, was used as an index of memory.

In the first study, puromycin was injected subcutaneously. The mice lost weight and became lethargic, but there were no effects on learning or memory. However, the subcutaneous injections are much less effective in inhibiting protein synthesis than are injections directly into the brain. Therefore, in subsequent studies, all injections were intracerebral. They were given bilaterally, in the hippocampal, frontal, and ventricular regions (see Fig. 11–1).

Frontal and ventricular injections did not disrupt the memory. The results were quite different when puromycin was injected, one day after completion of training, into the hippocampus. (The hippo-

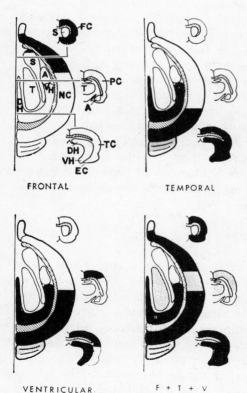

FRONTAL

TEMPORAL

VENTRICULAR

F + T + V

Figure 11–1 Spread of fluorescein after it is injected intracerebrally. The diagrams at the left indicate structures viewed from the top after removal of a horizontal section of the hemisphere; at the right, cross (frontal) sections of the hemisphere at the level indicated in the diagram for frontal injections. Relative intensity of staining is indicated by relative density of stippling. *A*, Amygdaloid nucleus; *DH*, dorsal hippocampus; *EC*, entorhinal cortex; *FC*, frontal cortex; *NC*, neocortex; *PC*, parietal cortex; *S*, corpus striatum; *T*, thalamus; *TC*, temporal cortex; *VH*, ventral hippocampus; $F + T + V$, frontal + temporal + ventricular injections. (From Flexner, L., Flexner, J., and Roberts, R. Memory in mice analyzed with antibiotics. Science, 1967, *155.* Copyright 1967 by the American Association for the Advancement of Science.)

campus is an area of the brain which has well documented involvement in memory). The mice retained the memory for 10 to 20 hours, but then became permanently amnesic. The effects of puromycin were blocked, i.e., there was no amnesia, if the mice were trained for 60 additional trials once the criterion had been reached.

When puromycin was injected into the hippocampus up to three days after training, it disrupted memory. With longer delays, injections into the hippocampus on both sides of the brain were insufficient; in order to disrupt the memory, it was necessary to inject at frontal and ventricular sites as well. When that was done, the injections were effective for as long as 60 days after training. Flexner et al. concluded that recent memory is localized primarily in the hippocampal area, and that as a memory grows older, it gets stored in an enlarged area of the neocortex.

The effects of puromycin were dose-dependent, and were correlated with the extent of inhibition of protein synthesis. While puromycin caused memory loss, it did not prevent the mice from relearning the maze. Substances which were structurally related to puromycin, but without its ability to inhibit protein synthesis, did not disrupt memory.

Barondes and Cohen (11) also used puromycin. They injected mice intracerebrally prior to training, and noted that their ability to learn in the maze was unimpaired. Fifteen minutes after training, their performance was still indistinguishable from that of controls. However, when the mice were tested three hours after having reached criterion, they had total amnesia. These results, along with those of Flexner and McGaugh, seemed to indicate that there are at least three stages in the permanent formation of memory:

1. The initial stage extends through training and for a few minutes beyond. It is readily disrupted by ECS and by several pharmacological agents; puromycin does not affect memory at this stage.

2. The second stage extends between about three hours and three days. It can be disrupted by bilateral hippocampal injections of puromycin.

3. Stage three lasts for at least 60 days after training. It is much less susceptible to disruption; amnesia can be produced only if puromycin is injected in other brain areas as well as in the hippocampus.

At this point an experiment by Cohen and Barondes (34), while in no way lessening the importance of the earlier results, demonstrated that the relatively coherent picture which they had suggested was illusory. Cohen and Barondes found that mice injected with puromycin have abnormal electrical activity within the hippocampus which persists for several hours after injection. The animals were more seizure-prone following subconvulsive doses of pentylenetetrazol. Moreover, when the anticonvulsant drug DPH was administered at the same time as the puromycin, no amnesia was observed. They therefore concluded that inhibition of protein synthesis may not be the important action of puromycin.

Another alternative to inhibition of protein synthesis was suggested by the observation that amnesic doses of puromycin caused swelling of neuronal mitochondria. There was no swelling when heximide was administered with the puromycin, nor does the combination of heximide and puromycin disrupt memory. It was therefore suggested that a toxic metabolic product of puromycin, possibly peptidyl-puromycin, was causing the neuronal swelling and the amnesia (61).

Flexner et al. reported an additional complication. Memories which had been disrupted by puromycin could be restored by injections of isotonic saline even 60 days after the original training. Thus, the effect of puromycin seems to be on retrieval rather than on memory formation. Saline may act to remove the peptidyl-puromycin.

The idea that inhibition of protein synthesis was the key to memory disruption seemed to be further discredited by studies with acetoxycycloheximide (AXM). Though AXM is an even more powerful protein inhibitor than puromycin, it does not cause abnormal electrical activity. In the early work, AXM was not shown to produce amnesic effects and, in fact, it protected against the effects of puromycin when administered concurrently with the latter (12). However, when Barondes and Cohen introduced a slight modification of procedure, the results were striking. Instead of training mice to a criterion of 9 correct responses out of 10, the mice were removed from the apparatus as soon as they had made 3 out of 4 correct responses (13).

Mice injected with AXM either subcutaneously or in the hippocampal region five hours prior to training were equal to control animals in their ability to learn the maze. There were still no differences between them when they were retested three hours later. However, when retesting was delayed six hours or more, the mice injected with AXM showed substantial deficits. Thus, the degree of original learning interacted with the administration of the drug. A second relevant factor in determining the effectiveness of AXM was task difficulty; the greater the difficulty, the greater the amnesic effect. The animals's state of arousal is also important; when mice were injected with amphetamine or subjected to electric shock, thereby increasing arousal, the effects of AXM were blocked (14). The amnesic effects of AXM, unlike those of puromycin, were not antagonized by intracerebral injections of saline (111).

None of the protein inhibitors disrupts synthesis totally, and it appears that even a little residual protein synthesis is sufficient to maintain the memory of tasks which have been well learned. Whatever the mechanism of action of AXM, that of puromycin is probably largely or completely unrelated to inhibition of protein synthesis.

Agranoff and Davis (reviewed in Ref. 2) have conducted a research program which largely parallels those of the Flexners and of Barondes and Cohen. Agranoff and Davis train goldfish to swim over a barrier to avoid shock; then, at varying time intervals, the fish are injected with puromycin or AXM. The fish are then retested for retention of the original learning. The results with goldfish have been essentially the same as those with mice, although the time constants have been somewhat different. When AXM preceded training, there was no change in ability to learn the avoidance response. However, the memory rapidly decayed until, after three days, the fish had almost total amnesia for the shock avoidance. When AXM was injected immediately after training, the decay process again took three days. When injections were delayed for three hours after training, AXM had no effect, either immediately or subsequently. From these latter results it was concluded that long-term memories are fully formed after about three hours, hence are resistant to the actions of AXM. Even though injections immediately after training block long-term memory, correct responses are emitted for a three day period; from these results it was deduced that short-term memory decays over a three day period.

In a further experiment, Agranoff and Davis found that short- and long-term memory processes display roughly complementary time constants. They used the short-acting protein inhibitor potassium chloride. Intracranial injections blocked the formation of long-term memory even when injected 18 hours after training; loss of short-term memory took about 12 hours. These results suggested that short-term memory is converted into long-term as it decays; perhaps the decay of the one and the formation of the other are both dependent on protein synthesis. The difference between AXM and potassium chloride is in duration of action. Because AXM inhibits protein synthesis for a much longer period of time, it blocks short-term memory loss for a longer period. An illuminating experiment offered dramatic confirmation of Agranoff and Davis' idea that the decay of short-term memory is dependent upon protein synthesis. Whereas a single injection of AXM immediately following training is associated with large retention deficits in fish tested three days afterward, three injections of the same dose, given one per day, result in much smaller decrements three days after original training. The interpretation is that both treatments block the formation of long-term memory, and the schedule of three injections prolongs the decay of short-term. The case would be even more convincing if it could be shown that long-term memory was in fact equally disrupted in the two groups. It would only be necessary to retest both groups after an interval greater than three days.

Even if short- and long-term memories do depend on similar processes, they are also considerably independent of each other. That is, although all short-term memories (by definition) decay over time, only some of them are converted to long-term memories.

Transfer Studies

In the early 1960's the scientific community was excited by the publication of several papers which collectively gave strong support to the hypothesis which pointed to chemical coding of permanent memory. The evidence seemed to favor RNA as the memory molecule. Hyden and Egyhazi (73) showed that the structure of cerebral RNA was changed by experience. Then followed McConnell's (86) exciting work with the common freshwater flatworms called planarians. He took advantage of two interesting properties of planarians: (a) when cut in half, both halves regenerate; (b) planarians are cannibalistic. McConnell et al. (87) found that when planarians which had been classically conditioned to light were bisected, and both halves allowed to regenerate, both new animals retained memory of the original conditioning. When, however, the two halves were incubated in a solution containing RNase, which destroys RNA, the memory was abolished (40). When naive worms were allowed to cannibalize trained ones, they showed much more "memory" in the apparatus than did naive worms which had dined on untrained donors. These reports came under heavy attack primarily because, it was argued, planarians are incapable of learning. Several caustic exchanges between McConnell and his critics appeared over the next few years, apparently resolved in favor of McConnell (41). In any event, the flatworm experiments were heuristic, and within a few years there were several reports of transfer of training in rats.

The first study with rats was published by Fjerdingstad et al. (56), and may be regarded as typical. The experimenters conditioned rats to approach either a light or dark alley for water reward. The animals were then killed and RNA extracted from their brains. This in turn was injected into naive animals. The recipients performed significantly better when tested in the alley than did rats which received RNA extracts from naive animals. Within a year at least five other positive reports from five different laboratories were published (3, 8, 55, 110, 128). Many other scientists began to work in this area, but the results were, on the whole, disappointing. In fact, in 1966, the prestigious journal *Science* carried a letter signed by 23 investigators stating that they had been unsuccessful in demonstrating memory transfer (24). Shortly thereafter, two of the signatories reported positive results.

An interesting positive chemical transfer experiment was recently reported by Braud and Braud (21). They employed a transposition paradigm in which rats trained to respond to the larger of two stimuli were tested in a situation involving choice between the originally larger stimulus and a new, even larger one. Under such conditions, rats typically show a preference for the new stimulus. Braud and Braud decapitated rats which had been trained to respond for food reward to the larger of two circles glued onto the arms of a maze. They then injected extracts from the brains of the trained rats into naive ones. Other rats received brain extract from untrained animals. At each of six test periods after the injections, during which time no rewards were given, recipients of brain extracts from trained donors made more responses to the larger test stimulus than did recipients of the control extract. They also learned more rapidly on training trials with the original stimuli.

The area of chemical transfer remains highly controversial, as witness the recent heated exchange in *Science* between Bryant et al. (22) and Stein and Rosen (119). They attacked and defended, respectively, a paper by Frank et al. (58) which seemed to indicate that what was actually being transferred in these experiments was a nonspecific factor caused by stress and not related to memory. In the paper under discussion, mice were injected with either brain or liver homogenate from donors that had been shocked in a box to which they had run in order to escape a mild stress; the mice took longer to enter the box than did recipients of extract from donors that had not been shocked. The criticisms of the study cited the following procedural flaws: improper statistical analysis of data; improper learning paradigm; insufficient dose of extract; and the testing of animals which were not fully recovered from the injection. In their rebuttal, Stein and Rosen noted that the critics themselves had previously used the procedures which they were attacking as being inadequate. One point about which all agreed was that nonspecific transfer effects do exist. Bryant et al. contended that the majority of transfer studies have not employed stress; consequently, the explanation by Stein and Rosen would be inadequate in any event.

Although detailed analysis of the present status of transfer work is beyond the scope of this book, a few general comments may serve to orient the interested reader.

The effect, if it is real, is very fragile. Slight changes in learning task, in extraction procedures, and in the species and even strain of animals being used have greatly altered results. In 1967, a symposium was called so that interested investigators might elaborate upon procedures which they had found successful, in order to make reliable replication possible (25). However, although several investigators provided detailed descriptions of their techniques, there are still none which are highly reliable outside the laboratories in which they originated.

The difficulty in replication creates a special problem, one which has also been faced by workers in the field of parapsychology; by chance alone, 1 of every 20 studies would be expected to yield results significant at the level generally acceptable to scientists (p = .05). The actual ratio of negative to positive transfer experiments might conceivably be greater than 19 to 1.

Although the impetus for the transfer research came from experimenters who believed that RNA is the memory molecule, they were probably wrong. That stimulation causes changes in RNA is not surprising, since RNA is so active in cellular processes. Stimulation also changes protein. A most convincing argument against the RNA hypothesis is that RNA does not penetrate the blood-brain barrier (84). Also, although extraction procedures vary, all of the extracts contain protein and other impurities (112).

Milner (95) has discussed the problems in a most enlightening way. He pointed out that synaptic transmission is effected through the release of neurotransmitters, the synthesis of which must be dependent upon RNA and DNA. Therefore, it is not surprising that interference with RNA or protein synthesis should interfere with learning and memory. He noted that the human brain contains approximately 10 billion neurons, each of which may synapse with as many as 2000 other neurons. Therefore, an obvious mechanism for memory storage would be in configurations of molecules, i.e., in synaptic relationships. The importance of RNA or protein might consist in their ability to effect changes in synaptic pathways.

THE CHOLINERGIC SYSTEM AND MEMORY

Scopolamine and other anticholinergic drugs induce confusion and disorientation of behavior. They impair learning of many different types of tasks. One of the simplest tests of memory is spontaneous alternation behavior. When rats are allowed to run down a T-maze which has no reward at the end of either arm, they typically alternate their first and second responses. Scopolamine blocks the alternation. Meyers and Domino (94) have attributed the block to a loss of memory for very recently learned material. The disruptive effect is not observed with methyl scopolamine, which differs from scopolamine primarily in that it does not enter the brain. Therefore, the site of action of scopolamine is probably central.

Scopolamine increases the number of responses made by rats when they are placed on extinction schedules (71). It impairs accuracy of discrimination in rhesus monkeys (75), and in rats it induces anterograde amnesia (68) — that is, amnesia which occurs for events that take place after the drug is administered. Scopolamine disrupts acquisition and retention of passive avoidance responses in rats (93). Other drugs which modify cholinergic mechanisms also affect memory. The actions of nicotine, which in small doses increases brain ACh and larger doses decreases it (134), have already been discussed. Physostigmine, which increases brain levels of acetylcholine (ACh), improves acquisition of avoidance responses, discrimination learning, and maze running (48, 125, 140).

The Berkeley Group

In Berkeley, a biochemist, a neuroanatomist, and two psychologists have been involved in a collaborative effort to determine the effects of conditions of rearing on the brain and on behavior (113). In their work, which was begun in 1958 and has continued to the present (although with some changes in the original group), rats are raised under one of three types of environmental conditions: impoverished, in which the animals live singly in quiet, dimly lit rooms and are handled by the experimenter only at weekly weighings; intermediate, in which they are kept three to a cage and are exposed to routine laboratory noises and routine care; and enriched, in which groups of 10 to 12 are housed in a large cage which includes constant access to novel, stimulating objects and periodic exposure to a series of mazes.

In the early work, the rats were assigned to their condition at weaning, when they were about 25 days of age, and kept for 80 days. (Later experiments showed that the same results were obtained with older animals as well.) They were then given several behavioral tests and were killed in order that their brains might be analyzed.

Several interesting findings emerged. Rats reared in enriched environments were superior to the other two groups in learning ability. Associated with the behavioral changes were changes in their brain biochemistry — specifically, in the activity of the cholinergic system. The enzyme AChE, which catalyzes the metabolism of ACh, was elevated, and its distribution through cortical and subcortical areas was altered. On the other hand, activity of protein and RNA was unchanged. The experimenters also found that genetically different strains of rats, which are unequal in learning ability, differ in brain AChE. The results further implicate cholinergic processes in learning and memory.

Carlton's Work

In 1962, Peter Carlton started a research program aimed at studying the effects of anticholinergic drugs. He distinguishes between three types of stimuli: those which are biological reinforcers, such as food; novel stimuli, such as flashing lights, to which an animal initially responds but to which it eventually habituates; and punishing stimuli, such as electric shock. Animals learn to inhibit responses to the latter two classes of stimuli, and Carlton's research has suggested to him that the inhibition is mediated by cholinergic processes. His hypothesis is based on the following types of evidence.

Carlton and Vogel (30) exposed rats treated with either scopolamine or saline to a complex stimulus consisting of a tone and two lights. At a later date they compared the disruptive effects of the stimulus on the same subjects, this time with no injection, while the rats were bar pressing for water reward. Rats which had received saline gave evidence of habituation to the stimulus and maintained their bar pressing, while the scopolamine group had its performance disrupted. Note: the data may be explained without the necessity of postulating cholinergic involvement in memory processes, merely by assuming that state dependent learning (discussed later) had occurred.

Rats that are given access to a bar which they can press in order to turn on a light typically have a high rate of responding which declines gradually over several test sessions. The rats probably stop responding because they become habituated to the light. Carlton (28) was able to reverse the decline by treating the rats with scopolamine. Several related experiments are summarized in Reference 29. Carlton argued that the seeming impairment of learning and memory stemming from scopolamine treatment results from the drug's disinhibition of responses to punishing stimuli or to stimuli to which the animal has already habituated. He cited an experiment in which the failure to habituate was separated from other types of memory loss. One arm of a maze led to a goal box which was filled with manipulable objects, while the goal box in the other arm was empty. Rats treated with scopolamine learned to respond to the toy-filled side 100 percent of the time, showing that they were capable of remembering. Undrugged rats ran to the toy-filled side only 65 percent of the time, which shows that they, unlike scopolamine-treated subjects, habituated to the novelty of the toys (83).

Although scopolamine blocks the suppression of responses

which have been punished, it does not affect the emission of responses which have had reward as a consequence (131). These differential effects of scopolamine on punished and rewarded behavior cannot be easily explained by those who contend that scopolamine disrupts memory. Carlton's explanation is that the hippocampus is under cholinergic control and functions to produce inhibition of unrewarded responses; both scopolamine and hippocampal lesions disinhibit the behavior. The explanation, while ingenious, seems incomplete. It does not account for the anterograde effects of scopolamine or the scopolamine-induced impairment of delayed matching.

Although Carlton stated that part of learning to go right in a maze involves learning not to go left, he failed to acknowledge that inhibition of inappropriate responses underlies all learning. Hence, the distinction between disinhibition and blockade of learning does not seem useful. Most importantly, Carlton's theory fails to account for the very exciting findings with anticholinesterases, to which we now turn.

Russell's Work

Russell et al. (114) injected the anticholinesterase drug 0,0-diethyl-S-ethylmercaptoethanol thiophosphate (Systox) into rats and then trained them to avoid shock. Drugged rats acquired the response as readily as controls. Hence, accumulation of brain ACh does not affect initial learning. However, extinction of the response was slower in the experimental animals. Glow and Rose (65), using a different type of anticholinesterase, diisopropylfluorophosphate (DFP), and a different training situation, reported similar findings. Banks and Russell (9) tested rats on a serial learning task which required the extinction of a response to one problem in order to be able to respond appropriately on the next problem. There was no effect of Systox on the first few problems, and no effect on any problems until doses were used which reduced AChE levels below a critical value of about 50 percent of normal. Then, there was a dose-related increase in the number of errors.

Deutsch's Work

Deutsch (42) hypothesized that learning involves changes in the amount of ACh emitted at synapses. He assumed that as a synapse increases in efficiency during continued exposure to a learning experience, increasing amounts of ACh are released until some maximal level is reached. The effects of a drug on an ACh-dependent system within the CNS would depend, therefore, on the efficiency of the synapse at the time the drug is injected. Such is the case in the peripheral nervous system. For example, injection of neostigmine into normal people leads to paralysis because it increases the level of ACh until the excess causes depolarization blockade. However, neostigmine improves muscular performance in people suffering from myaesthenia gravis, a disease characterized by muscular weakness resulting from an inadequate supply of ACh during repetitive stimulation at the neuromuscular junction. In other words, neostigmine improves the capacity of inefficient synapses but not that of normally functioning synapses.

The basic design in Deutsch's experiments involves training rats, then at some period thereafter injecting DFP, followed by testing of the animals 24 hours later when they are drug-free. The critical variable is the interval between training and drug injection. In most of his studies he used a maze which animals ran to avoid shock, but the same basic findings obtained for appetitive habits.

First, it was ascertained that DFP does not affect acquisition of an avoidance response in a maze when it is injected into naive rats. The animals were trained to a criterion of 10 consecutive correct responses, and there were no differences due to drugs. Under the conditions of testing, uninjected rats who have reached criterion retain the response almost perfectly through 14 days, but forget it almost completely by 28 days. Now, consider the strange results with DFP.

When the rats were injected 30 minutes after they had reached criterion, their retest performance one day later was considerably poorer than that of controls. But when injections were delayed for one to three days, there was no memory disruption. Injections given at 5 days and at 14 days produced near total amnesia. However, rats injected with DFP 28 days after training showed good retention. (The illustration of Deutsch's work reproduced as Fig. 11–2 extends to only 21 days).

The effects of scopolamine mirror those of DFP, which would be expected if the actions of the latter result from increased conduction at cholinergic synapses. Scopolamine had little effect at 30 minutes, profound disruptive effects at one to three days, and little thereafter. Both drugs modified retention only temporarily; the behavior soon returned to normal.

The results with DFP suggested an interesting experiment to Deutsch which did not involve the use of drugs. He reasoned that synaptic efficiency does not reach maximum until five days after training, because DFP produces amnesia when it is injected after five days, but not after three; only when synaptic efficiency has reached maximum would increased quantities of ACh be expected to impair efficiency. He trained rats to criterion and then retested

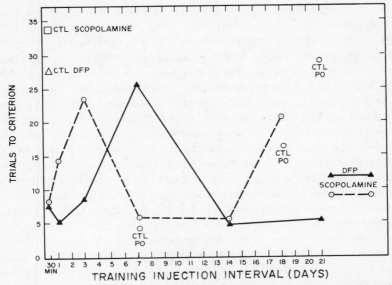

Figure 11–2 Mean number of trials to relearn after DFP and scopolamine when the original training-injection interval was varied. CTL PO refers to control animals which were injected with peanut oil. (From Wiener, N., and Deutsch, J. Temporal aspects of anticholinergic- and anticholinesterase-induced amnesia for an appetitive habit. J. Comp. Physiol. Psychol., 1968, *66*: p. 615.)

them after one, three, seven, or ten days. The latter two groups required about one-half the number of trials needed by the former to reach criterion. A comparable result, showing that memory increases for a while after a task is learned, with no additional training, had been reported several years earlier by Kamin (76). Nevertheless, the potential of pharmacological research for suggesting important psychological principles was clearly demonstrated.

There are two likely mechanisms by which the strength of a habit could be increased. First, a given synapse might increase in efficiency; and second, the total number of synapses might increase. Deutsch's early work favored the interpretation that increases in synaptic efficiency underlie memory improvements. He strengthened the conclusion by additional experiments in which he trained rats to high or low criteria of performance. The poorly learned habits were facilitated by DFP, and the well learned habits blocked. If the other alternative had been correct, it would be expected that each synapse, once operative, would be maintained at peak efficiency; then AChE would produce only deficits, regardless of degree of training.

In Deutsch's next experiment, he used the drug physostigmine to resolve the question of why animals stop emitting previously rewarded responses which no longer lead to reward. He recognized two possibilities: extinction of responding might result from weakening of the old habit, or from learning of a new one. He trained rats to criterion in the maze, then gave them extinction training soon afterwards. A second group received the original training but was not placed on extinction. Both groups were injected seven days later with physostigmine, and they showed amnesia to equal extent. The results favor the interpretation that extinction involves the learning of a new response, for if it consisted of a weakening of the original response, the physostigmine would have been expected to improve the performance of the group given extinction training. Remember, anticholinesterases facilitate weak habits (see preceding paragraph).

In another part of the experiment, rats were given extinction training four days after the original learning — three days before injection and retest. These animals took about twice as many trials to relearn the maze as did uninjected controls. Again, it is important to remember that physostigmine has little effect on three-day-old memories. The results suggest that the physostigmine blocked original learning, but left memory of the extinction trials relatively intact. They support the idea that extinction is the learning of a separate response.

RETRIEVAL

State Dependent Learning

A friend of the author once stayed up all night to study for a morning examination. He used amphetamines to help him keep awake. By morning, he felt that he knew the material perfectly. But when it came time to take the exam, he was a complete blank (which was what he got as a grade).

His predicament was anticipated by Lashley (80) who in 1917 reported that although acquisition of a maze was facilitated by prior administration of strychnine or caffeine, later performance of the rats without either drug was inferior to that of controls. The first explicit statement that learning while in a drugged state does not always transfer to the undrugged state was made by Girden (63). He classically conditioned dogs with curare and found that the conditioned response could only be elicited when they were again curarized. The findings parallel those from other kinds of research. Animals that learn a response in the presence of a particular stimulus complex often fail to emit the response when the stimulus complex is changed. Drugs constitute one important set of stimuli, and animals can discriminate between the drugged and undrugged states. For example, Conger (35) trained rats to run down an alley for food reward when they were drugged with alcohol, but to inhibit running when they were undrugged; in the latter case they were shocked when they ran. The animals readily learned. Responses which do not fully transfer from one state to another are called state dependent, and the phenomenon is called state dependent learning (STD).

STD is easily demonstrated for avoidance learning (100), but it is less apparent on discrimination tasks such as maze learning (cf. Refs. 18 and 101). Not all drug classes are equally effective; anesthetics and hypnotics are most powerful, although, as noted before, strychnine and caffeine were the first drugs for which the effect was shown. Amphetamine, chlorpromazine, and scopolamine also produce STD. The latter finding is relevant to some of Carlton's work (cited earlier) on interference with habituation by scopolamine.

Overton, who has been at the forefront of research on STD, discussed the need for appropriate experimental designs (100). Four groups are needed: D-D, D-ND, ND-D, and ND-ND, where D stands for drug and ND for no drug, first on training and then on test trials. If there are true state dependent effects, the D-D and ND-ND groups should outperform the other two on test days. Overton has noted that the effects are not symmetrical. That is, the decrements in going from a D to an ND state are generally greater than the decrements in the reverse direction. For example, rats trained in an avoidance conditioning situation while drugged with meprobamate performed poorly when tested without the drug. Rats trained without drug showed no decrements when tested with meprobamate (10).

Unfortunately, the term state dependent has been used in two different, although related, ways. The first use of the term has been in the manner described above—that is, to indicate failure to transfer training from one state to another; it has been used in a second way to indicate that animals are capable of being trained to emit different responses in different states. Thus, Stewart et al. (123) entitled their paper "State Dependent Learning," although they required that animals learn to discriminate between D and ND. Their paper is intriguing, because they showed that endogenous substances can produce STD. Specifically, high, nonphysiological doses of the hormone progesterone were discriminable by rats. The demonstration that hormonal status can be discriminated suggests the (admittedly wild) possibility that changes in hormonal status may produce true STD, as first defined above. In that case, memory in women may fluctuate with the menstrual cycle; events occurring during menstruation would be poorly remembered at midcycle, but would be retrievable during the next menstrual period.

Storm and Smart (124) proposed that the well-documented amnesia of the alcoholic may be an instance of STD. In a recent test of the hypothesis, Goodwin et al. (66) used the appropriate 2×2 design with medical student volunteers. They were tested on successive days with four tasks:

1. On day 1 they were required to learn the correct responses

to four patterns of light. They were punished for incorrect responses by a noxious tone. On the second day, the same patterns and responses were used, but the previous connections were now incorrect. Hence, the better the original relationships were remembered, the more they would be presumed to interfere with responding on day 2, and the more errors would be expected.

2. On day 1 the subjects memorized four sentences of varying difficulty, and on day 2 attempted to recall them.

3. Subjects were asked to free associate with the first word which came to mind upon presentation of stimulus words. On day two they were asked to recall their associations. (Note: this test is not exclusively one of memory; it is likely that patterns of associations differ for different states.)

4. On day 1 the subjects looked at 20 pictures, and on day 2 they tried to pick them out from a group of 40.

One clear-cut result was that sober subjects did better than drugged ones. In addition, STD was observed. D-D and ND-ND subjects made more errors on the noxious tone avoidance test than did the other two groups, indicating that they remembered more of the day 1 training. They made fewer errors on the sentence recall and word association tests, while the groups did not significantly differ on the picture recall test.

These results may partially explain why many alcoholics who manage to successfully practice total abstinence rapidly lose control of their drinking behavior if they are induced to take a single drink. Their learned behavior when they are sober is forgotten when blood alcohol concentration rises. In particular, their resolutions to abstain may be forgotten.

The phenomenon of STD may also account for the often observed differential effects of acute and chronic drug administration. The newly drugged animal has to relearn a great deal about its environment. One very important implication of STD concerns withdrawal from drugs prescribed for psychotherapeutic purposes. The problem is discussed on pp. 160 to 162.

Restoration of Repressed Memories

Barbiturates impair learning in many situations, but amobarbital has a special status. It was long reputed to be effective in restoring forgotten memories of painful experiences (67). In 1954 Bogoch demonstrated that amobarbital could restore some forgotten memories. He worked with hospitalized mental patients who had received electroconvulsive therapy during the course of their hospitalization, and had suffered memory loss as a consequence. Each patient was thoroughly questioned and, if the amnesia remained, was injected with amobarbital. The questioning was then repeated. Four of the patients had no memory improvement during the experiment, and two others improved prior to amobarbital treatment (they remembered even more after receiving the drug). Seventeen patients who had little or no recall during the initial interview registered significant gains during the question period with amobarbital. It would be worth repeating the experiment under double blind conditions, along with having some procedure for checking the accuracy of the restored memories.

More recently, Stein and Berger (121) reported an experiment which, they claimed, demonstrates that amobarbital is able to restore repressed memories in animals. They trained rats to drink milk solution from a tube, and then recorded how long it took to complete 100 licks. The time was progressively shortened over a training period of several days, until most of the rats completed their 100 licks within 50 seconds. The few who failed to meet the 50 second criterion were eliminated from the experiment. The successfully trained rats were then placed in the chamber, but without the drinking tube. After 15 seconds, electric shock was delivered through the floor. Control animals also spent 15 seconds in the chamber, but did not receive shock.

One week later, both control and experimental rats were retested in the chamber. Some were drugged and some were not. Consider first the results with the undrugged rats. Those which had not been shocked drank as rapidly as they had on the last day of training, while the previously shocked rats averaged about 200 seconds longer to make 100 licks. The obvious explanation is that the shock had made them fearful. Since tranquilizers reduce fear, it would have been reasonable to predict that the drinking times of the rats which had been shocked, and which were retested after having been injected with tranquilizer, would be intermediate between those of shocked and unshocked undrugged ones. Instead, shocked rats injected with amobarbital or the tranquilizer Wy 4036* had the longest drinking times of all. There was some drug specificity, because neither chlordiazepoxide nor chlorpromazine prolonged drinking time.

The prolongation of drinking times by amobarbital and Wy 4036 could not be accounted for by changes in thirst or in motor control, because it was not observed in the drugged but unshocked animals. General depressant side effects were also eliminated as a likely explanation by a modification of the experiment; the rats were given daily injections of oxazepam, a drug similar to Wy 4036, 30 minutes before each training and test session. By the end of the training

---

*The Wy comes from Wyeth Laboratories, where the drug was developed.

period, drinking was slightly elevated. Yet, drinking times of shocked animals were increased by oxazepam.

The explanation offered by Stein and Berger is that the drugs restored the memory of the shock, which had been partially repressed. To support their thesis, they reported that the drugged rats behaved in a fearful manner; they froze, defecated, and urinated more than did controls. In a further test of their hypothesis, they compared the effects of Wy 4036 and saline on suppression produced by different intensities of shock. They made the assumption that high levels of shock induce more repression than low levels, which counteracts the increased fear produced by the higher intensity; therefore, intensity of shock should not substantially influence suppression of drinking in rats treated with saline. On the other hand, amobarbital, by restoring the repressed memories, should have maximal effects in those instances where repression has been greatest. Hence, the longest drinking times should be exhibited in amobarbital-treated rats exposed to high intensity shock. The results were in the expected direction.

The experiments were carefully done. The data are fascinating. The explanation, however, does not necessarily follow from the data. The failure of shock intensity to affect drinking rate in saline-treated rats is at odds with much of the experimental literature. Stein and Berger's reasoning implies that once a period of time has elapsed for forgetting to take place, the original strength of an aversive stimulus is not a powerful determinant of behavior. Such is not the case, at least for some responses. For example, the magnitude of conditioned suppression is sensitive to the intensity of shock used in establishing the suppression (6).

There is an alternative explanation for the drug-induced increase in drinking time in the first part of the experiment. Since undrugged rats which had been shocked took longer to drink than did undrugged, unshocked rats, it is apparent that the animals retained at least partial memory of the shock and were fearful in the test chamber. But, small doses of barbiturates increase reactions to painful stimuli (15, 117), and when administered in the presence of severe pain or psychological disturbances sometimes cause delirium in man (117). Therefore, amobarbital probably increased drinking time not by restoring repressed memories, as the behavior of the shocked, undrugged rats shows that the memories were already present, but by interacting with the fear and potentiating it. The results would have much more convincingly fit the authors' interpretation had the interval between training and testing been sufficient to eliminate differences between shocked and unshocked undrugged animals.

In a further test of their hypothesis, Stein and Berger gave rats foot shock within the drinking chamber and then exposed one-half of them to ECS. Half of each of the two groups thus formed were treated with Wy 4036, the remainder with saline. When the rats were then tested for suppression of drinking, the most powerful effects were found in the drugged animals which had not received ECS. There was little suppression in the drug-ECS group, presumably because ECS had blocked consolidation of the painful memory, and it could not therefore be de-repressed. As evidence that ECS had blocked consolidation, the latencies of rats which had received saline-ECS were much shorter than the saline-no ECS rats.

The interpretation is not compatible with Bogoch's findings, cited earlier, that amobarbital restores memories lost after ECS. Stein and Berger concluded with the proposal that memory of a painful event stimulates the onset of a punishment process which shuts off the process of retrieval. Since tranquilizers block the punishment system, they facilitate the retrieval of painful memories. However, it seems illogical to say on the one hand that tranquilizers block the punishment system, and on the other to report that rats injected with the drugs and placed in the chamber in which they had received shock exhibit great fear. It would certainly be worthwhile to study the effects of amobarbital and Wy 4036 on forgotten events not associated with fear.

CONCLUSIONS

The reader should not be discouraged by the inadequacy of current theories to explain the actions of drugs on memory. Many conflicting reports have been presented, and the confusion is not likely to be eliminated in the foreseeable future. Several useful generalizations can, however, be made. The first is that there are drugs which improve learning under certain conditions. In fact, certain types of stimulants, such as strychnine in low doses, facilitate all aspects of learning and memory. Secondly, experiments from a variety of sources suggest that apparently lost memories can often be retrieved. A practical suggestion for retrieval is that attempted recall is most likely to be successful when conditions most closely approximate those under which the original learning occurred. Thirdly, the problem of task specificity must once again be stressed; Cook's experiments with yeast RNA illustrate that the nature of a task may determine to a great extent the action of a drug. Finally, and most importantly, the reader should be impressed with many of the experiments cited here, irrespective of the theories contrived to explain them. The theories may all eventually be discarded, but they are based on good, solid data. They certainly provide a rich lode of material, equal to the wildest imaginings of writers of science fiction.

REFERENCES

1. Abel, E. Marihuana and memory: acquisition or retrieval. Science, 1971, *173*: 1038–1040.
2. Agranoff, B. Recent studies on the stages of memory formation in the goldfish. In Byrne, W. (Ed.) *Molecular Approaches to Learning and Memory*. New York: Academic Press, 1970.
3. Albert, D. Memory in mammals: evidence for a system involving nuclear ribonucleic acid. Neuropsychologia, 1966, *4*:79–93.
4. Alpern, H., and Crabbe, J. Facilitation of the long-term store of memory with strychnine. Science, 1972, *177*:722–724.
5. Alpern, H., and Kimble, D. Retrograde amnesic effects of diethyl ether and bis (trifluorethyl) ether. J. Comp. Physiol. Psychol., 1967, *63*:168–171.
6. Annau, Z., and Kamin, L. The conditioned emotional response as a function of intensity of the US. J. Comp. Physiol. Psychol., 1961, *54*:428–432.
7. Astin, A., and Ross, S. Glutamic acid and human intelligence. Psychol. Bull., 1960, *57*:429–434.
8. Babich, F., Jacobson, A., Bubash, S., and Jacobson, A. Transfer of a response to naive rats by injection of ribonucleic acid extracted from trained rats. Science, 1965, *144*:656–657.
9. Banks, A., and Russell, R. Effects of chronic reductions in acetylcholinesterase activity on serial problem-solving behavior. J. Comp. Physiol. Psychol., 1967, *64*:262–267.
10. Barnhart, S., and Abbott, D. Dissociation of learning and meprobamate. Psychol. Rep., 1967, *20*:520–522.
11. Barondes, S., and Cohen, H. Puromycin effect on successive phases of memory storage. Science, 1966, *151*:594–595.
12. Barondes, S., and Cohen, H. Comparative effects of cycloheximide and puromycin on cerebral protein synthesis and consolidation of memory in mice. Brain Research, 1967, *4*:44–51.
13. Barondes, S., and Cohen, H. Delayed and sustained effect of acetoxycycloheximide on memory in mice. Proc. Nat. Acad. Sci., 1967, *58*:157–164.
14. Barondes, S., and Cohen, H. Arousal and the conversion of "short-term" to "long-term" memory. Proc. Nat. Acad. Sci., 1968, *61*:923–929.
15. Barry, H., III, and Miller, N. Comparison of drug effects on approach, avoidance, and escape motivation. J. Comp. Physiol. Psychol., 1965, *59*:18–24.
16. Bauer, R., and Duncan, N. Proactive facilitation of learning. J. Comp. Physiol. Psychol., 1971, *77*:521–527.
17. Beach, G., and Kimble, D. Activity and responsivity in rats after magnesium pemoline injections. Science, 1967, *155*:698–701.
18. Bindra, D., and Reichert, H. The nature of dissociation: effects of transitions between normal and barbiturate-induced states on reversal learning and habituation. Psychopharmacologia, 1967, *10*:330–344.
19. Bogoch, S. A preliminary study of postshock amnesia by amytal interview. Am. J. Psychiat., 1954, *111*:108–111.
20. Bovet, D., Bovet-Nitti, F., and Oliverio, A. Effects of nicotine on avoidance conditioning of inbred strains of mice. Psychopharmacologia, 1966, *10*:1–5.
21. Braud, L., and Braud, W. Biochemical transfer of relational responding. Science, 1972, *176*:942–944.
22. Bryant, R., Golub, A., McConnell, J., and Rosenblatt, F. Nonspecific behavioral effects of substances from mammalian brain. Science, 1972, *178*:521–522.
23. Burns, J., House, R., Fensch, F., and Miller, J. Effects of magnesium-pemoline and dextroamphetamine on human learning. Science, 1967, *155*:849–851.
24. Byrne, W. et al. Memory transfer. *Science*, 1966, *153*:658.
25. Byrne, W. In: Byrne, W. (Ed.) *Molecular Approaches to Learning and Memory*. New York: Academic Press, 1970.
26. Byrne, W., and Samuel, D. Behavioral modification by injection of brain extract prepared from a trained donor. Science, 1966, *154*:418.
27. Cameron, D., and Solyom, L. Effects of ribonucleic acid on memory. Geriatrics, 1961, *16*:74–81.

28. Carlton, P. Scopolamine, amphetamine, and light-reinforced responding. Psychon. Sci., 1966, 5:347–348.
29. Carlton, P. Brain-acetylcholine and inhibition. In: Tapp, J. (Ed.) *Reinforcement and Behavior*. New York: Academic, 1969.
30. Carlton, P., and Vogel, J. Studies of the amnesic properties of scopolamine. Psychon. Sci., 1965, 3:261–262.
31. Cherkin, A., and Lee-Teng, E. Interruption by halothane of memory consolidation in chicks. Fed. Proc., 1965, 24:328.
32. Chisholm, D., and Moore, J. Effects of chlordiazepoxide on the acquisition of shuttle avoidance in the rabbit. Psychon. Sci., 1970, 19:21–22.
33. Cicala, J., and Hartley, D. The effects of chlordiazepoxide on the acquisition and performance of a conditioned escape response in rats. Psychol. Rec., 1965, 15:435–440.
34. Cohen, H., and Barondes, S. Puromycin effect on memory may be due to occult seizures. Science, 1967, 157:333–334.
35. Conger, J. The effect of alcohol on conflict behavior in the albino rat. Quart. J. Stud. Alcohol, 1951, 12:1–29.
36. Conner, R., and Levine, S. The effects of adrenal hormones on the acquisition of signaled avoidance behavior. Hormones Behav., 1969, 1:73–83.
37. Cook, L., and Davidson, A. Effects of yeast RNA and other pharmacological agents on acquisition, retention and performance in animals. *In* Efron, D. (Ed.) *Psychopharmacology: A Review of Progress*. U.S. PHS Pub. No. 1836, 1968.
38. Cook, L., Davidson, A., Davis, D., Green, H., and Fellows, E. Ribonucleic acid: effect on conditioned behavior in rats. Science, 1963, 141:268–269.
39. Cooper, B., Potts, W., Morse, D., and Black, W. The effects of magnesium pemoline, caffeine and picrotoxin on a food-reinforced discrimination task. Psychon. Sci., 1969, 14:225–226.
40. Corning, W., and John, E. Effect of ribonuclease on retention of conditioned response in regenerated planarians. Science, 1961, 34:1363–1365.
41. Corning, W., and Riccio, D. The planarian controversy. *In* Byrne, W. *Molecular Approaches to Learning and Memory*. New York: Academic, 1970.
42. Deutsch, J. The cholinergic synapse and the site of memory. Science, 1971, 174: 788–794.
43. DiMascio, A. Drug effects on competitive-paired associate learning: relationship to and implications for the Taylor manifest anxiety scale. J. Psychol., 1963, 56:89–97.
44. Dingman, W., and Sporn, M. Molecular theories of memory. Science, 1964, 144: 26–29.
45. Domino, E. Some behavioral actions of nicotine. *In* von Euler, U. (Ed.) *Tobacco Alkaloids and Related Compounds*. Oxford: Pergamon, 1965.
46. Doty, B., and Doty, L. Effect of age and chlorpromazine on memory consolidation. J. Comp. Physiol., 1964, 57:331–334.
47. Doty, B., and Doty, L. Facilitation effects of amphetamine on avoidance conditioning in relation to age and problem difficulty. Psychopharmacologia, 1966, 9:234–241.
48. Doty, B., and Johnston, M. Effects of post-trial eserine administration, age and task difficulty on avoidance conditioning in rats. Psychon. Sci., 1966, 6: 101–102.
49. Enesco, H. Effect of vitamin B_{12} on neuronal RNA and on instrumental conditioning in the rat. *In* Wortis, J. (Ed.) *Recent Advances in Biological Psychiatry*, 10. New York: Plenum, 1968.
50. Enesco, H. RNA and memory: a re-evaluation of present data. J. Canad. Psychiat. Assoc., 1967, 12:29–33.
51. Erickson, C. Studies on the mechanism of avoidance facilitation by nicotine. Psychopharmacologia, 1971, 22:357–368.
52. Essman, W. Purine metabolites in memory consolidation. *In* Byrne, W. (Ed.) *Molecular Approaches to Learning and Memory*. New York: Academic Press, 1970.
53. Essman, W. Drug effects and memory and learning processes. Advan. Pharmacol. Chemother., 1971, 9:241–330.

54. Essman, W. Some neurochemical correlates of altered memory consolidation. Trans. N.Y. Acad. Sci., 1971, 32:948–973.

55. Essman, W., and Lehrer, G. Is there a chemical transfer of training? Fed. Proc., 1966, 25:208.

56. Fjerdingstad, E., Nissen, T., and Roigaard-Petersen, H. Effect of ribonucleic acid (RNA) extracted from the brain of trained animals on learning in rats. Scand. J. Psychol., 1965, 6:1–6.

57. Flexner, L., Flexner, J., and Roberts, R. Memory in mice analyzed with antibiotics. Science, 1967, 155:1377–1383.

58. Frank, B., Stein, D., and Rosen, J. Interanimal "memory" transfer: results from brain and liver homogenates. Science, 1970, 169:399–402.

59. Franks, C., and Trouton, D. Effects of amobarbital sodium and dexamphetamine sulfate on the conditioning of the eyeblink response. J. Comp. Physiol. Psychol., 1958, 51:220–222.

60. Frey, P., and Polidora, V. Magnesium pemoline: effect on avoidance conditioning in rats. Science, 1967, 155:1281–1282.

61. Gambetti, P., Gonatas, M., and Flexner, L. Puromycin: action on neuronal mitochondria. Science, 1968, 161:900–902.

62. Garg, M., and Holland, H. Consolidation and maze learning: a further study of posttrial injections of a stimulant drug (nicotine). Int. J. Neuropharm., 1968, 7:55–59.

63. Girden, E. The dissociation of blood pressure conditioned response under erythroidine. J. Exp. Psychol., 1942, 31:219–231.

64. Glasky, A., and Simon, L. Magnesium pemoline: enhancement of brain RNA polymerases. Science, 1966, 151:702–703.

65. Glow, P., and Rose, S. Cholinesterase levels and operant extinction. J. Comp. Physiol. Psychol., 1966, 61:165–172.

66. Goodwin, D., Powell, B., Bremer, D., Hoine, H., and Stern, J. Alcohol and recall: state-dependent effects in man. Science, 1969, 163:1358–1360.

67. Grinker, R., and Spiegel, J. War Neuroses in North Africa. New York: Josiah Macy, 1943.

68. Gruber, R., Stone, G., and Reed, D. Scopolamine-induced anterograde amnesia. Int. J. Neuropharm., 1967, 6:187–190.

69. Hanson, L. Evidence that the central action of (+)-amphetamine is mediated via catecholamines. Psychopharmacologia, 1967, 10:289–297.

70. Hardy, T., and Wakely, D. The amnesic properties of hyoscine and atropine in pre-anesthetic medication. Anaesthesia, 1962, 17:331–336.

71. Hearst, E. Effects of scopolamine on discriminated responding in the rat. J. Pharmacol. Exp. Ther., 1959, 126:349–358.

72. Hernandez-Peon, R., Scherrer, H., and Jouvet, M. Modification of electric activity in cochlear nucleus during "attention" in unanesthetized cats. Science, 1956, 123:331–332.

73. Hyden, H., and Egyhazi, E. Nuclear RNA changes of nerve cells during a learning experiment in rats. Proc. Nat. Acad. Sci., 1962, 48:1366–1373.

74. Jarvik, M. The influence of drugs on memory. In Steinber, H., de Reuck, A., and Knight, J. (Eds.) Animal Behavior and Drug Action. Boston: Little, Brown, 1964.

75. Jarvik, M. Effects of drugs on memory. In Black, P. (Ed.) Drugs and the Brain. Balt.: Johns Hopkins, 1969.

76. Kamin, L. The retention of an incompletely learned avoidance response. J. Comp. Physiol. Psychol., 1957, 50:457–460.

77. Katz, J., and Halstead, W. Protein organization and mental function. Comp. Psychol. Monogr., 1950, 20:1–38.

78. Keleman, K., and Bovet, D. Effects of drugs upon the defensive behavior of rats. Acta Physiol. Acad. Sci. Hung., 1961, 19:143–154.

79. Kornberg, A. Biologic synthesis of deoxyribonucleic acids. Science, 1960, 131:1503–1508.

80. Lashley, K. The effect of strychnine and caffeine upon rate of learning. Psychobiology, 1917, 1:141–170.

81. Latane, B., and Schachter, S. Adrenalin and avoidance learning. J. Comp. Physiol. Psychol., 1962, 55:369–372.
82. Laties, V., and Weiss, B. Behavioral mechanisms of drug action. In Black, P. (Ed.) Drugs and the Brain. Baltimore: Johns Hopkins University Press, 1969.
83. Leaton, R. The effects of scopolamine on exploratory motivated behavior in the rat. Paper presented at Eastern Psychol. Assoc. Meetings, 1967.
84. Luttges, M., Johnson, T., Buck, C., Holland, J., and McGaugh, J. An explanation of "transfer of learning" by nucleic acid. Science, 1966, 151:834–837.
85. Magoun, H. Research with implications for learning. In Pribram, K. (Ed.) On the Biology of Learning. New York: Harcourt Brace Jovanovich, 1969.
86. McConnell, J. Memory transfer through cannibalism in planarians. J. Neuro-psychiat., 1962, 3:42–48.
87. McConnell, J., Jacobson, A., and Kimble, D. Effects of regeneration upon retention of a conditioned response in the planarian. J. Comp. Physiol. Psychol., 1959, 52:1–5.
88. McGaugh, J. Time-dependent processes in memory storage. Science, 1966, 153: 1351–1358.
89. McGaugh, J., and Petrinovich, L. The effect of strychnine sulphate on maze learning. Am. J. Psychol., 1959, 72:99–102.
90. McGaugh, J., and Petrinovich, L. Effects of drugs on learning and memory. Int. Rev. Neurobiol., 1965, 8:139–196.
91. Melges, F., Tinklenberg, J., Hollister, L., and Gillepspie, H. Temporal disintegration and depersonalization during marihuana intoxication. Arch. Gen. Psychiat., 1970, 23:204–210.
92. Mendenhall, M. The effect of sodium phenobarbital on learning and reasoning in white rats. J. Comp. Psychol., 1940, 29:257–276.
93. Meyers, B. Some effects of scopolamine on a passive avoidance response in rats. Psychopharmacologia, 1965, 8:111–119.
94. Meyers, B., and Domino, E. The effect of cholinergic blocking drugs on spontaneous alternation in rats. Arch. Int. Pharmacodyn. Ther., 1964, 150:525–529.
95. Milner, P. Physiological Psychology. New York: Holt, Rinehart and Winston, 1970.
96. Moore, K. Effects of α-methyltyrosine on brain catecholamines and conditioned behavior in guinea pigs. Life Sci., 1966, 5:55–65.
97. Moran, G., Ahmad, S., and Meagher, R. Adrenalin and avoidance learning: partial replications. J. Exper. Res. Personal., 1970, 4:84–89.
98. Nash, H. Alcohol and Caffeine; A Study of Their Psychological Effects. Springfield, Ill.: Charles C Thomas, 1962.
99. Nash, H. Psychological effects of amphetamines and barbiturates. J. Nerv. Ment. Dis., 1962, 134:203–217.
100. Overton, D. Dissociated learning in drug states (state dependent learning). In Efron, D. (Ed.) Psychopharmacology: A Review of Progress. U.S. PHS Pub. No. 1836, 1968.
101. Overton, D. State-dependent or "dissociated" learning produced with pentobarbital. J. Comp. Physiol. Psychol., 1964, 57:3–12.
102. Pearlman, C., Sharpless, S., and Jarvik, M. Retrograde amnesia produced by anesthetic and convulsant agents. J. Comp. Physiol. Psychol., 1961, 54:109–112.
103. Petrinovich, L. Drug facilitation of learning: strain differences. Psychopharmacologia, 1967, 10:375–378.
104. Plotnikoff, N. Magnesium pemoline: enhancement of learning and memory of a conditioned avoidance response. Science, 1966, 151:703–704.
105. Plotnikoff, N. Learning and memory enhancement by pemoline and magnesium hydroxide (PMH). In Wortis, J. (Ed.) Recent Advances in Biological Psychiatry, 10. New York: Plenum Publishing Corp., 1968.
106. Plotnikoff, N., and Evans, A. Enhancement of conditioned photic evoked responses in the rabbit by pemoline and magnesium hydroxide. Int. J. Neuropsychiat., 1967, 3:263–267.
107. Quarton, G., and Talland, G. The effects of methamphetamine and pentobarbital on two measures of attention. Psychopharmacologia, 1962, 3:66–71.
108. Quatermain, D., McEwen, B., and Azmitia, E. Amnesia produced by electro-

convulsive shock or cycloheximide: conditions for recovery. Science, 1970, 17:683–686.

109. Rech, R., Borys, H., and Moore, K. Alterations in behavior and brain catecholamine levels in rats treated with α-methyltyrosine. J. Pharmacol. Exp. Ther., 1966, 153:412–419.

110. Reinis, S. The formation of conditioned reflexes in rats after the parenteral administration of brain homogenate. Activitas Nervosa Super., 1965, 7:167–168.

111. Rosenbaum, M., Cohen, H., and Barondes, S. Effect of intracerebral saline on amnesia produced by inhibitors of cerebral protein synthesis. Comm. Behav. Biol., 1968, 2:47–50.

112. Rosenblatt, F. In Ungar, G. (Ed.) Molecular Mechanisms in Memory and Learning. New York: Plenum Publishing Corp., 1970.

113. Rosenzweig, M. Effects of environment on development of brain and behavior. In Tobach, E., Aronson, L., and Shaw, E. (Eds.) The Biopsychology of Development. New York: Academic Press, 1971.

114. Russell, R., Watson, R., and Frankenhaeuser, M. Effects of chronic reductions in brain cholinesterase activity on acquisition and extinction of a conditioned avoidance response. Scand. J. Psychol., 1961, 2:21–29.

115. Russell, W., and Nathan, P. Traumatic amnesia. Brain, 1946, 69:280–300.

116. Scheckel, C., Boff, E., Dahlen, P., and Smart, T. Behavioral effects in monkeys of racemates of two biologically active marijuana constituents. Science, 1968, 160:1467–1469.

117. Sharpless, S. Hypnotics and sedatives I. the barbiturates. In Goodman, L., and Gilman, A. The Pharmacological Basis of Therapeutics. New York: Macmillan Publishing Co., 1965.

118. Smith, R. Magnesium pemoline: lack of facilitation in human learning, memory, and performance tests. Science, 1967, 155:603–605.

119. Stein, D., and Rosen, J. Letter to editor. Science, 1972, 178:522–523.

120. Stein, H., and Yellin, T. Pemoline and magnesium hydroxide: lack of effect on RNA and protein synthesis. Science, 1967, 157:96–97.

121. Stein, L., and Berger, B. Paradoxical fear-increasing effects of tranquilizers: evidence of repression of memory in the rat. Science, 1969, 166:253–256.

122. Stevens, D., Resnick, O., and Krus, D. The effects of p-chlorophenylalanine, a depletor of brain serotonin, on behavior: facilitation of discrimination learning. Life Sci., 1967, 6:2215–2220.

123. Stewart, J., Krebs, W., and Kaczender, E. State-dependent learning produced with steroids. Nature, 1967, 216:1223–1224.

124. Storm, T., and Smart, R. Dissociation; a possible explanation of some features of alcoholism, and implication for its treatment. Quart. J. Stud. Alcohol, 1965, 26:111–115.

125. Stratton, L., and Petrinovich, L. Post-trial injection of an anticholinesterase drug and maze learning in two strains of mice. Psychopharmacologia, 1963, 5:47–54.

126. Taber, R., and Banuazizi, A. CO_2-induced retrograde amnesia in a one-trial learning situation. Psychopharmacologia, 1966, 9:382–391.

127. Talland, G., and McGuire, M. Test of learning and memory with Cylert. Psychopharmacologia, 1967, 10:445–451.

128. Ungar, G. Role of proteins and peptides in learning and memory. In Ungar, G. (Ed.) Molecular Mechanisms in Memory and Learning. New York: Plenum Publishing Corp., 1970.

129. Ungar, G., and Oceguera-Navarro, C. Transfer of habituation by material extracted from brain. Nature, 1965, 207:301–302.

130. Varner, W. The effects of alcohol on two maze habits of albino rats. Psychol. Bull., 1933, 30:616.

131. Vogel, J. The differential effect of scopolamine on rewarded and punished behavior. Unpublished doctoral dissertation, Rutgers University, 1968.

132. Vogel, W., Broverman, D., Draguns, J., and Klaiber, E. The role of glutamic acid in cognitive behaviors. Psychol. Bull., 1966, 65:367–382.

133. Waelsch, H., and Lajtha, A. Protein metabolism in the nervous system. Physiol. Rev., 1961, 41:709–736.

134. Warwick, K., and Eysenck, H. Experimental studies of the behavioural effects of nicotine. Pharmakopsychiat., 1968, 1:145–169.
135. Weil, A., and Zinberg, N. Acute effects of marihuana on speech. Nature, 1969, 222:434–437.
136. Weissman, A. Effect of anticonvulsant drugs on electroconvulsive shock-induced retrograde amnesia. Arch. Intern. Pharmacodyn., 1965, 154:122–130.
137. Weissman, A. Drugs and retrograde amnesia. Int. Rev. Neurobiol., 1967, 10: 167–198.
138. Weitzner, M. Manifest anxiety, amphetamine, and performance. J. Psychol., 1965, 60:71–79.
139. Wenzel, B., and Jeffrey, D. The effect of immunosympathectomy on the behavior of mice in aversive situations. Physiol. Behav., 1967, 2:193–202.
140. Whitehouse, J. The effects of physostigmine on discrimination learning. Psychopharmacologia, 1966, 9:183–188.
141. Zimmerman, F., and Ross, S. Effect of glutamic acid and other amino acids on maze learning in the rat. Arch. Neurol. Psychiat., 1944, 51:446–451.
142. Zinkin, S., and Miller, A. Recovery of memory after amnesia induced by ECS. Science, 1967, 155:102–104.

CHAPTER 12

CREATIVITY

The problem of generalization from rat to man, which complicates the interpretation of experimental findings in many areas, is of no concern to researchers in the field of creativity. Even the best of animal trainers are unable to teach rats to write sonnets (although members of several primate species, including chimpanzees, gorillas, orangutans, and cebus monkeys, have produced paintings which were judged by critics to be of very high caliber [32]). For the most part, products which are of esthetic interest to man are created by man. Therefore, research on drug-induced modifications of creative potential has been conducted solely with human volunteers.

The field is plagued by many serious problems, foremost of which is inadequate criteria for evaluating creative efforts. There is little agreement on this point in texts on esthetics (19, 37, 41). Nor do psychologists agree. One of the more popular tests for measuring creativity was designed by Mednick (31). The subject is required to find a word which provides an effective link between three others. For example, he might be given "rat," "blue," and "cottage." The correct answer is "cheese." Mednick claimed that scores on his test correlated with ratings of creativity of architectural and psychology graduate students. However, Jackson and Messick (21) argued that since there is only one correct answer for each item, the test reflects intelligence rather than creativity. They suggested four criteria for judging creative products: unusualness, appropriateness to the demands of the situation, power to transform the reality of the observer, and condensation in meaning. Whether or not the criteria are meaningful, they are difficult to apply.

Four of the many other tests in current use are as follows:

Word Association Test

Subjects are asked to respond with the first word which comes into their minds when they are presented with a stimulus word. Unusual responses are scored positively.

Mosaic Design Test

Subjects provided with a box of mosaic tiles create a design which is judged on the basis of originality, organization, and esthetic appeal.

Unusual Uses Test

The subject must list various uses to which each of several common objects, such as bricks and toothpicks, could be put. Both quantity and quality of responses are scored.

Productive Thinking

Hypothetical conditions, such as the synthesis of a new gas with unusual properties, are described, and subjects are asked to discuss what the consequences might be.

Art Critics

The proliferation of tests of creativity underscores the lack of unanimity among psychologists. Nor do painting, drama, literature, or music critics agree on criteria by which works of art can be judged. Many works which are now highly regarded were accorded hostile receptions by the critics of their day. Just a few of the more prominent artists whose works were received harshly are van Gogh, Picasso, Cézanne, Kokoschka, Racine, Beethoven, Stravinsky, and Mozart. However, although perfect consensus among psychologists and among art critics may never be reached, they are probably capable of making generally reliable estimates of the merits of works of art.

A PRIORI REASONS FOR BELIEVING THAT DRUGS MIGHT ENHANCE CREATIVITY

There are many reasons why some drugs in some circumstances might enhance creativity. Some people are so beset by personal problems that they are incapable of behaving in constructive ways. In such cases, creative expression may be facilitated indirectly by the use of drugs which have as their primary action the relief of anxiety, depression, or psychotic agitation. Perhaps the role of alcohol in the lives of such literary giants as F. Scott Fitzgerald, Tennessee Williams, Thomas Wolfe, and William Faulkner can be attributed to its ability to release creative expression by relieving anxiety.

Stimulant drugs such as caffeine and amphetamine might occasionally be useful in sustaining a person during an outpouring of creative effort, where failure to remain alert would result in loss of motivation or of valuable ideas. However, routine reliance on stimulants for the purpose of improving creativity is probably unwise. There is an extensive literature which shows that high doses of amphetamine produce stereotyped behavior, the antithesis of creativity. Rats, guinea pigs, pigeons, and cats repeat the same behaviors for hours at a time (36). Amphetamine psychosis in man is a predictable consequence of high dose use, and in many respects resembles schizophrenic behavior; in particular, there are elements of compulsivity such as repetition of single words or phrases (11). Amphetamine increases ability to attend to dull tasks which have already been well learned, such as naming colors; it reduces effectiveness when the requirement is to view things from new perspectives (discussed in 7). It would appear, therefore, that the amphetamines are poor prospects for enhancing creativity.

The class of drugs which has been most thoroughly studied for ability to modify creative expression is the hallucinogens, which includes LSD, mescaline, psilocybin, marijuana, morning-glory seeds, the *Amanita muscaria* mushroom, peyote, dimethyltryptamine, and diethyltryptamine. They are all capable of altering consciousness, a process which often precedes creative acts. Hallucinatory episodes may have much in common with creative thinking. See Table 12.1 for some examples of altered states of consciousness during which were formulated many important ideas and inventions.

Harman et al. (18) have constructed a table (reprinted as Table 12.2) which indicates specific ways in which hallucinogenic drugs might act to modify creative output. Points number 2 and 9 are especially worth emphasizing because of their similarity to the rules for successful brainstorming, a technique developed by Osborn (33) which is still widely used in courses on creative thinking.

Brainstorming usually requires group participation. A problem is presented to a group and the members are instructed to follow three simple rules:

1. Criticism of ideas is not permitted.
2. Quantity of ideas is desired.
3. Remote, bizarre, and wild ideas are encouraged.

TABLE 12.1 Altered States of Consciousness and Creativity

INDIVIDUAL	ALTERED STATE	ACCOMPLISHMENT
Robert Louis Stevenson	dreaming	dreamed and remembered complete stories, e.g., "Dr. Jekyll and Mr. Hyde"
Wagner	dreaming	Rheingold theme
Tartini	dreaming	"heard" sonata, which gave inspiration for "Devil's Trill"
Mozart, Schumann, and Saint-Saens	dreaming	all first heard some of their music during dreams
Niels Bohr	dreaming	conceptual model of atom
Otto Loewi	dreaming	concept of transmission in nervous system is chemical, not electrical
Elias Howe	dreaming	sewing machine
Kekulé	dreaming	discovery of structure of benzene ring
A. R. Wallace	malarial fever	theory of evolution by natural selection
Tissot	daydream	painting: "The Ruins"
Rachmaninoff	hypnosis	Concerto No. 2 in C Minor for Piano and Orchestra

Someone is appointed to keep a verbatim record of attempts at solution. Then, sometime after the termination of the session, the proposed solutions are evaluated.

There have been several modifications of the brainstorming method, most notably the technique devised by Gordon (16). However, the basic rules remain unchanged, and brainstorming and its variants have proved successful (9, 34). It should be noted that brainstorming sessions give rise to many ideas which are of little value and must be discarded. The crucial consideration is that there are some good ideas which might not have otherwise occurred. Similarly, the creation of many inferior artworks does not invalidate the claim that hallucinogenic drugs foster creativity. The relevant question is whether or not some superior works owe their existence to the drugs.

Hallucinogens may provide an impetus to creativity by supply-

TABLE 12.2   Some Reported Characteristics of the Psychedelic Experience*

THOSE SUPPORTING CREATIVITY	THOSE HINDERING CREATIVITY
1. Increased access to unconscious data	1. Capacity for logical thought processes may be diminished.
2. More fluent free association; increased ability to play spontaneously with hypotheses, metaphors, paradoxes, transformations, relationships, and so forth.	2. Ability to consciously direct concentration may be reduced.
3. Heightened ability for visual imagery and fantasy.	3. Inability to control imaginary and conceptual sequences.
4. Relaxation and openness.	4. Anxiety and agitation.
5. Sensory inputs more acutely perceived.	5. Outputs (verbal and visual communication abilities may be constricted).
6. Heightened empathy with external processes, objects, and people.	6. Tendency to focus upon "inner problems" of a personal nature.
7. Aesthetic sensibility heightened.	7. Experienced beauty may lessen tension to obtain aesthetic experience in the act of creation.
8. Enhanced "sense of truth" and ability to "see through" false solutions and phony data.	8. Tendency to become absorbed in hallucinations and illusions.
9. Lessened inhibition and reduced tendency to censor own creations by premature negative judgment.	9. Finding the best solution may seem unimportant.
10. Motivation may be heightened by suggestion and providing the right set.	10. "This-worldly" tasks may seem trivial, and hence motivation may be decreased.

*Reprinted with permission of author and publisher: Harman, W., McKim, R., Mogar, R., Fadiman, J., and Stolaroff, M. Psychedelic agents in creative problem solving—a pilot study. Psychological Reports, 1966, 19:211–277. (Table 1: "Some reported characteristics of the psychedelic experience", p. 214.)

ing the artist with a unique, rich, and emotionally intense experience. The value of experience to artists was expressed by Nietzsche: "Poets act shamelessly towards their experiences: they exploit them."

Hallucinogens may affect physiological systems which influence creativity. For example, LSD (and many other drugs with no proposed effects on creativity) increases body temperature, and performance on a wide variety of complex tasks is greatest when body temperature is high (22). Green et al. (17) have adduced evidence that an EEG pattern of low frequency alpha and theta rhythms often accompanies creativity. LSD *increases* alpha frequency, and marijuana decreases it slightly. (See Chapter 1 for an explanation of EEG patterns.)

STATEMENTS BY AUTHORITIES

Partially as a result of uncertain criteria, but for other reasons as well (discussed later), there is a wide range of opinion concerning the efficacy of hallucinogenic drugs in enhancing creativity, as the following sampling reveals:

Donald Louria: LSD-induced creativity is a myth (27, p. 142).

Timothy Leary: Psychedelic drugs. . . enhance the creative perspective, but the ability to convert your new perspective, however
glorious it may be, into a communication form still requires
the technical skill of a musician or a painter or a composer (26,
p. 143).

James Goddard: Mind-stretching claims for LSD are "pure bunk"
(quoted in 6).

John Finlater: Creatively, LSD is a complete bust. Users talk about
creativity, but they don't do anything about it. The painter stops
painting and fantasy replaces reality (35).

Alan Watts: Having seen some of the more recent works that have
come out of the psychedelic experience, I think that LSD has
been very beneficial (to the creative experience). These works
have returned the glory to Western art. We haven't had anything
like it since illuminated manuscripts and stained glass windows.
It's difficult to estimate its value in literature. I can only say
from my own point of view that I have derived all kinds of ideas
for lectures and writings from it (35).

Sidney Cohen: An overestimate of one's capabilities is not infrequent. Often mental productions are not as highly assessed
when they are later examined in the sober state (10).

Stanley Yolles: It may. . . lead to heightened suggestibility and a
faulty perception, really an exaggerated notion of thinking more
clearly, profoundly, and creatively (50).

Differences of opinion, as exemplified by the above statements,
must be frustrating to those who believe that a dispassionate view-
ing of the evidence should produce consensus. Of course, the view-
ing is anything but dispassionate. In addition, the field is beset by
several complex methodological problems which allow for alternative
interpretations of data.

PSYCHOMETRIC DATA

The Studies

There have been only a few studies for which the dependent
variable has been score on an objective psychological test. Aldrich
(1) tested claims that marijuana improves the ability of jazz musicians by giving a synthetic marijuana-like compound to 12 musicians
who were experienced users. Their performance was unchanged or
impaired on a test which involved making judgments about which
of two musical notes was higher in pitch, louder in intensity, richer

in timbre, and so on. Significantly, 8 of the 12 believed that their scores had improved.

Zegans et al. (51) administered tests of personality and of creativity to 31 paid male volunteers, who then drank glasses of water which, for 20 of them, contained 0.5 $\mu g/kg$ LSD. The men were retested two hours later, when the drug had taken effect. There were only small differences on the various measures of creativity between men given a placebo and those given the drug. However, those subjects who were judged on the basis of the pre-drug personality tests to have an "integrated mixture of affect and intelligence" showed the greatest improvements upon retesting. The poorest showings of drugged subjects were on tests requiring visual attention.

McGlothlin et al. (30) used male volunteers who had had no prior experience with LSD. They were randomly assigned to 3 groups which received either 25 μg LSD, 200 μg LSD, or 20 mg amphetamine. The drugs were given on three separate occasions, with unspecified intervals between them. The groups which received amphetamine and the low dose of LSD served as controls. Many tests, including seven measures of creativity, were administered two weeks and again six months after the third drug session. The tests did not distinguish between the three groups, indicating that there are no residual effects of LSD on tests of creativity. No data were reported on acute effects of LSD on creativity. McGlothlin et al., and several other investigators as well (4, 49), found that skill at freehand drawing was impaired.

Shortcomings of the Studies

The Zegans et al. and McGlothlin et al. studies suffer from many serious shortcomings, some of which were recognized by the authors themselves. They are detailed here because the studies are often cited as evidence that LSD does not improve creativity. Studies in which no differences between groups are found are always somewhat inconclusive, because the results might have been caused by insensitive tests or inadequate control of the relevant variables. In the Zegans et al. study, only eight of the men who scored well on the pre-drug personality test were given LSD, yet these were the men who showed the greatest improvements with LSD; the drug would have had to exert a very powerful effect in order for the results to have been significant. In both studies, the chance of getting powerful effects was minimized by the authors' reliance on tests which put a premium on speed of response. Reference to Table 12.2 will show that the claims of enhanced creativity from LSD do not have increased speed of response as one of the bases.

A very serious problem is that the typical laboratory setting, which is appropriate for most scientific work, is hardly ideal for studies of creativity. Consider the comment of Simon Vinkenoog, a Dutch poet, who described an experiment in which he served as subject (24, p. 166): "In 1959, LSD was inflicted on me by a team of unqualified doctors-to-be who messed up some of my most beautiful experiences ever by having me fill in silly forms, by hooking me up to an electroencephalograph going momomomomomomomomo, etc." Poetic expression is not fostered by the filling in of forms.

When amphetamines are tested for their effects on motor performance, significant improvements are rarely observed except when the participants are highly skilled (42). By the same token, hallucinogenic drugs may improve the creativity only of already highly creative persons. In neither study were subjects selected on such a basis.

In both studies, subjects were given a battery of tests prior to taking LSD, then were retested some time after ingestion. Changes in performance between pre- and post-drug tests furnished the basis of comparison between drug and placebo subjects. This paradigm biases the results against LSD, for subjects in the placebo group would be expected to derive the most benefit from their first exposure to the test; subjects in the LSD group would be hampered by the phenomenon called state dependent learning (discussed earlier on pp. 274 to 276). Briefly, state dependent learning is said to occur when a subject who learns a task in one state (e.g., a drug condition) fails to recall it when tested in another state.

It is inappropriate to test drugs just once—or even a few times. The drug state involves many profound perceptual, motor, and cognitive changes, so much so that users may be unable or unwilling to ignore them completely in order to give full attention to paper and pencil tests. In addition, they may suffer considerable anxiety, which can interfere with performance. With respect to this point, it is worth noting that people who use marijuana for the first time show impaired performance on several tests, whereas chronic users do not (48).

Positive Psychometric Data

Harman et al. (18) provided an environment more conducive to creative efforts. They picked creative people from a variety of professions who had been stymied in their work by problems which demanded creative solutions. The subjects received 200 mg of mescaline, and then relaxed and listened to quiet music while they waited for it to take effect. They were then retested on three tests of creativity—the first tests had been administered a few days prior to the drug experience—and they improved on all. The improvement may be accounted for simply by virtue of prior exposure to the tests. A more serious flaw in the experiment is that it lacked a group of subjects given the same instructions to relax and listen to music in comfortable surroundings. At present, the only safe conclusion is that some aspect(s) of the procedure, not necessarily involving mescaline, facilitates test-taking performance. Other parts of the experiment are considered below.

CREATIVE PRODUCTS

Because of the dearth of well-controlled laboratory studies, and as a result of the interest in the question of possible induction of creative states by hallucinogenic drugs, it is necessary to seek information from sources outside the laboratory. The approach is a dangerous one. For one thing, the capacity for self-criticism is often blunted while the drug is acting, so that first-person accounts are unreliable. A particularly interesting example of self-deception has been described by William James (reported in 14, p. 77). He had been experimenting with nitrous oxide, and had on several occasions experienced mystic revelations. However, he had been unable to record his moments of illumination, or remember them when he awoke, until one night he managed to write down his monumental thoughts before losing consciousness. Upon arising, he rushed to his paper, to find written:

Hogamus, Higamous
Man is polygamous,
Higamous, Hogamous,
Woman is monogamous.

First-person accounts are those of successful artists. Even if noncreative people have benefited from drug experiences, their improved work has still not been of high enough quality to merit attention. Exceptions are the paintings of many psychiatric patients undergoing LSD therapy, which were "far above average for the beginning art student" (43, p. 54); and Boszormenyi's finding (5) that subjects who had taken diethyltryptamine reported awakened interest in art and writing. Exceptions aside, the fact that proven artists have been creative while in the drug state hardly points to the drug as the causative agent. To cite an obvious example, much has been made of the fact that Aldous Huxley wrote parts of three books, *Heaven and Hell, The Doors of Perception,* and *Island,* while under the influence of mescaline. To say that he was helped by the drug ignores his prior standing as one of the most important and prolific writers of the twentieth century. *Brave New World* and several other of Huxley's novels have received greater critical acclaim than any of the three books associated with his use of mescaline. At the least, the three books do show that a drug habit is not totally incompatible with creative acts.

The writing of a novel, the composition of a symphony, or the execution of a major painting occupies a much greater time span than the duration of a single drug trip. Yet accounts of drug-induced creativity are generally not explicit about specific aspects which are and are not due to drugs. Can a drug be said to have important effects on creativity if it inspires the conception of a work of art, but nothing more?

One of the most famous poems in the English language is Coleridge's "Kubla Khan." Its purported genesis is well known. Coleridge was ill and had received an anodyne, most probably opium, from which he fell into a profound sleep in the midst of reading a passage about the emperor Kubla Khan. He had very vivid dreams and awakened with full recollection of them. He began writing them down, but was interrupted by a visitor. When he returned to writing he was able to recontruct only the fragment which still survives. More recently, Robert Graves wrote poetry after ingesting the *Psilocybe* mushroom. Peyote is the muse of poet Michael McClure, while Henri Michaux uses marijuana.

Many other writers have used hallucinogenic drugs. Ken Kesey took peyote and LSD just prior to writing several passages of *One Flew Over the Cuckoo's Nest.* LSD was used by Allan Ginsberg in writing poems for *Kaddish and Other Poems;* and by Alan Watts, who also used mescaline and psilocybin while writing *The Joyous Cosmology.* William Burroughs attributed much of his *Naked Lunch* to marijuana.

Masters (44, p. 286) tried a novel approach to induce creative writing. He used a male psychologist as his subject. The psychologist was given LSD and was then told that he would have one minute to construct a story; he was further instructed that a minute was all that he would need because his subjective experience of time would be much longer. The subject's comments follow:

By God, it was strange. I have never had an experience like that. Well, it seemed to be the beginning of a novel. It was an English country estate and there was a car. It had a woman sitting in it, a rather middle-aged attractive but not beautiful woman, and a little dog, and the chauffeur came up to her and—but this is why I laughed. Talk about a writer "getting inside" his characters! First I was inside of this woman, then I was inside the chauffeur, and then I was inside of the dog, and I really could feel my body and my personality change in each case as I became first one and then the other. I tell you, I was really getting into those characters in a very literal sense but it would take forever, in that way, to do a novel. I recognized this and so I kind of pulled back and the rest of the time I just observed what was happening, as if I were watching a film. But it wasn't a novel, it was kind of a little, strange vignette, very poignant, and very curious. This woman, you see, was going down to the pier where the body of her husband was being returned to her from some place where he had died. He had been in the diplomatic service. All of the time she is driving down to pick up the body, this little dog is sitting there with her in the back seat of the big old touring car and is looking from side to side. Both the woman and the dog have perfectly inscrutable faces, so one has no idea at all what she is thinking or feeling. And she meets the ship where her husband's body is being brought off and a lot of dignitaries are on hand to posthumously give him medals and there are salutes being fired and evidently he has performed some great act that this country is honoring him for. She attends the ceremony. Through it all she just stands there, and it isn't possible at all to guess what she is thinking or feeling, and when it is over she gets back into her car. The chauffeur is driving her back to the estate, the little dog is sitting there as before, looking from side to side impassively, not very interested in anything. But then suddenly a rabbit jumps alongside the road. The dog gets very, very excited and causes this woman to notice the rabbit. And then, in an instant, this same woman seems to display a kind of murderous fury and she reaches down and picks up a gun and shoots the rabbit right through the head — and everything freezes for a minute right there — the excited expression on the face of the dog, the curious look of fury on the face of the woman, the rabbit just as its brains are blasted out, only the chaffeur as he was before. This scene just hangs together for a strange, terrible few moments, and then time and movement go back to their normal pace, the face of the woman is entirely inscrutable again, the dog looks from side to side impassively. They turn up into her driveway and the car stops at her house. But you have this strange, frightening sense of that one instance when she and the dog came to life and she blew the rabbit's brains out — that just for a moment something awful had been revealed about this woman and possibly about her relationship to her husband. Although what was revealed is left undefined, you know that there is something latent in her and the inscrutable face and the utterly conventional manner cover something that has the possibility of breaking through.

It would be necessary to give the subject the same instructions without the drug, and to test others as well, before the significance of the findings could be assessed. Even then, their relevance for the production of meaningful works of art would still have to be demonstrated.

The procedures and objective data from the Harman et al. study have been described and criticized. In the main part of the study, 27 professional people worked for four hours while they were under the influence of mescaline on problems whose solution had been eluding them. They were requested to answer a questionnaire six to eight weeks later. The results were impressive. Of 44 problems attempted, there were:

20   new avenues for investigation opened
2   working models completed

1	developmental model to test solution authorized
6	solutions accepted for construction or production
10	partial solutions obtained, being developed further or being applied
1	no further activity since session
4	no solutions obtained

The subjects also listed benefits of a more general nature, such as increased ability to communicate and to respond to pressure. Four architects who participated in the study agreed that LSD aided them in visualizing three-dimensional space and heightened their perceptivity.

Kiyo Izumi is an architect who was commissioned to design a building for the mentally ill. By way of preparation, Izumi took LSD and then visited with and spoke to mental patients confined in various hospitals; he believed that he would thus be enabled to achieve the patients' perspectives. He constructed plans according to several guiding principles which were developed from his experience. These were the more important of his goals (20):

1. To provide as much privacy as practicable.
2. To minimize ambiguity in architectural design and detail.
3. To create an environment without intimidating qualities.
4. To create spatial relationships that reduce the frequency and intensity of undesirable confrontations.

The completed building, which is now the Yorkton Psychiatric Center, has many innovative design features. Izumi said ". . . it is my firm conviction that, without my LSD experience, many of these insights might not have been possible." Of course, the results may have limited applicability to the general problem of creativity.

Barron (3) administered psilocybin to a ballet dancer and then filmed her actions during the next five hours. The members of her troupe later viewed the film and they felt that she had done some unusual and worthwhile movements. The report would have been more convincing if she had also been filmed while performing without the drug but with instructions to be innovative. If the troupe members were not told which was the psilocybin segment, and still offered the same comments about that segment, it might be concluded that psilocybin helps interpretive dancers.

Berlin et al. (4) tested four well-known graphic artists after they had ingested either LSD or mescaline. Their motor skills, as measured by an objective test (Draw-A-Person), were impaired; however, the consequence of the impairment was judged to be desirable, in that their use of lines was much freer. They also used more vivid colors and were more acutely aware of dead spaces on the canvas. Their work was judged by other qualified artists to have greater esthetic value than their earlier works. The study is subject to the same criticism as the previous report, namely, that the judges were not blind as to the source of inspiration for the artwork. Experimenter bias is an insidious factor. People who are biased in favor of a particular outcome tend to make errors in favor of that outcome, even when they are dealing with objective data (38); subjective judgments are much more easily influenced by experimenter bias.

There have been several reports on the response of painters to LSD or mescaline. Tonini and Montanari (46) gave several different drugs, at various times, to a 30-year-old painter who was judged to be in good physical and emotional health. His drawings were then collected and analyzed. After 500 mg of mescaline he had compelling hallucinations, illusions, and synesthesia. As a result, he did not paint much; vivid colors were heavily emphasized in

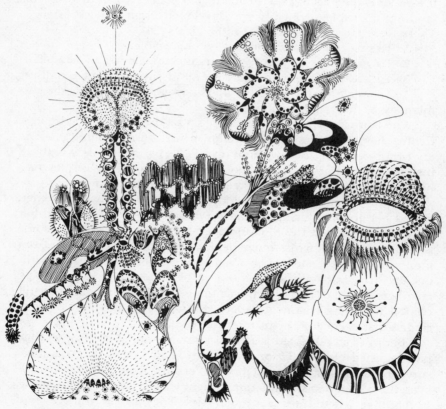

Figure 12–1 Untitled ink on paper drawing by Isaac Abrams done in 1966. 11″ × 14″. Abrams had never painted until taking LSD in 1965. (From *Psychedelic Art,* by Robert E. L. Masters and Jean Houston, 1968, Balance House, p. 39.)

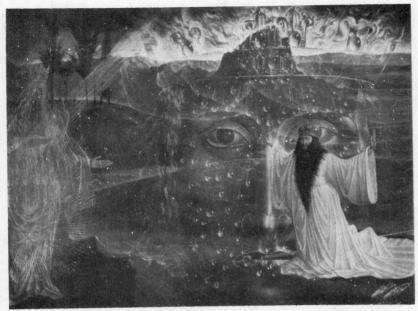

Figure 12-2   Painting by Ernst Fuchs (as it appears in *Psychedelic Art,* by Robert E. L. Masters and Jean Houston, 1968, Balance House, p. 31).

those works which he did complete. The authors felt that 60 μg of LSD or 30 mg of amphetamine, or the combination of amphetamine with mescaline or LSD, did not greatly affect the quality of his work for better or worse.

Hartmann (45) observed that nearly all of 34 artists whom he tested declined in skill after receiving 100 μg of LSD, and that most of them overestimated the worth of their productions while in the drug state. Matefi (29) described the effects of LSD on the paintings of a physician as leading to expansion, whereas mescaline paintings indicated withdrawal.

A common finding in the experiments with the graphic artists and painters was that their work was similar in many respects to that done by schizophrenics. All of the studies except Hartmann's were done in the 1950's. During that period, LSD was called a psychotomimetic because many researchers believed that its acute effects resembled those of a psychotic state. These expectations on the part of both experimenters and subjects undoubtedly influenced the outcomes of the investigations. More recently, the consciousness-expanding properties of LSD have been emphasized. Masters and Houston (28) published a book which describes the works of artists with this orientation. Many feel that they have been profoundly influenced by experiences with hallucinogenic drugs. An interesting example is that of Isaac Abrams, who had never painted prior to 1965. Then he took LSD, and has since achieved some prominence as a painter. Many other examples are given in *Psychedelic Art,* and three of the paintings are reproduced in Figures 12–1 to 12–3. Figures 12–4 and 12–5 are reproductions from the latter part of Van Gogh's life, when he was frankly psychotic. They are given as contrast. It should be obvious that, without appropriate controls, no firm

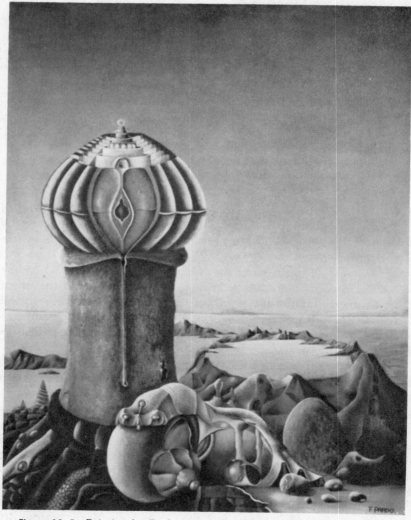

Figure 12–3 Painting by Frederick Pardo (as it appears in *Psychedelic Art,* by Robert E. L. Masters and Jean Houston, 1968, Balance House, p. 78).

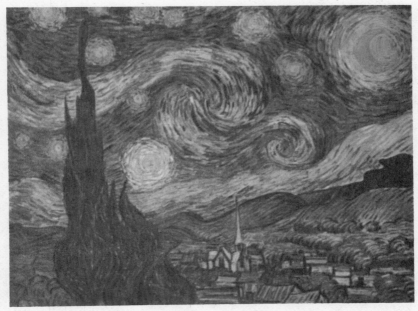

Figure 12–4 *The Starry Night,* by Vincent van Gogh (1889). Oil on canvas, 29″ × 36¼″. This painting and the self-portrait in Figure 12–5 were painted during the latter years of van Gogh's life, when the artist suffered from psychosis. (Collection, The Museum of Modern Art, New York. Acquired through the Lillie P. Bliss Bequest.)

conclusions can be drawn about the effects of psychedelic drugs on painting.

Krippner (24) surveyed 91 unnamed artists, many said by him to be prominent, and all known to have had one or more experiences which they regarded as psychedelic. Of these, four used induction procedures other than drugs: self-hypnosis, yoga, prayer, and spontaneous experience of a psychedelic state. Several fields of creative activity were represented: painting, light shows, mixed media, films, prose, photography, instrumental music, poetry, collage, sculpture, theater, and happenings. Many different types of drugs had been used, with LSD and marijuana being the most popular. Eighty-two of the artists said that their psychedelic experiences were pleasurable, and five more agreed with some qualifications. None felt that their work had suffered, although several admitted that others did not share their view. Forty-nine believed that their techniques had improved. Many, but not all, worked during the duration of action of the drug.

It is worth noting that many creative people develop ritualistic acts which they invariably perform prior to or during any attempts

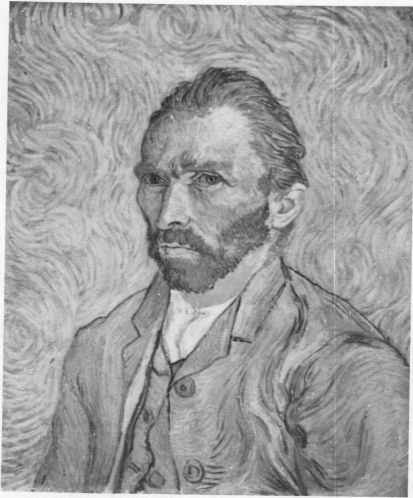

Figure 12–5 *Portrait of the Artist,* by Vincent van Gogh (November, 1889). (Collection, Musée du Jeu de Paume.)

at creative thinking. A few interesting ones are described by Vornoff (47):

1. Schiller, while writing, kept his feet in ice to diminish the circulation of blood there and to increase it in his head. André Créty, the French composer, did the same.
2. Bossuet stood in a cold room and covered his head with fur.
3. Descartes, Leibniz, Milton, and Rossini meditated under piles of blankets.

4. Rousseau bared his head to the sun, and felt that certain odors inspired him.
5. The French naturalist Buffon donned ceremonial apparel. His countryman poet Gérard de Naval wrote only while dressed in pearl-gray clothing.
6. Tycho Brahe required total silence.
7. Balzac and Poincaré needed coffee.

It is unlikely that anyone would seriously argue that the particular acts enhanced creativity. Rather, the belief in the efficacy of the acts, and the rituals themselves, were important. It is conceivable that hallucinogenic drugs serve the same function. The more distinctive the effects of a ritual, the more effective it is likely to be. Hallucinogens may be especially valuable in this respect.

INTERESTING CLAIMS WHICH HAVE NOT BEEN VERIFIED

Krippner (24, p. 178) quoted a "well-known pop recording artist" as saying that most of the top rock-'n'-roll groups use marijuana regularly and have tried LSD at least once. This echoes the claim of Rosevear (39), who said that marijuana was and still is extremely popular among musicians. In a *Playboy* interview, Richard Alpert made the claim that 90 percent of the rock industry is linked to LSD (35). Timothy Leary (26) said that over 70 percent of nonacademic artists have used psychedelic drugs, and Allen Ginsberg (15, p. 245) maintained that most of the major poets, painters, musicians, cineastes, sculptors, singers, and publishers in America and England are long-time users of marijuana.

ESTHETIC SENSIBILITIES

Among the most prominent acute effects of many hallucinogenic drugs is an appreciation of music and color. The architect Kiyo Izumi claimed that after taking LSD he began to appreciate certain qualities in the paintings of El Greco and Utrillo for the first time (20). Ballet music also affected him profoundly. Burroughs (8) claimed that after using mescaline he acquired a permanent ability to see a painting fully. Korngold (23) said that patients given LSD reported frequent occurrences of feelings of intense beauty and creative originality. Barron (2) abstracted from subjective reports of many people who had used mescaline, LSD, or psilocybin:

Colors become more vivid and glowing; the play of light on objects is enchanting; surface details become sharply defined; sensual harmonies, of sound, light, color, become marked. There are beautiful synesthesias, in which patterns of association usually confined to a single sense modality may cross over to others; music is "heard" as colored light, for example.

In some cases, ugliness will become intensified. A garish light may seem horrible, an unmusical sound unbearable; a false tone in a human may seem like a shriek; a false expression on a face may make it into a grotesque mask.

Both beauty and ugliness in objects thus are more than usually important and the esthetic qualities of the perceived world take on much greater value.

Allen Ginsberg wrote (15):

Marijuana is a useful catalyst for specific optical and aural aesthetic perceptions. I apprehended the structure of certain pieces of jazz and classical music in a new manner under the influence of marijuana, and these apprehensions have remained valid in years of normal consciousness. I first discovered how to see Klee's *Magic Squares* as the painter intended them (as optically three-dimensional space structures) while high on marijuana. I perceived ("dug") for the first time Cézanne's "petit sensation" of space achieved on a two-dimensional canvas (by means of advancing and receding colors, organization of triangles, cubes, etc., as the painter describes in his letters) while looking at *The Bathers* high on marijuana. And I saw anew many of nature's panoramas and landscapes that I'd stared at blindly without even noticing before; thru the use of marijuana, awe and detail were made conscious. These perceptions are permanent—and deep aesthetic experience leaves a trace, and an idea of what to look for that can be checked back later. I developed a taste for Crivelli's symmetry; and saw Rembrandt's *Polish Rider* as a sublime Youth on a Deathly horse for the first time—saw myself in the rider's face, one might say—while walking around the Frick Museum high on pot. These are not "hallucinations"; these are deepened perceptions that one might have catalyzed not by pot but by some *other* natural event (as natural as pot) that changes the mind, such as an intense love, a death in the family, a sudden clear dusk after rain, or the sight of the neon spectral reality of Times Square one sometimes has after leaving a strange movie. So it's all *natural*.

In three different studies (12, 30, 40), participants who took LSD were requested to fill out questionnaires some time later. To the question "Was the LSD experience a thing of great beauty?" 66 percent in one study (by Ditman et al.) and 81 percent in another (by Savage et al.) opted for the choices "quite a bit" or "very much." The other alternatives were "a little" and "not at all." In the Ditman study, 38 percent reported increased interest in nature, 34 percent in art, 33 percent in music. In the six-month questionnaire by McGlothlin et al., 62 percent reported a greater appreciation of music, and 46 percent a greater appreciation of art. In addition, the subjects spent more time than previously—and more time than controls who had not taken LSD—in museums, attending musical events, and buying records. Although the results of the three studies are impressive, it is worth pointing out a second study by Ditman and his colleagues (13) involving responses to the statement "I felt the beauty and meaning of music as never before." Subjects who were told that they might receive LSD but who actually received the minor tranquilizer chlordiazepoxide gave as many positive responses to the statement as did subjects who actually received LSD.

CONCLUSIONS

It is safe to conclude that users of hallucinogens *believe* that the drugs improve their creative talents. Also indisputable is that, during drug states, they become more interested in esthetic pursuits. As a result they increase their likelihood of favorable exposure to artworks, which may in turn form the basis for lasting attention to and appreciation of art.

Beyond the above, there is little agreement. The data are sufficiently ambiguous so that reviews of identical material have spawned diametrically opposed conclusions. No study has met all the criteria for a good scientific experiment; controls have been lacking, or the designs were such as to minimize the possibility that the effect which was being tested would be seen. Experimenters with strong beliefs about the efficacy of hallucinogenic drugs for enhancing creativity, and hence strong stakes in the outcomes of their experiments, have made subjective evaluations about the worth of the products of the psychedelic experience. Subjects have been of two types: (1) naive volunteers, not selected for special creative abilities, who would be expected to be somewhat apprehensive about the experience (and a high proportion of whom probably suffered from severe emotional disturbances); or (2) creative people who enjoyed using drugs, and who were probably highly motivated to "prove" that the drugs were useful. Clearly, authors of statements such as were quoted earlier in the chapter have judged the case prematurely.

A few words should be said about alternatives to drugs. Many methods are used to foster creativity: brainstorming and its variants, meditation, biofeedback conditioning, courses in painting and creative writing, and several more. All of these have the virtue of being legal and probably safe, and some are of proven effectiveness. Results are not immediate, which is one of the attractions of the claims for hallucinogens. A more important difference between drugs and alternatives to them is that the latter are concerned primarily with improving technique; hallucinogens on the other hand, if they have any value, are effective by virtue of providing new perspectives which provide challenges to basic assumptions about the nature and function of art. This is reflected, for better or worse, in the book on psychedelic artists by Masters and Houston.

REFERENCES

1. Aldrich, C. The effect of a synthetic marihuana-like compound on musical talent as measured by the Seashore test. Pub. Health Rep., 1944, 59:431–433.
2. Barron, F. The psychology of creativity. In Newcomb, T. (Ed.) New Directions in Psychology II. New York: Holt, Rinehart and Winston, 1965.
3. Barron, F. The relationship of ego diffusion to creative perception. In Taylor, C. (Ed.) Widening Horizons in Creativity. New York: John Wiley and Sons, 1964.
4. Berlin, L., Guthrie, T., Weider, A., Goodell, H., and Wolff, H. Studies in human cerebral function: the effects of mescaline and lysergic acid on cerebral processes pertinent to creative activity. J. Nerv. Ment. Dis., 1955, 122:478–491.
5. Boszormenyi, Z. Creative urge as an after effect of model psychoses. Conf. Psychiat., 1960, 3:117–126.
6. Braden, W. In Aronson, B., and Osmond, H. (Eds.) Psychedelics. New York: Doubleday and Co., Inc., 1970.
7. Broverman, D., Klaiber, E., Kobayashi, Y., and Vogel, W. Roles of activation and inhibition in sex differences in cognitive abilities. Psychol. Rev., 1968, 75:23–50.
8. Burroughs, W. Points of distinction between sedative and consciousness-expanding drugs. In Solomon, D. (Ed.) The Marihuana Papers. New York: Signet Books, 1966.
9. Clark, C. Brainstorming. New York: Doubleday and Co., Inc., 1958.
10. Cohen, S. Pot, acid, and speed. Med. Sci., 1968, 19:30–35.
11. Connell, P. Amphetamine Psychosis. London: Chapman and Hall, 1958.
12. Ditman, K., Hayman, M., and Whittlesey, J. Nature and frequency of claims following LSD. J. Nerv. Ment. Dis., 1962, 134:346–352.
13. Ditman, K., Moss, T., Forgy, E., Zunin, L., Lynch, R., and Funk, W. Dimensions of the LSD, methylphenidate, and chlordiazepoxide experiences. In Matheson, D., and Davison, M. (Eds.) The Behavioral Effects of Drugs. New York: Holt, Rinehart and Winston, 1972.
14. Gibbons, D., and Connelly, J. (Eds.) Selected Readings in Psychology. St. Louis: Mosby, 1970.
15. Ginsberg, A. First manifesto to end the bringdown. In Solomon, D. (Ed.) The Marihuana Papers. New York: Signet Books, 1966.
16. Gordon, W. An operational approach to creativity. Harvard Bus. Rev., 1957, Dec./Jan., 41–51.
17. Green, E., Green, A., and Walters, E. Voluntary control of internal states: psychological and physiological. J. Transpers. Psychol., 1970, 2:1–26.
18. Harman, W., McKim, R., Mogar, R., Fadiman, J., and Stolaroff, M. Psychedelic agents in creative problem solving: a pilot study. Psychol. Rep., 1966, 19:211–227.
19. Hofstadter, A., and Kuhns, R. (Eds.) Philosophies of Art and Beauty. New York: Random House, 1964.
20. Izumi, K. LSD and architectural design. In Aaronson, B., and Osmond, H. (Eds.) Psychedelics. Garden City: Doubleday and Co., 1970.
21. Jackson, P., and Messick, S. The person, the product, and the response: conceptual problems in the assessment of creativity. J. Personal., 1965, 33:309–329.
22. Kleitman, N. Diurnal variation in performance. Am. J. Physiol., 1933, 104:449–456.
23. Korngold, M. LSD and the creative experience. Psychoanal. Rev., 1963, 50:682–685.
24. Krippner, S. The psychedelic artist. In Masters, R., and Houston, J. Psychedelic Art. New York: Grove Press, 1968.
25. Krippner, S. The psychedelic state, the hypnotic trance, and the creative act. In Tart, C. (Ed.) Altered States of Consciousness. New York: John Wiley and Sons, 1969.
26. Leary, T. The Politics of Ecstasy. New York: G. P. Putnam's Sons, 1968.
27. Louria, D. The Drug Scene. New York: McGraw-Hill Book Co., 1968.
28. Masters, R., and Houston, J. Psychedelic Art. New York: Grove Press, 1968.
29. Matefi, L. Mezcalin-und Lyergsaurediathylamid-Rausch. Confin. Neurol., 1952, 12:146–176.

30. McGlothlin, W., Cohen, S., and McGlothlin, M. Long-lasting effects of LSD on normals. *In* Cole, J., and Wittenborn, J. (Eds.) *Drug Abuse.* Springfield, Ill.: Charles C Thomas, 1969.

31. Mednick, S. The associative basis of the creative process. Psychol. Rev., 1962, 69:220–232.

32. Morris, D. *The Biology of Art.* New York: Alfred A. Knopf, Inc. 1962.

33. Osborn, A. *Applied Imagination.* New York: Charles Scribner's Sons, 1957.

34. Parnes, S., and Meadow, A. Effects of "brain-storming" instructions on creative problem-solving by trained and untrained subjects. J. Educ. Psychol., 1959, 50:171–176.

35. *Playboy.* The drug revolution. Feb., 1970, 53–74.

36. Randrup, A., and Munkvad, I. Stereotyped activities produced by amphetamine in several animal species and man. Psychopharmacologia, 1967, 11:300–310.

37. Read, H. *The Philosophy of Modern Art.* New York: Fawcett World Library, 1967.

38. Rosenthal, R. *Experimenter Effects in Behavioral Research.* New York: Appleton-Century-Crofts, 1966.

39. Rosevear, J. *Pot: A Handbook of Marijuana.* New York: University Books, Inc. 1967.

40. Savage, C., Harman, W., Fadiman, J., and Savage, E. A follow-up note on the psychedelic experience. Cited in Psychedelic Review, 1963, 1:18–26.

41. Shaw, T. *Don't Get Taught Art This Way.* Boston: Lyle Stuart Inc., 1967.

42. Smith, G., Weitzner, M., and Beecher, H. Increased sensitivity of measurement of drug effects in expert swimmers. J. Pharmacol. Exp. Ther., 1963, 139:114–119.

43. Stafford, P., and Golightly, B. *LSD: The Problem Solving Psychedelic.* New York: Award Books, 1967.

44. Tart, C. *Altered States of Consciousness.* Garden City: Doubleday and Co., 1972.

45. *Time.* Painting under LSD. Dec. 5, 1969, 88.

46. Tonini, G., and Montanari, C. Effects of experimentally induced psychoses on artistic expression. Conf. Neurol., 1955, 15:225–239.

47. Vornoff, S. *From Cretin to Genius.* New York: Alliance, 1941.

48. Weil, A., Zinberg, N., and Nelsen, J. Clinical and psychological effects of marihuana in man. Science, 1968, 162:1234–1242.

49. Wilson, R., and Shagass, C. Comparison of two drugs with psychotomimetic effects (LSD and Ditran). J. Nerv. Ment. Dis., 1964, 138:277–286.

50. Yolles, S. Recent research on LSD, marijuana, and other dangerous drugs. Statement before Committee on the Judiciary, U.S. Senate, March, 1968.

51. Zegans, L., Pollard, J., and Brown, D. The effects of LSD-25 on creativity and tolerance to regression. Arch. Gen Psychiat., 1967, 16:740–749.

CHAPTER 13

SEX AND REPRODUCTION

The alchemist's search for a means to transmute lead to gold was never more diligent than the quest of men everywhere for a reliable aphrodisiac. The results, so far, have been comparable. A partial listing of substances reputed to have aphrodisic properties, taken from Borelli (9), includes celery, parsley, asparagus, yohimbine, Spanish fly, strychnine, wild oats, certain orchids, irises, cola nuts, and many kinds of herbs and shrubs. Appel, writing in *Playboy* (3), offered his own extensive list of reputed aphrodisiacs.

A valuable offshoot of the search for aphrodisiacs was a burgeoning interest in the then little known science of endocrinology, following the claim in 1889 by a 72-year-old man that his sexual vigor was renewed after self-administration of extracts of dog testes (87, p. 23). The claim was a valid one, in that the treatment did restore sexual vigor, but as with any of the above mentioned substances, the important component was not the pharmacological effect but the faith in the efficacy of the treatment.

The word aphrodisiac is defined in the *American College Dictionary* as a drug which arouses sexual desire. It is often used in two additional ways to refer to drug-induced increases in sexual performance and in sexual enjoyment. All three aspects of sexual function are considered in this chapter, with much of the information deriving from work with laboratory animals. However, although the sexual desire and performance of laboratory animals can be measured and evaluated, subject to the same limitations as any other types of animal experiments, it is much more difficult to measure their enjoy-

308

ment. One solution would be to ignore laboratory data, and to focus attention on subjective reports of people who use drugs. However, although the subjective data are important, they are difficult to interpret. The major problem, which is foreshadowed by the many false claims about aphrodisiacs, is that people who report on the enhancement of sexual pleasure through the use of drugs do not use placebo controls. Foulds (29) has reported that four times as many studies without placebo controls get positive findings as when controls are instituted. Sexual behavior, perhaps more than any other form of behavior, is influenced by expectations. Any substance or ritual which is believed to enhance enjoyment of the sexual act is likely to do so. The placebo effect is especially powerful.

COPULATION IN FEMALE MAMMALS

The sexual receptivity of female subprimates is regulated largely or entirely by gonadal hormones. The ovaries secrete both estrogen and progesterone, and when estrogen levels are high relative to progesterone, the animal becomes receptive, i.e., it is in estrus. Rodents in estrus are indiscriminate about accepting males; they respond sexually to all males which display the species-specific sexual patterns. Dogs in estrus show preference for some males over others (5). Primate females are further emancipated from hormones, but even humans are considerably influenced by hormonal levels. Udry and Morris (88) found via questionnaire that frequency of intercourse and orgasm is greater in women during midcycle than just prior to or just after menstruation. In contrast, Hart (42) reported that libido was greater during the premenstruum. It is possible that both sets of findings are better explained by cultural factors than by biological ones; some proof for the assertion is that Kinsey et al. (48) reported that ovariectomy does not affect the sexual responsiveness of most women.

The all-or-none aspect of rodent female receptivity greatly limits their usefulness to researchers interested in the sexuality of women. The reader who desires information on induction or suppression of estrus behavior by drugs is referred to Meyerson (59). In female rhesus monkeys, ovarian hormones are necessary for normal sexual functioning; ovariectomy greatly reduces receptivity, and replacement therapy with estrogen restores it. In one study, the receptivity of ovariectomized females was restored to an even greater extent by the male hormone testosterone than by estrogen (85). Unfortunately for the females, the testosterone reduced their attractiveness, so males were unresponsive to their solicitations.

Testosterone may increase libido in women, perhaps by height-ening clitoral sensitivity. Testosterone has been used to treat breast cancer and certain gynecological disorders. There have been several reports of increased sexual arousal following treatment (38, 44, 68), and there have even been some successes in the treatment of frigidity with testosterone (80). The hormones cortisone and corticosterone, both secreted by the adrenal glands, may also contribute to female eroticism. Waxenberg et al. (90) removed the adrenals from 14 women suffering from breast cancer; there was substantial improvement of the cancerous condition, but the women all indicated depressed sexuality.

COPULATION IN MALE MAMMALS

The forms of copulation in male mammals are impressive in their diversity. Some of the various patterns have been described by Dewsbury (23) and by Hediger (43). There are certain characteristics which are of necessity common to all, and which have therefore been subject to extensive analysis. The speed with which a male approaches and mounts a receptive female has been taken as an index of desire. The speed with which he effects an intromission, or insertion of the penis into the vagina, indicates potency. The importance of distinguishing between desire and potency can be appreciated by considering an early study by Stone (78), in which he reported that castration does not affect the ability of male rats to copulate. The conclusion is misleading, because Stone's criterion for sexual responsiveness was one "copulation" per test. Subsequent research (4) has shown that mounting behavior is initially affected only slightly by castration, but the frequency of intromissions and ejaculations drops precipitously. Although Beach and Holz were the first scientists to make use of the distinction between the forms of sexual response, they were anticipated by Shakespeare, for in *Macbeth*, the gatekeeper says that alcohol "provokes the desire, but it takes away the performance."

Another frequently used measure in rats is the number of intromissions which precede each ejaculation. The importance of intromissions was demonstrated by Adler (1). He allowed some pairs of copulating rats to achieve a single ejaculation undisturbed, and separated others when an ejaculation appeared imminent. In the latter case a second female was immediately introduced, and the new pair copulated to ejaculation. The procedure resulted in the formation of two groups of females, distinguished by the number of intromissions they had received prior to deposition of the ejaculate. When the ejaculation occurred after three or fewer intromissions, only 22 percent of the females became pregnant. The figure was 90 percent for the high (at least four) intromission group. The stimulation from a series of intromissions apparently triggers the release of hormones which are essential to successful implantation.

Still another measure of sexual activity is the length of time following ejaculation before the resumption of sexual behavior. This is taken to indicate recovery from sexual fatigue. Although all of the measures are useful, their very number does not allow for simple interpretation. Whether sexual behavior is judged to be facilitated or retarded by a drug depends on the measure used, and the interpretation of it.

DRUGS AND SEXUALITY

Presumptive Aphrodisiacs

Yohimbine has long enjoyed a reputation as an aphrodisiac. Sulman and Black (79) failed to find any differences between yohimbine-treated male rats and controls in sex glands, sexual organs, descent of testes, or frequency of spontaneous erections. Danowski and Price (19) were also disappointed in tests with reputed aphrodisiacs; neither bois cochon bark nor pega palo vine altered the weight of the testes, prostate, or seminal vesicles of male rats.

Cantharidin, also called Spanish fly because of its derivation from certain insects, has a centuries-old reputation as an aphrodisiac (37, p. 983). It has an irritant action on the bladder which causes urgency of urination and, occasionally, persistent erections. It is used infrequently in veterinary medicine as a local irritant. Spanish fly is highly toxic, and several deaths from its improper use have been reported (11, 17, 63). Leavitt (52) tested 12 male rats with 0.67 mg/kg Spanish fly. Eight of them died during the course of testing. There were no differences in the sexual behavior of the four survivors when they were tested in both cantharidin and control sessions.

Leslie and Bruhl (54) worked with impotent men. They reported that a commercial preparation consisting of equal portions of nux vomica (strychnine is the active ingredient), yohimbine, and methyltestosterone (a testosterone compound which is effective orally) was effective in increasing the potency of their patients. The study was conducted in double blind fashion, with one-half of the men receiving an inert placebo. The basis of the success of the mixture is an interesting problem, since the individual components have been shown to be ineffectual. (Testosterone improves sexual functioning in men who are impotent because of hypoactive gonads. However, only a small proportion of impotent men have this problem.) One possibility is that the central stimulating effects of strychnine, the antidiuretic action of yohimbine, and the anabolic effects of methyltestosterone make the preparation easily discriminable from inert substances. Its effectiveness as a placebo would thereby be considerably enhanced, and not necessarily adequately controlled by the double blind technique.

Dubin (27) and Montesano and Evangelista (61) also claimed to have cured impotent men. They both worked with a methyltestosterone-thyroid compound. The rationale for its use was that testosterone restores sexual functioning in hypogonadal males, and a healthy thyroid gland is important for normal testosterone production. There were 58 patients in the Dubin study, 10 of whom left before its completion. There were 40 patients in the Montesano and Evangelista study. Eighteen of 24 and 14 of 20 patients in the respective drug groups exhibited substantial improvement in sexual functioning, as compared with only 1 of 24 and 3 of 20 who received placebos. Men whose impotence was of short duration were helped most by the treatments. Montesano and Evangelista reported that improvements were maintained even after treatment was discontinued, although they did not offer any data to support their conclusion.

The explanation proffered by the authors, that the methyltestosterone-thyroid combination acts by synergistically increasing levels of circulating testosterone, is insufficient. Most impotent men have normal gonadal function and are not greatly influenced by the administration of testosterone (76). The animal work is relevant. Grunt and Young (39) ranked male guinea pigs on the basis of sexual activity, then castrated them and injected all with equal amounts of testosterone. When they were retested, all with the same amount of circulating testosterone, their rankings were unchanged. Grunt and Young suggested that some animals are better able to utilize testosterone than others. As part of the same study, the guinea pigs received, progressively increasing dosages; there were no changes in rankings. Champlin et al. (13), using mice, obtained similar findings.

Neither Dubin nor Montesano and Evangelista gave any indication of the methods by which subjects were assigned to groups. Nonrandom assignment, such as placing more men whose impotence was of short duration and whose prognosis was therefore most favorable into the drug group, would obviously have biased the results. The very fact that such individuals responded best increases the plausibility of an explanation in terms of expectational rather than pharmacological effects, since impotence of short duration is the type most readily cured by psychotherapy.

One additional factor which must be considered is that many patients reported a lessening of fatigue after drug treatment, which suggests that they were not in peak health prior to treatment. Their impotence may have been caused by poor physical health, which might have been improved by methyltestosterone-thyroid. Nevertheless, further investigations are certainly warranted.

Increases in the sense of physical well-being probably account in large part for the apparent aphrodisic effects of L-DOPA. L-DOPA is a recently discovered drug used to treat Parkinson's disease, previously a fatal ailment characterized by progressively severe tremor and speech impairment. Physicians who worked with L-DOPA noticed that some treated patients reported striking increases in sexual activity. However, the changes are more easily explained by remission of disabling symptoms than by increased libido and potency.

Benkert et al. (6) administered L-DOPA to 10 impotent men. There was some increase in the frequency of spontaneous erections during the night, but erectile function was not sufficiently improved during the day to enable the men to have normal sexual intercourse. Only two of the eight who finished the treatment reported any increases in libido.

Hormones

The effects of testosterone have been described. Soulairac and Soulairac have done extensive work on hormones and the sexual behavior of rats, which they reviewed in 1965 (74). ACTH, a hormone synthesized in the pituitary which influences the production of corticosteroids by the adrenal glands, and deoxycorticosterone, one of the adrenal hormones, decreased both intromission frequency (IF) and ejaculatory latency (EL). Corticosterone, another adrenal hormone, decreased IF but increased EL. The thyroid hormones thyroxine and thiouracil and the synthetic estrogen diethylstilbesterol all decreased ejaculation frequency (EF). Melin and Kihlstrom (58) reported that oxytocin, a hormone synthesized in the hypothalamus, had a facilitatory effect on several aspects of sexual performance in male rabbits, including EL, EF, and volume of ejaculate. The result is difficult to explain, since Cross and Glover (18) had previously failed to find an oxytocic effect on either seminal vesicle contractility or semen emission in rabbits. Leavitt (52) did not observe any enhancement of sexual behavior following oxytocin administration in rats.

CNS Stimulants

Silverman (70) found that "mating" of male rats was unaffected by doses of 1.0 to 5.0 mg/kg amphetamine. However, in his work *male* rats were tested in pairs, and mating consisted of such elements as following, sniffing, mounting, and attempted mounting. Soulairac observed a biphasic response to amphetamine; for the first three test periods, low doses shortened refractory periods and increased EF, but sexual behavior was frequently disrupted during later administrations. Bignami likewise reported an acceleration of sexual behavior after small doses (8). Leavitt criticized their experimental designs, but nevertheless found a similar pattern of results after injections of methamphetamine, thus indicating that the effect is a robust one. Leavitt also tested cocaine and found a facilitatory effect.

Observations with humans extend the animal research. Rylander, who works with people addicted to central stimulating drugs, reported that when the drugs are taken intravenously, they are the most powerful aphrodisiacs known (66). They produce very strong sexual stimulation. One addict was quoted as saying about phenmetrazine that "the shot goes straight from the head to the scrotum." Another claimed that sex stimulation is 50 percent the cause of drug abuse. Bejerot (91, p. 65) quoted this remark by a phenmetrazine addict: "Those who haven't had intercourse when high, they don't know what sexual life is."

Neither small doses of strychnine nor nicotine changed mating behavior in male rats, but larger doses of nicotine impaired behavior (8). Caffeine, which belongs to yet another class of central stimulants, improved performance when given in doses of 20 or 30 mg/kg (93).

CNS Depressants

Alcohol increases ejaculation latency in both dogs (31) and rats (21), and is capable of blocking erection in man. Yet, in man, the effects of alcohol are more complex than they are in laboratory animals. Inability to have an erection may result from physiological causes, as during the refractory period following ejaculation, but also is commonly caused by insufficient arousal or by anxiety in the presence of arousing stimuli. Alcohol reduces anxiety, and when taken in small doses that do not impair the physiological mechanisms for maintaining erection, it may increase both sexual desire and performance in people otherwise disabled by anxiety. Brady (10) has confirmed that some mild forms of sexual disorder are benefited by alcohol, barbiturates, or meprobamate.

Drugs Used in Psychiatric Practice

Several drugs used routinely in psychiatric practice have as undesirable side effects the inhibition of ejaculation. Men treated with guanethidine, thioridazine, chlordiazepoxide, and chlorprothixene have reported failure to ejaculate and, in some cases, impotence (26, 40, 45, 60). Guanethidine-treated rats do not differ from normal rats in their copulatory pattern, but their ejaculates lack sperm (7). Acetophenazine blocks mating in male rats (53). The drugs, which are used to treat hypertension, anxiety, and related states, may owe their common action to sympathetic blockade. Yet yohimbine, which has a similar sympatholytic action, induces ejaculations in mice (55).

Diazepam

Diazepam, an antianxiety drug, had unusual effects on mating behavior in rats (52). In many respects the animals acted as though they were highly motivated. They mounted females sooner than they did on control days, and they continued mounting at markedly elevated rates throughout the testing sessions. Yet they were unable to achieve intromission, with the result that 4 of 16 tests at low dose and 13 of 16 at high dose ended in failure to ejaculate. There were only 3 of 32 control trials which ended in failure.

Reserpine

Studies with reserpine, a drug which produces degenerative histological changes in the testes upon prolonged administration (86), yielded mixed results. Fuller (30) reported inhibition of sexual behavior in male rats, while the Soulairacs (73), Dewsbury (20), and Dewsbury and Davis (24) all reported reduced IF at low doses. High doses suppressed sexual behavior. A major procedural difference is that Fuller's rats were tested over a period of seven months, while the other experimenters used much shorter durations. In man, there are clinical reports of reduced sexual desire and impotence following use of reserpine (56).

Chlorpromazine

Chlorpromazine, the most widely used antipsychotic drug, was tested in rats by Soulairac (72), who found an increase in IF. Both Gillett (34) and Zimbardo and Barry (93), using much smaller doses, reported a decrease. Soulairac failed to distinguish between mounts and intromissions, but that alone does not account for the disparate results. Both mounts and intromissions were decreased in the Zimbardo and Barry study. Chlorpromazine has been reported in rare instances to increase sexual urges, primarily in women (16). As with alcohol, increased libido may not be a direct pharmacological effect but a secondary one resulting from diminution of anxiety.

Monoamine Oxidase Inhibitors

Wide variations in procedure and dosage complicate interpretations of findings with MAOI's. High doses of pargyline (33, 82) reduced sexual behavior of male rats; iproniazid increased it (75); and tranylcypromine (52) and nialamide (12) had little effect. Dewsbury et al. (25) tested three different MAOI's—iproniazid, pargyline, and nialamide—and found that all three retarded sexual behavior. Their interpretation that the effects were due to high levels of biogenic amines is questionable on several counts. First, Soulairac, Leavitt, and Butcher all obtained different patterns of results with MAOI's. Secondly, the differences between low and high dose effects in the study by Dewsbury et al. were impressive. For example, the most powerful drug in altering sexual behavior was pargyline. In two separate replications they found 13 significant differences between pargyline- and saline-treated rats. In 6 of the 13 cases the response to a low dose of pargyline was in the opposite direction from the response to a high dose. Yet both low and high doses raise levels of biogenic amines. Three of twenty-four animals injected with the high dose of nialamide died, raising the possibility that the others did not perform well because they were sick.

A final point is that authorities do not agree on the significance of certain changes in the sexual pattern. Dewsbury et al. interpreted the increased intromission frequencies of their rats as indicating retardation of sexual behavior. Yet Adler's work, cited previously, demonstrated that too few intromissions reduce the likelihood of successful pregnancy in rats. Rats which have large numbers of intromissions prior to ejaculation also tend to have many ejaculations (unpublished observations). Furthermore, rats which are permitted to copulate without interference have more intromissions before they achieve the first ejaculation, when they are most highly motivated and most potent, than they have with later ones. Therefore, it seems at least as justifiable to interpret increased IF as augmenting rather than retarding copulatory behavior.

Illicit Drugs

Opiates

One of the major reasons for use of some illicit drugs is to enhance sexual enjoyment, but opiates are different in this respect from illegal stimulants or hallucinogens. Nearly half of 100 heroin users studied by Chein et al. (14, p. 166) were sexually impotent, and Seevers (69) reported a depression of sexual behavior in morphine-treated monkeys. It has even been claimed that heroin is used as a substitute for sex (51, p. 22). During withdrawal from opiates there are powerful rebound effects, and frequently ejaculations occur during sleep, as well as in response to minimal stimulation of the genitalia (32, p. 494).

Marijuana

Sex was mentioned as a reason for starting marijuana use by 10 percent of those surveyed in one sampling (15) and by 30 percent in a second (71). When Goode (36) surveyed 200 marijuana users, 44 percent replied that their sexual desires were increased, and frequent users agreed that enjoyment was also increased. The comments of students questioned by Tart (83, 84) and Haines and Green (cited in 47, p. 78) give rise to similar conclusions. In Tart's studies, substantial proportions of respondents agreed with statements to the effect that "My sex drive goes up when I'm stoned"; "I have more need for sex, but only in situations in which I'd normally be aroused"; "My orgasms have new, pleasurable qualities"; and "I'm a better lover when I'm stoned."

LSD

Work with LSD clearly illustrates the limitations of animal studies. It was first tested for its effects on sexual behavior by Gillett (34), who found that high doses impaired or completely disrupted sexual behavior in male rats. In later studies, with smaller doses, sexual behavior was accelerated (8). Thus, there is a nice dose-response curve. However, the work with rats gives no hint of the paeans of praise which have been sung to LSD as an enhancer of sexual pleasures. Wakefield (89) offered two quotes:

(1) While these drugs are not actually aphrodisiacs—that is they don't specifically stimulate the user to sexual activity—a good experience with the drugs heightens and intensifies all experience, and just as one can enjoy music and art during the experience with a new and deeper appreciation, so one can do the same with sex—it can be a beautiful experience under the drug.
(2) The early studies from psychological laboratories and psychiatric clinics reported that psychedelic drugs were not aphrodisiac. More recently, evidence obtained from more than 25 married couples taking psilocybin or LSD in their homes seems to indicate that psychedelic substances can provide extraordinary intensification and broadening of all types of sensory experience, including the sexual.

Stafford and Golightly (77) quoted several psychiatrists who believe that LSD is an extremely effective agent in the cure of homosexuality, frigidity, and impotence. Until formal studies with placebo control groups are run, the supposed curative powers of LSD must be treated warily.

Peyote

Fernberger (28) reported that the ability of his subjects—nine university professors—to become erotically aroused was greatly reduced by peyote. Kluver (49), who has worked extensively with the drug, feels that it has no effect on sexual desire or performance.

NEUROTRANSMITTER MECHANISMS

Adrenergic System

Sympatholytic compounds may interfere with erectile capability and with the ejaculatory mechanism (as previously discussed). Sympathomimetics may have the opposite effect: Cross and Glover (18) reported that both epinephrine and norepinephrine produced contractions of the seminal vesicles of male rabbits, and emission of semen. Orbach (64) found that male rats ejaculate, even in the absence of females, soon after epinephrine injection. When receptive females are present, small doses of epinephrine increase EF. Norepinephrine, on the other hand, inhibits sexual behavior. The effects of other compounds which affect the adrenergic system—reserpine, cocaine, amphetamine, LSD, and MAOI's—have been discussed earlier.

Cholinergic System

Bignami (8) systematically investigated the effects of various antagonists of the neurotransmitter acetylcholine upon the sexual behavior of male rats. All but adiphenine were disruptive; the others, in decreasing order of strength, were scopolamine, benactyzine, atropine, and methylatropine. The central anticholinergic activities of the drugs follow the same pattern, with benactyzine differing from adiphenine only in that the latter does not penetrate the blood-brain barrier. Bignami's results have been confirmed in other studies (52, 75).

Nicotine and physostigmine represent the other side of the cholinergic-anticholinergic coin. Nicotine, which first stimulates and then depresses transmission in automatic ganglia, had little effect upon copulatory behavior except at doses which produced motor impairment (8). By contrast, even low doses of physostigmine produced severe decrements in rats (52). The combined results suggest that all modifications of cholinergic functioning interfere with sexual behavior. Yet several cholinergic drugs, including ACh, pilocarpine, and physostigmine, elicited ejaculations in mice when they followed in close temporal sequence the administration of pernostone

(55); in addition, methacholine was even more powerful than epine-phrine in inducing ejaculations in rats (64). Perhaps the data with physostigmine should be reevaluated, and tests with other cholino-mimetic compounds should be made.

Serotonergic System

It has recently been proposed that brain serotonin acts to in-hibit sexual behavior (24). As evidence was cited the finding that reserpine and parachlorophenylalanine, both of which deplete brain serotonin, also facilitate sexual behavior, while MAOI's increase brain serotonin and retard sexual behavior. The cumulative evi-dence is, however, equivocal. With respect to the reserpine and MAOI data, an important measure of sexual change was intromis-sion frequency and, as discussed above, the meaning of changes in IF is unclear. The data are not wholly uniform, either; when Fuller (30) administered reserpine to rats, she did not obtain the same pat-tern of results as Dewsbury did. The same situation obtains with tetrabenazine, a drug which is similar in action to reserpine. Dewsbury (22) reported that tetrabenazine reduced IF, while Butcher et al. (12) found that it eliminated copulatory behavior. A precursor of serotonin, 5-hydroxytryptophan, reduced IF and increased EF (74).

Results with parachlorophenylalanine are interesting. Gessa (3, p. 86), one of a team of scientists who discovered it, said, "We are optimistic that our work may lead to the development of a true aphrodisiac." The statement was based on studies with both rats and rabbits, in which groups of males mounted each other repeat-edly (33). However, additional research has been sobering. Although there have been several positive studies of heterosexual behavior (2, 67, 82), there have been negative ones as well (94). Zitrin et al. (94) emphasized the need for appropriate controls in research on sexuality. They noted that a substantial proportion of normal, un-treated male cats exhibit homosexual behavior, and attempt to copu-late with members of other species and with inanimate objects.

Once again, it must be emphasized that all drugs have many actions. To attribute a drug-induced change in sexual activity to a particular action on neurotransmitter mechanisms is, given our current state of knowledge, premature.

HOMOSEXUALITY

Until very recently there was no evidence to support the once popular but then discredited hypothesis that homosexuality is the result of an endocrine imbalance. In fact, clinical reports indicate that treatment of homosexuals with sex hormones intensifies homosexual behavior (41). Swyer (81) was unable to discriminate between homosexual and heterosexual men on the basis of androgen level; nor is female homosexual behavior caused by excessive androgen. Margolese (57) has now offered the first evidence that homosexuality may have an endocrine basis. He analyzed urine samples from heterosexual men, both in good and in poor health, and from healthy homosexual men. The ratio of androsterone to etiocholanolone—two urinary excretion products of testosterone which may be derived from either the testis or the adrenal cortex, and which are excreted by women as well as men—was the highest in the healthy heterosexuals. The ratio was about equal in the other two groups. Since unhealthy heterosexuals had low ratios, it may be concluded that hormonal status is not a sufficient cause of direction of sex drive. In addition, the findings do not exclude the possibility that sexual preferences determine hormone output rather than the other way around. If the behavior is causally affected by the hormones, it might be simple to treat pharmacologically those homosexuals who want therapy.

ORAL CONTRACEPTIVES

Various orally administered combinations of estrogen and progesterone are highly effective in preventing pregnancy.* Although there have been recurring reports of toxic side effects from these formulations, Swyer (80), Pincus (65), and the Scientific Study Group of the World Health Organization (92) have all concluded that they are safe. Inman and Vessey (46) accumulated data which show that oral contraceptives increase the user's chances of suffering occluded blood vessels; however, the risk is less than that incurred during pregnancy.

While some pill users become depressed, others report a reduction in premenstrual and menstrual anxiety and tension (35). Their increase in emotional well-being may relate directly to their reduced fear of becoming pregnant (62). Kutner and Duffy (50) found that women whose fear of pregnancy was reduced by the pill also reported fewer minor side effects such as swollen and sore breasts. They also noted that many of the symptoms reported by pill users were similar to those of pregnancy. They offered as a tentative explanation for the variability in symptoms among users the idea that response to an estrogen-progesterone combination is greatest in those women in whom the normal levels of estrogen and progesterone are least. The soreness in the breasts is then easily explained, because the breasts are very sensitive to estrogen.

---

*As indicated above, sexual desire may be greatly influenced by level of estrogen. Therefore, the particular pill prescribed for a woman may have important implications for her libido.

Kutner and Duffy tested their hypothesis by administering a personality inventory which is designed to measure degree of femininity to women for whom the pill was being prescribed. Seven of eight of the women who received the lowest scores of femininity, and only one of eight of the most feminine, reported an increase in swollen and sore breasts after three months of an oral contraceptive regimen. The data are interesting, but there is an important empirical link which must be made before much credence can be placed in the explanation, namely, it must be shown that scores on the personality inventory are related to levels of circulating hormones.

REFERENCES

1. Adler, N. The role of the male's copulatory behavior in successful pregnancy of the female rat. Ph.D. Dissertation, University of California, Berkeley, 1967.
2. Ahlenius, S., Eriksson, H., Larsson, K., Modigh, K., and Sodersten, P. Mating behavior in the male rat treated with p-chlorophenylalanine methyl ester alone and in combination with pargyline. Psychopharmacologia, 1971, 20: 383–388.
3. Appel, F. Just slip this into her drink. Playboy, August, 1970, 82–176.
4. Beach, F., and Holz, M. Mating behavior in male rats castrated at various ages and injected with androgen. J. Exp. Zool., 1946, 101:91–142.
5. Beach, F., and LeBoeuf, B. Coital behavior in dogs. I. Preferential mating in the bitch. Anim. Behav., 1967, 15:546–598.
6. Benkert, O., Crombach, G., and Kockott, G. Effect of L-DOPA on sexually impotent patients. Psychopharmacologia, 1972, 23:91–95.
7. Bermant, G., and Westbrook, W. Peripheral factors in regulation of sexual contact by female rats. J. Comp. Physiol. Psychol., 1966, 61:244–250.
8. Bignami, G. Pharmacological influences on mating behavior in the male rat. Psychopharmacologia, 1966, 10:44–58.
9. Borelli, S. Die Wirksamkeit der Sexualanregungsmittel. Archiv Fur Klinisohe und Experimentelle Dermatologie, 1960, 211:147–149.
10. Brady, J. Frigidity. Med. Aspects Human Sex., 1967, 1:42–48.
11. Browne, S. Cantharidin poisoning due to a "blister beetle." Brit. Med. J., 1960, part 2: 1290–1291.
12. Butcher, L., Butcher, S., and Larsson, K. Effects of apomorphine, (+)-amphetamine, and nialamide on tetrabenazine-induced suppression of sexual behavior in the male rat. Europ. J. Pharmacol., 1969, 7:283–288.
13. Champlin, A., Blight, W., and McGill, T. The effects of varying levels of testosterone on the sexual behavior of the male mouse. Anim. Behav., 1963, 11:244–245.
14. Chein, I., Gerard, D., Lee, R., and Rosenfeld, E. Narcotics, Delinquency, and Social Policy. London: Tavistock, 1964.
15. Chopra, R., and Chopra, G. The present position of hemp-drug addiction in India. Indian Med. Res. Mem., 1939, 31:1–119.
16. Cohen, I. Complications of chlorpromazine therapy. Am. J. Psychiat., 1956, 113: 115–121.
17. Craven, J., and Polak, A. Cantharidin poisoning. Brit. Med. J., 1954, 2:1386–1388.
18. Cross, B., and Glover, T. The hypothalamus and seminal emission. J. Endocrinol., 1958, 16:385–395.
19. Danowski, T., and Price, L. Organ weights of animals maintained on alleged aphrodisiacs: "Pega Palo" and "Bois Cochon." Endocrinol., 1960, 66:788–790.
20. Dewsbury, D. Copulatory behavior of male rats following reserpine administration. Psychon. Sci., 1971, 22:177–179.
21. Dewsbury, D. Effects of alcohol ingestion on copulatory behavior of male rats. Psychopharmacologia, 1967, 11:276–281.

22. Dewsbury, D. Effects of tetrabenazine on the copulatory behavior of male rats. Europ. J. Pharmacol., 1972, 17:221–226.
23. Dewsbury, D. Patterns of copulatory behavior in male mammals. Quart. Rev. Biol., 1972, 47:1–33.
24. Dewsbury, D., and Davis, H. Effects of reserpine on the copulatory behavior of male rats. Physiol. Behav., 1970, 5:1331–1333.
25. Dewsbury, D., Davis, H., and Jansen, P. Effects of monoamine oxidase inhibitors on the copulatory behavior of male rats. Psychopharmacologia, 1972, 24: 209–217.
26. Ditman, K. Inhibition of ejaculation by chlorprothixene. Am. J. Psychiat., 1964, 120:1004–1005.
27. Dubin, M. Treatment of impotence with a methyltestosterone-thyroid compound. West. Med., 1964, 5:67–68.
28. Fernberger, S. Further observations on peyote intoxication. J. Ab. Soc. Psychol., 1932, 26:367–378.
29. Foulds, G. The design of experiments in psychiatry. In Sainsbury, P., and Kreitman, N. (Eds.) Methods of Psychiatric Research. London: Oxford, 1963.
30. Fuller, R. Sexual changes in the male rat following chronic administration of reserpine. Nature, 1963, 200:585–586.
31. Gantt, W. Acute effects of alcohol on autonomic (sexual, secretory, cardiac) and somatic responses. In Himwich, H. (Ed.) Alcoholism: Basic Concepts and Treatment. Washington, D.C., A.A.A.S., 1957.
32. Gebhard, P. In Beach, F. (Ed.) Sex and Behavior. New York: John Wiley and Sons, 1965.
33. Gessa, G. Brain serotonin and sexual behavior in male animals. Ann. Intern. Med., 1970, 73:622–626.
34. Gillett, E. Effects of chlorpromazine and D-lysergic acid diethylamide on sex behavior of male rats. Proc. Soc. Exper. Biol. Med., 1960, 103:392–394.
35. Glick, I. Mood and behavioral changes associated with the use of the oral contraceptive agents. Psychopharmacologia, 1967, 10:363–374.
36. Goode, E. The Marijuana Smokers. New York: Basic Books, 1970.
37. Goodman, L., and Gilman, A. The Pharmacological Basis of Therapeutics. New York: The Macmillan Publishing Co., 1965.
38. Greenblatt, R. Testosterone propionate pellet implantation in gynecic disorders. J.A.M.A., 1943, 121:17–24.
39. Grunt, J., and Young, W. Differential reactivity of individuals and the response of the male guinea pig to testosterone propionate. Endocrinol., 1952, 51: 237–248.
40. Haider, I. Thioridazine and sexual dysfunctions. Int. J. Neuropsychiat., 1966, 255–257.
41. Hampson, J., and Hampson, J. The ontogenesis of sexual behavior in man. In Young, W. (Ed.) Sex and Internal Secretions. Baltimore: Williams and Wilkins Co., 1961.
42. Hart, R. Monthly rhythm of libido in married women. Brit. Med. J., 1960, 1:1023–1024.
43. Hediger, H. Environmental factors influencing the reproduction of zoo animals. In Beach, F. (Ed.) Sex and Behavior. New York: John Wiley and Sons, 1965.
44. Herrmann, J., and Adair, F. The effect of testosterone propionate on carcinoma of the female breast with soft tissue metastases. J. Clin. Endocr. Metab., 1946, 6:769–775.
45. Hughes, J. Failure to ejaculate with chlordiazepoxide. Am. J. Psychiat., 1964, 121: 610–611.
46. Inman, W., and Vessey, M. Investigation of death from pulmonary, coronary, and cerebral thrombosis and embolism in women of child-bearing age. Brit. Med. J., 1968, 2:193–199.
47. Kaplan, J. Marijuana—The New Prohibition. New York: World Publishing Co., 1970.
48. Kinsey, A., Pomeroy, W., Martin, C., and Gebhard, P. Sexual Behavior in the Human Female. Philadelphia: W. B. Saunders Co., 1953.
49. Kluver, H. Mescal, The "Divine" Plant and Its Psychological Effects. London: K. Paul, Trench, Trubner and Co., 1928.

50. Kutner, S., and Duffy, T. A psychological analysis of oral contraceptives and the intrauterine device. Contraception, 1970, 2:289–296.
51. Laurie, P. *Drugs.* Baltimore: Penguin Books, Inc., 1967.
52. Leavitt, F. Drug-induced modifications in sexual behavior and open field locomotion of male rats. Physiol. Behav., 1969, 4:677–683.
53. Leavitt, F. Drug-induced modifications in the sexual behavior of male rats. Ph.D. Dissertation, University of Michigan, 1968.
54. Leslie, C., and Bruhl, D. An effective anti-impotence agent; statistical evaluation of 1000 reported cases. Memphis and Mid-South Med. J., 1963, 38:379–385.
55. Loewe, S. Influence of autonomic drugs on ejaculation. J. Pharm. Exp. Ther., 1938, 63:70–75.
56. Luby, E. Reserpine-like drugs—clinical efficacy. *In* Efron, D. (Ed.) *Psychopharmacology: A Review of Progress.* U.S. PHS Pub. No. 1836, 1968.
57. Margolese, M. Homosexuality: a new endocrine correlate. Hormones Behav., 1970, 1:151–155.
58. Melin, P., and Kihlstrom, J. Influence of oxytocin on sexual behavior in male rabbits. Endocrinol., 1963, 73:433–435.
59. Meyerson, B. Central nervous monoamines and hormone induced estrus behavior in the spayed rat. Acta Physiol. Scand., 1964, 63: supp. 241.
60. Money, J., and Yankowitz, R. The sympathetic-inhibiting effects of the drug Ismelin on human male eroticism with a note on Mellaril. J. Sex Res., 1967, 3:69–82.
61. Montesano, P., and Evangelista, I. Methyltestosterone-thyroid treatment of sexual impotence. Clin. Med., 1966, 12:69–71.
62. Moos, R. Psychological aspects of oral contraceptives. Arch. Gen. Psychiat., 1968, 19:87–94.
63. Nickolls, L., and Teare, D. Poisoning by cantharidin. Brit. Med. J., 1954, part 2, 1384–1386.
64. Orbach, J. Spontaneous ejaculation in rat. Science, 1961, 134:1072.
65. Pincus, G. Control of conception by hormonal steroids. Science, 1966, 153:493–500.
66. Rylander, G. Clinical and medico-criminological aspects of addiction to central stimulating drugs. *In* Sjoqvist, F., and Tottie, M. (Eds.) *Abuse of Central Stimulants.* New York: Raven Press, 1969.
67. Salis, P., and Dewsbury, D. P-chlorophenylalanine facilitates copulatory behaviour in male rats. Nature, 1971, 232:400–401.
68. Salmon, U., and Geist, S. Effect of androgens upon libido in women. J. Clin. Endocrinol. 1943, 3:235–238.
69. Seevers, M. Opiate addiction in the monkey. II: Dilaulid in comparison with morphine, heroin, and codeine. J. Pharmacol., 1936, 56:157–165.
70. Silverman, A. The social behaviour of laboratory rats and the action of chlorpromazine and other drugs. Behaviour, 1966, 27:1–38.
71. Soueif, M. Hashish consumption in Egypt with special reference to psychosocial aspects. UN Bull. on Narcotics, 1967, 19:1–12.
72. Soulairac, A. La signification physiologique de la période réfractaire dans le comportement sexuel du rat mâle. J. Physiol., 1952, 44:99–113.
73. Soulairac, A., and Soulairac, M. Action de la reserpine sur le comportement sexuel du rat mâle. C. R. Soc. Biol., 1961, 155:1010–1013.
74. Soulairac, A., and Soulairac, M. Effect of certain steroid hormones on the sexual behaviour of the male rat and an analysis of their effect on the central nervous system. *Hormonal Steroids, Biochemistry, Pharmacology and Therapeutics; Proceedings of the First International Congress on Hormonal Steroids, Vol. 2.* New York: Academic Press, 1965.
75. Soulairac, M. Etude expérimentale des regulations hormononerveuses du comportement sexuel du rat mâle. Ann. Endocrinol., 1963, 24:1–98.
76. Spence, A. Testosterone propionate in functional impotence. Brit. Med. J., 1940, 2:411–413.
77. Stafford, P., and Golightly, B. *LSD: The Problem-Solving Psychedelic.* New York: Award Books, 1967.
78. Stone, C. Copulatory activity in adult male rats following castration and injections of testosterone propionate. Endocrinol., 1939, 24:165–174.

79. Sulman, F., and Black, B. The alleged endocrine effect of Yohimbine. Endocrinol., 1945, 36:70–72.
80. Swyer, G. Clinical effects of agents affecting fertility. In Michael, R. (Ed.) Endocrinology and Human Behaviour. London: Oxford University Press, 1968.
81. Swyer, G. Homosexuality: the endocrinological aspects. Practit., 1954, 172:374–377.
82. Tagliamonte, A., Tagliamonte, P., Gessa, G., and Brodie, B. Compulsive sexual activity induced by p-chlorophenylalanine in normal and pinealectomized rats. Science, 1969, 166:1433–1435.
83. Tart, C. Marijuana intoxication: common experiences. Nature, 1970, 226:701–704.
84. Tart, C. On Being Stoned. Palo Alto: Science and Behavior Books, Inc., 1971.
85. Trimble, M., and Herbert, J. The effect of testosterone or oestradiol upon the sexual and associated behaviour of the adult female rhesus monkey. J. Endocrinol., 1968, 42:171–185.
86. Tuchmann-Duplessis, H., and Mercier-Parot, L. Action de la reserpine sur la glande mammaire du rat mâle et femelle. C.R. Soc. Biol., 1957, 151:656–658.
87. Turner, C. General Endocrinology. Philadelphia: W. B. Saunders Company, 1966.
88. Udry, J., and Morris, N. Distribution of coitus in the menstrual cycle. Nature, 1968, 220:593–596.
89. Wakefield, D. The hallucinogens: a reporter's objective view. In Solomon, D. (Ed.) LSD: The Consciousness-Expanding Drug. New York: G. P. Putnam's Sons, 1964.
90. Waxenburg, S., Drellich, M., and Sutherland, A. The role of hormones in human behaviour. I. Changes in female sexuality after adrenalectomy. J. Clin. Endocr. Metab., 1959, 19:193–202.
91. Wilson, C. Adolescent Drug Dependence. Oxford: Pergamon Press, 1968.
92. World Health Organization. Clinical aspects of oral gestagens. WHO Rep. Ser. No. 326, 1966.
93. Zimbardo, P., and Barry, H. Effects of caffeine and chlorpromazine on the sexual behavior of male rats. Science, 1958, 127:84–85.
94. Zitrin, A., Beach, F., Barchas, J., and Dement, W. Sexual behavior of male cats after administration of parachlorophenylalanine. Science, 1970, 170:868–870.

CHAPTER 14

AGGRESSION

Neurosurgery, which is a dangerous and irrevocable procedure, has been proposed by some as a means of eliminating tendencies toward violence in perennial criminals. Fortunately, protests that the treatment would be inhumane have so far prevailed, and consequently it has not yet been implemented on a wide scale. Scientists are trying to find more practical methods for curbing violence, and pharmacologists are in the forefront among them. However, although several drugs have been proved capable of reducing aggression in the laboratory, their significance for use with overly aggressive people is not yet established. For one thing, the emphasis in animal studies has been on the acute effects of drugs, whereas the control of aggression in man must be of long duration. A more serious difficulty is that aggressive behavior is a very complex phenomenon. Many laboratory procedures are effective in eliciting some forms of aggression, but whether or not any of them have relevance for any of the varied forms of aggression in man is questionable. One indication of the complexity of aggressive behavior was given by Moyer in 1968 (65). He reviewed evidence which showed that aggression is not a unitary trait; rather, different forms of aggression have different physiological bases.

There is no standardized procedure for scoring an aggressive response. Some experimenters merely count the number or duration of fights. Others, e.g. Charpentier (17), have analyzed aggression into components which are not always similarly affected by drugs. The latter approach is more sophisticated, because changes in fighting behavior may be secondary to other changes which have little to do with aggression. For example, a drug may increase aggression

325

by interfering with an animal's capacity for emitting or responding to a stereotyped appeasement gesture. There is no evidence that drugs selectively influence areas of the brain which control aggression.

In this chapter, work with hormones will be considered first, followed by a discussion of the most popular animal models of aggression. The chapter concludes with a few studies of drug effects on social interaction in man.

HORMONES

Males of most mammalian species are more combative than are females. The fighting does not appear until puberty (75), but can be advanced by injecting immature males with testosterone (60). Neonatal castration of males converts their aggressive behavior to the female pattern; however, when they reach adulthood, the animals, unlike normal adult females, do not respond to testosterone with increased aggression (11). Castration of adult males abolishes fighting, and testosterone replacement therapy restores it (26). One effect of testosterone is to increase muscular strength (91, p. 56), which may indirectly increase fighting.

There are cases in which androgen levels in man have been directly manipulated. Dehydroisoandrosterone was administered to adolescents who suffered from feelings of inadequacy, and a side effect was that their levels of aggression increased (72). The largest increases were in patients with a prior history of aggression. Castration is an old and effective technique for reducing aggression in man. The synthetic estrogen stilbestrol has been used to the same end (72). One exception to the rule that the level of testosterone influences aggressive tendencies in male rats comes from the work of Karli (51), who showed that it is irrelevant to the readiness with which rats kill mice. The muricidal behavior of rats has received extensive study, even though its physiological substrate is obviously different from that which underlies aggression between conspecifics (as will be seen).

Hormonal levels also affect aggression in females. Neonatal testosterone increases aggression (10). The effects of levels of circulating estrogens in adult females vary among species. The aggressiveness of mice is unaffected (41, 61), but that of monkeys, baboons, and hamsters (7, 8, 54) is elevated by estrogen. On the other hand, hostility in women is least at midcycle, when estrogen levels are highest (39). In one study (25) it was found that 49 percent of 156 newly convicted women prisoners had committed their crimes during the premenstruum or menstruation. Cooke (24) compiled figures on violent crimes by women in France and found that 84 percent of them were committed during the premenstruum or menstruation.

ANIMAL MODELS OF AGGRESSION

Animals show aggression in many experimental situations, as when they are isolated or are given painful shocks. When the effects of drugs on such aggression are studied, results are not necessarily applicable to human aggression. It is important to realize that most of the methods for inducing aggression in animals produce very high baseline rates. Therefore, it is not surprising that most drugs reduce fighting in these situations: the only possible direction of change is downward. This will be borne out in the tables and text which follow.

Isolation

When male mice are caged in isolation for longer than two or three weeks, they become aggressive. Part of the reason for such behavior is that they become hypersensitive to all physical stimuli. They attack without provocation and continue fighting even if their attacks are not returned. Yet the fighting is directed; they only attack other males, never females or inanimate objects. Welch and Welch (101) reviewed evidence which showed that the isolation procedure induces changes in many physiological systems, including the synthesis and utilization of brain norepinephrine, dopamine, and serotonin, all of which are decreased. The mice became supersensitive to catecholamines; large doses of MAOI plus DOPA were more lethal to isolates than to grouped mice, even when all were individually housed after the drugs were administered. The changes often enable previously subordinate mice to become dominant when they are paired with previously dominant mice which have been living in groups. The technique of isolation is simple and is popular among researchers. Table 14.1, taken largely from Valzelli et al. (97), summarizes selected drug studies on isolation-induced aggression. Note that, with one exception, drugs from all classes reduce aggression. Acetophenazine was the only drug tested which increased aggression. In all of the tables in this chapter, where a drug produced dose-dependent directional effects, acetophenazine has been listed as increasing aggression.

TABLE 14.1 Effects of Drugs on Isolation-Induced Aggression in
Mice and Rats

DRUG	EFFECT*	REFERENCE	DRUG	EFFECT*	REFERENCE
Antidepressants			*Barbiturates*		
amitriptyline	D	97	hexobarbital	D	97
imipramine	D	97	phenobarbital	D	97
desipramine	D	97	pentobarbital	D	97
MAOI's			*Stimulants*		
phenelzine	D	97	amphetamine	D	97
pheniprazine	D	97	magnesium pemoline	D	97
tranylcypromine	D	97	methylphenidate	D	97
Tranquilizers			*Psychotomimetics*		
meprobamate	D	97	LSD	D	97
tybamate	D	97	marijuana	D	73
trioxazine	D	97	mescaline	D	97
chlordiazepoxide	D	97	hybogaine	D	97
diazepam	D	97			
oxazepam	D	97	*Inhibitors of the ANS*		
nitrazepam	D	97	atropine	D	97
			methysergide	D	97
Antipsychotics			propranolol	D	97
acetophenazine	I	55	phentolamine	D	97
chlorpromazine	D	97			
levomepromazine	D	97	*Miscellaneous*		
propericiazine	D	97	ampyzine	D	97
reserpine	D	97	opipramol	D	97
			gamma amino butyric acid	D	97
			yohimbine	D	97
			probenecid	D	97

*I = increase; D = decrease; N = no change.

Pain-Induced Aggression

In their natural habitats, animals fight over food, territory, and mates, and nonaggressive individuals do not enjoy great reproductive success. Pain, which is most often inflicted by an animal's conspecifics, is a powerful stimulus for aggression. In the laboratory, aggression is readily provoked by the administration of a painful stimulus to one or both of a pair of subjects (rats, snakes, turtles, chickens, hamsters, cats, monkeys [95]). The aggression is not long lasting. It is usually limited to the duration of the shock.

Drugs may reduce fighting by reducing the impact of the shocks, either by analgesic action or by reducing the emotional component of the pain. On the other hand, animals which are hypersensitive to pain may rapidly become submissive, thus also reducing observed aggression. Another mechanism which is often applicable is depression of activity, which would reduce the likelihood that the animals would come into contact with each other. Fighting is an inverse function of cage size, and depression of activity may work in the same way as increases in cage size. More generally, any agent which debilitates is likely to have a suppressant effect on aggression, which is a behavior requiring alertness, coordination, and direction.

Rats, and probably other animals as well, are attracted more to moving objects than to inanimate objects (14). Drugs, by reducing an animal's activity, may reduce its stimulus value as an object of attack to a second animal. Drug-induced changes in odor may also account for the observation (79) that other animals often react differently to drugged animals than they do to controls. Table 14.2 summarizes studies on drugs and pain-induced aggression.

The implications of findings with shock-induced aggression should be recognized by scientists who attempt to elicit aggression by other means. They must be sure to control for the possibility that their techniques cause pain. In particular, those who use electrical stimulation of the brain should be aware that their results may in

TABLE 14.2 Effects of Drugs on Pain-Induced Aggression in Rats and Mice

DRUG	EFFECT*	REFERENCE	DRUG	EFFECT*	REFERENCE
Antidepressants			*Barbiturates*		
imipramine	D	82	hexobarbital	D	13
lithium	D	77	pentobarbital	D	20
MAOI's			*Stimulants*		
iproniazid	I	88	amphetamine	D	57
isocarboxazid	D	88	cocaine	I	13
phenelzine	D	88	methamphetamine	I	13
tranylcypromine	D	88	pentylenetetrazol	I	88
Tranquilizers			*Psychotomimetics*		
chlordiazepoxide	D	82	LSD	I	13
diazepam	D	82			
mephenesin	D	89	*Inhibitors of the ANS*		
meprobamate	D	89	benactyzine	D	13
Antipsychotics			*Miscellaneous*		
chlorpromazine	D	89	clomacran	D	82
perphenazine	D	88	diphenylhydantoin	D	89
prochlorperazine	D	89	morphine	D	13
promazine	D	88	p-chlorophenylalanine	N	23
reserpine	D	89	rubidium	I	86
thioridazine	D	82	serotonin	D	13
trifluoperazine	D	89			
tetrabenazine	D	45			

*I = increase; D = decrease; N = no change.

some cases be attributable not to excitation of specific brain circuits but to pain.

Muricide

About 1 to 20 percent of laboratory rats kill mice or other small animals independently of hunger (52, 56). The appearance of this muricidal response depends on the integrity of the amygdala, a group of a dozen or more nuclei in the temporal lobe. Hunger is of course a regularly recurring motivator in all animals, and one source of food for rats *is* other animals. Therefore, even though other types of aggression are affected by castration, it is understandable that behaviors related to food getting are more resistant to disruption. Table 14.3 summarizes studies involving drugs and muricide. Sofia (83) noted that drugs which reduced muricide at doses which did not produce apparent toxicity were related to amphetamine.

While muricide is an interesting phenomenon, and is readily susceptible to laboratory manipulations, its relevance to human aggression is not apparent.

TABLE 14.3   Effects of Drugs on Muricide in Rats

Drug	Effect*	Reference	Drug	Effect*	Reference
Antidepressants			*Barbiturates*		
amitriptyline	D	47, 83	pentobarbital	D	47
desipramine	D	83			
imipramine	D	83	*Stimulants*		
thiazesim	D	47	amphetamine	D	83
			methamphetamine	D	83
MAOI's			methylphenidate	D	83
iproniazid	D	47, 83	pipradrol	D	47, 83
pargyline	D	83	caffeine	D	83
phenelzine	D	47, 83			
tranylcypromine	D	83	*Inhibitors of the ANS*		
			atropine	D	47
Tranquilizers					
chlordiazepoxide	D	48	*Antihistaminics*		
diazepam	D	47	chlorpheniramine	D	83
meprobamate	D	47	diphenhydramine	D	83
Antipsychotics			*Miscellaneous*		
fluphenazine	D	47	norepinephrine		
			p-chlorophenylalanine	I	76
			physostigmine†		

*I = increase; D = decrease; N = no change.
†Administered in microgram quantities through bilateral cannulae placed in the amygdala, a brain area known to be important for muricidal behavior.

TABLE 14.4   Effects of Drugs on Taming of Cynomolgus and
Squirrel Monkeys

Drug	Effect*	Reference
Tranquilizers		
chlordiazepoxide	D	43
diazepam	D	43
meprobamate	N	43
Antipsychotics		
chlorpromazine	N	43
Barbiturates		
pentobarbital	N	43
phenobarbital	N, D	43
Stimulants		
amphetamine	N	74

*I = increase; D = decrease; N = no change.

Aggression of Monkeys and Other Animals Toward Man

Heise, Scheckel, and Boff (43, 74) have worked with various species of monkeys which are normally hostile toward humans. Table 14.4 summarizes the results of their studies on the taming effects of various drugs. The information that monkeys are tamed by a particular drug may be utilized by people who must handle the monkeys; again, however, the relevance of the information to aggression in man must be questioned. The aggression of the monkeys undoubtedly depends to a great extent on their level of fear, and may be altered by drugs which allay fear.

Ginsburg (35) worked with a wolf which had received little exposure to humans and was fearful of them. Treatment with methaminodiazepoxide, reserpine, or chlorpromazine made it much bolder and more aggressive. Heuschele (44) used chlordiazepoxide, shown by Heise et al. to be effective in monkeys, in 22 different species of zoo animals. It reduced aggression in 18 of them.

Brain Stimulation and Lesions

Stimulation of certain portions of the hypothalamus and other areas of the brain through implanted electrodes elicits rage responses in many mammalian species (31, 66, 70). The behaviors resemble natural aggressive responses, and they can be provoked in both sexes and in inexperienced as well as experienced animals. Brain lesions, too, can increase aggressiveness; cerebral dysfunction under-

TABLE 14.5 Effects of Drugs on Hypothalamic-Induced Hissing in Cats*

Drug	Effect[†]	Reference
Antidepressants		
amitriptyline	D	33
desipramine	D	33
imipramine	D	33
Tranquilizers		
chlordiazepoxide	D	5
Antipsychotics		
chlorpromazine	I	33
ethomoxane	D	33
perphenazine	I	98
reserpine	D	1
trifluoperazine	I	33
triperidol	I	33
Barbiturates		
amobarbital	D	62
pentobarbital	N	33

*Brain stimulation-induced hissing probably produces aggression motivated by fear rather than by rage.
[†]I = increase; D = decrease; N = no change.

lies many instances of violent behavior in man (87). Lesions of certain brain structures within the limbic system may transform previously docile animals into raging beasts. Influences of drugs on aggression provoked by stimulation are summarized in Table 14.5. Drug effects on aggression caused by lesions are not given, because Sofia (82) has shown that drugs reduce such aggression only at doses which have some toxic effects.

Spontaneous Fighting

The popular laboratory animals have been bred for docility. They have low baseline rates of spontaneous fighting. Therefore, in contrast to the other situations, spontaneous fighting is increased by many drugs, as indicated in Table 14.6.

Problems Arising from the Use of Animal Models

Animal models of aggression are of doubtful validity for understanding aggression in man. Human aggression takes many forms, some of which undoubtedly play a role in our highest forms of crea-

TABLE 14.6   Effects of Drugs on Spontaneous Aggression in Rats and Mice

Drug	Effect*	Reference
Tranquilizers		
diazepam	I	32
Antipsychotics		
chlorpromazine	D	99
reserpine	D	22
Stimulants		
caffeine	I	14
Psychotomimetics		
marijuana	N, I[†]	15
Miscellaneous		
apomorphine	I	63
DOPA	I	67
reserpine + amphetamine	N	100
reserpine + apomorphine	I	63
reserpine + LSD	I	100

*I = increase; D = decrease; N = no change.
[†]Marijuana increased aggression in rats only when the animals were starved.

tive expression. Even in animals, aggressive responses have their roots in behaviors which are desirable. Many species are characterized by cohesive social groups, which have obvious adaptive functions. Cappell and Latane (14), on the basis of their findings that gregariousness in rats is increased by caffeine and epinephrine and reduced by alcohol and chlorpromazine, suggested that the changes were produced by modifications of level of arousal. Gregariousness is desirable, but a consequence of increased arousal and greater frequency of interactions is increased fighting. No animal model is an obvious analogue to any type of undesirable aggression in man, and the various procedures for inducing aggression are differentially sensitive to pharmacological interventions.

Drugs which reduce aggression act by diverse mechanisms, few at doses which do not also produce ataxia. There is no evidence to support the conclusion that they selectively depress neural substrates which mediate aggression. One additional difficulty in interpreting animal drug experiments is that the injection procedure, which involves removal of the animals from their cages, handling, and insertion of needles, is stressful. Even injections of inert substances affect behavior (6). Superimposed on the handling stress, which of itself modifies aggression, is the disorientation produced by many psychoactive drugs. Differences between drugged and control animals therefore may in some instances be accounted for by the action of the drug on responsivity to stress or confusion. The drug might have very different effects in humans, who self-administer it under comfortable circumstances.

Perhaps a better animal model will be developed. An appropriate species would be one which normally lives, like man, in cohesive social groups. Many primates have such well developed societies, but rats and mice, although they live in colonies, do not. The most meaningful measure of aggression, if relevance to man is the criterion, is spontaneous fighting over long periods of time, provided the animals are not deprived of any commodity essential to life. Simultaneous measures of health and activity would be necessary in order to exclude the possibility that reductions in aggression are secondary to the debilitating effects of a drug. Finally, it would be important to test drugged animals in interactions with nondrugged ones.

NEUROTRANSMITTER MECHANISMS

Catecholamines

In 1961, Everett (30) reported that mice, rats, dogs, cats, and monkeys injected with DOPA after treatment with MAOI showed extremely high amounts of spontaneous aggression. Randrup and Munkvad (67) replicated the findings in rats. Since DOPA is a precursor to both norepinephrine and dopamine, and since MAOI blocks their metabolism, Everett interpreted his findings as indicating that high brain levels of norepinephrine and/or dopamine increase fighting. However, Randrup and Munkvad also observed rage reactions after MAOI plus scopolamine. They also tested four drugs in combination: MAOI plus DOPA, to increase levels of norepinephrine and dopamine; and diethyldithiocarbamate (DDC) plus reserpine, to inhibit the synthesis and deplete the stores of norepinephrine. The four-drug treatment led to high brain levels of dopamine but not of norepinephrine. Under these conditions, aggression was strongly reduced. Yet DDC plus MAOI, a combination that also blocks norepinephrine synthesis, resulted in increased aggression. Rats injected with 3,4-dihydroxyphenylserine, a precursor of norepinephrine, did not show rage. Their findings may be summarized by saying that aggression has not yet been shown to depend on specific types of changes in brain catecholamines.

Welch and Welch (101) noted three types of drug effects which could act to reduce fighting:

1. General reactivity to stimuli might be decreased.

2. Specific neural mechanisms which control fighting might be lowered in activity.

3. The animal might be rendered incapable of making the appropriate coordinated responses.

Welch and Welch pointed out that the aggression of isolates is reduced by both parachlorophenylalanine and 5-hydroxytryptophan, even though the former reduces and the latter augments brain levels of serotonin. Conner et al. (23) found no effect of parachlorophenylalanine on shock-induced aggression, even though the drug has been shown to increase shock thresholds (90).

Welch and Welch administered MAOI plus DOPA, the combination that was reported by Everett and Randrup and Munkvad to increase fighting. They found that the mice only appeared aggressive, and that despite a great deal of jumping and squealing, there was no coordinated aggressive activity. Reis et al. (68) arrived at a somewhat similar conclusion after administering MAOI plus DOPA to cats. They said that the cats hissed and snarled, but that the behavior appeared to be motivated more by fear than by attack. Defensive postures and flight were predominant.

Thoa and his colleagues (28, 92) have worked with two relatively new drugs, 6-hydroxydopamine, which produces a long-lasting depletion of brain catecholamines, and 6-hydroxydopa, which selectively depletes brain norepinephrine while leaving dopamine unaffected. A single dose of the first drug produced a progressive increase in shock-induced aggression for durations of up to six months. A similar pattern prevailed after 6-hydroxydopa, with no increase in fighting during the first three days after administration, but with substantial increases starting on day 4. The authors noted that since norepinephrine levels are as low on day 2 as they are on day 7, norepinephrine depletion cannot be the sole cause of the fighting. They also reported that the rats did not fight among themselves in their home cages, which indicated that the increases were specific to the shock procedure. In addition to the last two qualifications and those expressed by the Welches, there is a problem when fighting behavior is repeatedly elicited; previous outcomes of fights greatly alter current behavior (36). Thus, in Thoa's studies, small differences in rats due to drug dose on day 1 may have become progressively greater even if there were no drug effects after the first day.

The Cholinergic System

Electrical stimulation of the lateral hypothalamus induces killing behavior in several species of animals (31, 70). Cholinergic stimulation has much the same effect. Bandler (4) injected carbachol through implanted cannulae directly into the lateral hypothalamus of rats. Those rats which normally killed mice were tested with mice, and the rest were tested with frogs, which they invariably killed. The rats responded by killing much more rapidly than they did under control conditions. Norepinephrine, when placed in some brain sites, suppressed the killing response. Sodium chloride, strychnine, and methylphenidate did not affect the response, which indicates that the carbachol effect is not likely to have been mediated by non-specific stimulation.

Smith et al. (81) worked with nonkiller rats. They too injected carbachol into the lateral hypothalamus and tested the response of the rats to mice. There was a clear-cut effect: the rats killed them. Neostigmine had the same effect, but sodium chloride, norepine-phrine, serotonin, and 5-hydroxytryptophan did not stimulate the nonkillers. The authors further tested that the killing response is cholinergically mediated by injecting the muscarinic blocker atro-pine into the lateral hypothalamus of killers. In this case, they did not kill. Injections of carbachol outside the lateral hypothalamus did not affect killing behavior.

As mentioned above, predatory aggression may bear little re-lationship to other forms of aggression. Carbachol and other drugs placed within the lateral hypothalamus have significant effects on eating and drinking behavior. It would be of considerable interest to know if drugs within the lateral hypothalamus affect intraspecific fighting, a type of aggression which is not usually followed by eating.

STUDIES OF HUMAN AGGRESSION

Effects of Various Drugs

Amphetamines

It is important to distinguish between low and high dose usage of the amphetamines. High dose users are at times hyperactive, hyperexcitable, and paranoid (80). The combination is a very danger-ous one. Lemere (59) reported that amphetamine addicts become ag-gressive and often violent. On the other hand, several authors (53, 58) have found that low doses of amphetamine, alone or in combination with secobarbital, increase feelings of friendliness and cooperation.

Phenmetrazine

Rylander (71) reported on the problem of phenmetrazine abuse in Sweden. Phenmetrazine is an amphetamine-like stimulant, but it gives a more agreeable euphoria. According to Rylander, paranoid psychoses eventually strike all advanced addicts and make them extremely dangerous.

Cocaine

The response to cocaine is similar to that seen with amphetamine and phenmetrazine. Cocaine acts as a stimulant, and it induces paranoia. The addict often carries weapons to use against his alleged persecutors. Jaffe (37, p. 299) said that cocaine addicts often fit the otherwise inappropriate stereotype of the "depraved dope fiend."

LSD

Edwards et al. (27), in a study discussed on p. 114, found that LSD users scored higher than nonusers on a questionnaire designed to measure hostility. Cheek and Holstein (18), on the other hand, found that the effects varied with the subject population. They rated interactions among groups of reformatory inmates, alcoholics, and schizophrenics. The total number of social interactions was increased by 25 μg or 50 μg of LSD but was reduced by 200 μg. For reformatory inmates, the increases were all in a negative direction, with many more disagreements and instances of overt hostility. The increase in the alcoholic group was positive, with more praise of others and more joking. The schizophrenics increased in both positive and negative interactions.

Tinklenberg and Stillman (93) believe that the fear which accompanies bad LSD trips makes assaultive behavior unlikely, and, if it does occur, poorly enacted.

Marijuana

Kaplan (50) and Grinspoon (40) have both adduced evidence which clearly demonstrates that the link between marijuana usage and crime is at best tenuous. For example, in one study of 8280 naval and marine prisoners, only 40 used marijuana; of those, only two became more aggressive during marijuana intoxication (9). Chopra and Chopra (21) suggested that marijuana may be a deterrent to crimes of violence, and that excessive use reduces the likelihood of serious crime. Charen and Perelman (16) reached a similar conclusion. One reason may be that marijuana produces muscular weakness and reduced expenditure of physical energy (46).

Alcohol

Kaplan (50) has pointed out two factors which would, a priori, be expected to increase the likelihood of aggressiveness in users of alcohol. First, alcohol lowers inhibitions. Second, the popular stereotype of the drunkard, which is generally accepted by alcoholics and which may therefore contribute to their behavior, includes swaggering toughness. The stereotype also serves to free the alcoholic from responsibility for his actions. The alcohol, not he himself, is to blame. The intuitive arguments are supported by data. In three separate studies of homicide offenders (78, 84, 102), the proportion of those who had been drinking just prior to the crime ranged from 43 to 87 percent. Medina (64), working in Chile, found that 35 percent of crimes of violence were committed by people under the influence of alcohol; moreover, 62 percent of men and 35 percent of women brought in as *victims* of homicide had high blood levels of alcohol. The use of alcohol is also associated with arrests for assault and nonfatal shootings (78).

Opiates

Narcotic addicts lose their vitality (19). They become drowsy and apathetic, and they fight less than previously. Their criminal activity increases because they need money to obtain drugs, but they commit fewer crimes against persons, such as rape and assault, than do people in the population at large (19).

Verbal Output as a Measure

Gottschalk (38) has devised a procedure whereby subjects are asked to speak for about five minutes on topics of personal interest. He claims that content analysis enables experimenters to score hostility, both inwardly and outwardly directed. He has shown that the scores are related to other measures of hostility. Gottschalk found that perphenazine and chlordiazepoxide reduced both types of hostility, whereas imipramine and secobarbital increased outwardly directed hostility. LSD did not influence hostility scores.

Haward (42) also used verbal output to measure aggression. He found some interesting patterns. In one study, both chlorpromazine and haloperidol reduced outwardly directed aggression; however, while haloperidol also reduced aggression directed inwardly, chlorpromazine increased it. In a second study, Haward made use of a typology formulated by Ax (2). Ax had produced evidence that people respond to stressful situations in one of two ways: some show elevated heart rate, respiration rate, and systolic blood pressure, whereas others respond with lowered heart rate, no change in respiration rate, and an increase in diastolic pressure. Ax called the first type norepinephrine dominant and the second epinephrine dominant. Elmadjian (29) postulated that norepinephrine dominant people would be more predisposed to aggressive behavior, a finding which was borne out in Haward's study. In addition, the antiepileptic drug diphenylhydantoin (DPH) reduced outwardly directed verbal hostility in the norepinephrine dominant group, while having no effect on either inwardly directed hostility or outward hostility in the epinephrine dominant group.

Treatment of Aggression

The term hyperkinetic has been applied to children who have been hyperactive and aggressive since birth. In many cases the symptoms derive from slight brain damage. The aggression is effectively controlled by stimulants such as amphetamine and methylphenidate, whereas barbiturates exacerbate it. The effect is paradoxical, but well documented (see Chap. 7). Amphetamines have also been used successfully for the control of aggression in psychopaths.

DPH is a popular antiepileptic drug which was used to curb temper flare-ups in delinquent boys as long ago as 1942 (12). Several other studies since then have shown it to be an effective drug in controlling outbursts of temper and in inducing greater cooperation in refractory patients (3, 85, 104). Resnick (69) described several patients who responded well to DPH treatment, and emphasized that many of them did not have discernible epileptic foci. They did have in common "explosiveness, low frustration tolerance, irritability, impulsive behavior, compulsive behavior, aggressive behavior, erratic behavior, inability to delay gratification, mood swings, short attention spans, undirected activity, and the like." Richmond (cited in Ref. 34) acknowledged that he administers DPH daily to between one-third and one-half of the more aggressive prisoners at Oakalla Prison Farm in British Columbia. The number of aggressive incidents has been enormously reduced by the treatments. Turner (94), too, has reported on the use of DPH as an antiaggressive agent.

It is surprising that diazepam has not received more widespread trials for controlling violent behavior in man, as it effectively reduces animal aggression elicited by a variety of means. Kalina (49) did find it to be of value with psychotic criminals. Their episodic outbursts were efficiently controlled by small doses.

REFERENCES

1. Alcocer-Cuaron, C., Bach y Rita, P., Brust-Carmona, H., and Hernandez-Peon, R. Efectos de la reserpina sobre las respuestas emocionales producidas por estimulcion del sistema limbico. Acta Neurol. Latinoam., 1958, 4:288–293.

2. Ax, A. Physiological differentiation between fear and anger in humans. Psychosom. Med., 1953, 15:433–442.

3. Baldwin, R. Behavior disorders in children. Maryland Med. J., 1969, 18:68–71.

4. Bandler, R. Facilitation of aggressive behaviour in the rat by direct cholinergic stimulation of the hypothalamus. Nature, 1969, 224:1035–1036.

5. Baxter, B. The effect of chlordiazepoxide on the hissing response elicited via hypothalamic stimulation. Life Sci., 1964, 3:531–537.

6. Beaton, J., and Gilbert, R. Injection controls for drug studies. Nature, 1968, 218: 391–392.

7. Birch, J., and Clark, G. Hormonal modification of social behavior. II: The effects of sex-hormone administration on the social dominance status of the female-castrate chimpanzee. Psychosom. Med., 1946, 8:320–331.

8. Bolwig, N. A study of the behaviour of the chacma baboon, Papio ursinus. Behaviour, 1959, 14:136–163.

9. Bromberg, W., and Rogers, T. Marihuana and aggressive crime. Am. J. Psychiat., 1946, 102:825–827.

10. Bronson, F., and Desjardins, C. Aggression in adult mice: modification by neonatal injections of gonadal hormones. Science, 1968, 161:705–706.

11. Bronson, F., and Desjardins, C. Aggressive behavior and seminal vesicle function in mice: differential sensitivity to androgen given neonatally. Endocrinol., 1969, 85:971–974.

12. Brown, W., and Solomon, C. Delinquency and the electroencephalograph. Am. J. Psychiat., 1942, 98:499–503.

13. Brunaud, M., and Siou, G. Action of psychotropic substances on an induced aggressive state in rats. Neuro-psychopharmacology, 1959, 1:282–286.

14. Cappell, H., and Latane, B. Effects of alcohol and caffeine on the social and emotional behavior of the rat. Quart. J. Studies Alc., 1969, 30:345–356.

15. Carlini, E., and Masur, J. Development of aggressive behavior in rats by chronic administration of Cannabis sativa (marihuana). Life Sci., 1969, 8:607–620.

16. Charen, S., and Perelman, L. Personality studies of marihuana addicts. Am. J. Psychiat., 1946, 102:674–682.

17. Charpentier, J. Analysis and measurement of aggressive behavior in mice. In Garattini, S., and Sigg, E. (Eds.) Aggressive Behaviour. New York: John Wiley and Sons, 1969.

18. Cheek, F., and Holstein, C. Lysergic acid diethylamide tartrate (LSD-25) dosage levels, group differences, and social interaction. J. Nerv. Ment. Dis., 1971, 153:133–147.

19. Chein, I., Gerard, D., Lee, R., and Rosenfeld, E. Narcotics, Delinquency and Social Policy. London: Tavistock, 1964.

20. Chen, G., Bohner, B., and Bratton, A. The influence of certain central depressants on the fighting behavior of mice. Arch. Intern. Pharmacodyn., 1963, 142: 30–34.

21. Chopra, R., and Chopra, G. The present position of hemp drug addiction in India. Indian Med. Res. Mem., 1939, 31:1–119.

22. Christian, J. Reserpine suppression of density-dependent adrenal hypertrophy and reproductive hypoendocrinism in populations of male mice. Am. J. Physiol., 1957, 187:353–356.

23. Conner, R., Stolk, J., Barchas, J., Dement, W., and Levine, S. The effect of para-chlorophenylalanine (PCPA) on shock-induced fighting behavior in rats. Physiol. Behav., 1970, 5:1221–1224.

24. Cooke, W. Presidential address: differential psychology of American women. Am. J. Obstet. Gynecol., 1945, 49:457–472.

25. Dalton, K. Menstruation and crime. Brit. Med. J., 1961, 2:1752–1753.

26. Davis, D. The physiological analysis of aggressive behavior. In Etkin, W. (Ed.) Social Behavior and Organization Among Vertebrates. Chicago: University of Chicago Press, 1964.

27. Edwards, A., Bloom, M., and Cohen, S. The psychedelics: love or hostility potion? Psychol. Rep., 1969, 24:843–846.

28. Eichelman, B., Thoa, N., and Ng, K. Facilitated aggression in the rat following 6-hydroxydopamine administration. Physiol. Behav., 1972, 8:1–3.

29. Elmadjian, F. *Symposium on Catecholamines.* Baltimore: Williams & Wilkins, 1959.
30. Everett, G. Some electrophysiological and biochemical correlates of motor activity and aggressive behavior. Neuro-psychopharmacology, 1961, *2*:479–484.
31. Flynn, J. The neural basis of aggression in cats. *In* Glass, D. (Ed.) *Neurophysiology and Emotion.* New York: Rockefeller University Press, 1967.
32. Fox, K., and Snyder, R. Effect of sustained low doses of diazepam on aggression and mortality in grouped male mice. J. Comp. Physiol. Psychol., 1969, *69*: 663–666.
33. Funderbunk, W., Foxwell, M., and Hakala, M. Effects of psychotherapeutic drugs on hypothalamic-induced hissing in cats. Neuropharmacol., 1970, *9*:1–7.
34. Garattini, S., and Sigg, E. (Eds.) *Aggressive Behaviour.* New York: John Wiley and Sons, 1969.
35. Ginsburg, B. Coaction of genetical and nongenetical factors influencing sexual behavior. *In* Beach, F. (Ed.) *Sex and Behavior.* New York: John Wiley and Sons, 1965.
36. Ginsburg, B., and Allee, W. Some effects of conditioning on social dominance and subordination in inbred strains of mice. Physiol. Zool., 1942, *15*:485–506.
37. Goodman, L., and Gilman, A. *The Pharmacological Basis of Therapeutics.* New York: The Macmillan Co., 1965.
38. Gottschalk, L. The measurement of hostile aggression through the content analysis of speech — some biological and interpersonal aspects. *In* Garattini, S., and Sigg, E. (Eds.) *Aggressive Behaviour.* New York: John Wiley and Sons, 1969.
39. Gottschalk, L., Kaplan, S., Gleser, G., and Winget, C. Variations in magnitude of emotion: a method applied to anxiety and hostility during phases of the menstrual cycle. Psychosom. Med., 1962, *24*:300–310.
40. Grinspoon, L. *Marihuana Reconsidered.* Cambridge: Harvard University Press, 1971.
41. Gustafson, J., and Winokur, G. The effect of sexual satiation and female hormone upon aggressivity in an inbred mouse strain. J. Neuropsychiat., 1960, *1*: 182–184.
42. Haward, L. Differential modifications of verbal aggression by psychotropic drugs. *In* Garattini, S., and Sigg, E. (Eds.) *Aggressive Behaviour.* New York: John Wiley and Sons, 1969.
43. Heise, G., and Boff, E. Continuous avoidance as a base-line for measuring behavioral effects of drugs. Psychopharmacologia, 1962, *3*:264–282.
44. Heuschele, W. Chlordiazepoxide for calming zoo animals. J. Am. Vet. Med. Assoc., 1961, *139*:996–998.
45. Hingtgen, J., and Hamm, H. Modification of tetrabenazine effects following pain-induced aggression in rats. Life Sci., 1969, *8*:1–7.
46. Hollister, L., Richards, R., and Gillespie, B. Comparison of tetrahydrocannabinol and synhexyl in man. Clin. Pharmacol. Ther., 1968, *9*:783–791.
47. Horovitz, Z., Piala, J., High, J., Burke, J., and Leaf, R. Effects of drugs on the mouse-killing (muricide) test and its relationship to amygdaloid function. Int. J. Neuropharmacol., 1966, *5*:405–411.
48. Horovitz, Z., Ragozzino, P., and Leaf, R. Selective block of rat mouse-killing by antidepressants. Life Sci., 1965, *4*:1909–1912.
49. Kalina, R. Use of diazepam in the violent psychotic patient: a preliminary report. Colorado GP, 1962, *4*:11.
50. Kaplan, J. *Marijuana: The New Prohibition.* New York: World Publishing Co., 1970.
51. Karli, P. Hormones steroides et comportement d'aggression interspecifique Rat-Souris. J. Physiol., 1958, *50*:346–347.
52. Karli, P., Vergnes, M., and Didiergeorges, F. Rat-mouse interspecific aggressive behaviour and its manipulation by brain ablation and by brain stimulation. *In* Garattini, S., and Sigg, E. (Eds.) *Aggressive Behaviour.* New York: John Wiley and Sons, 1969.
53. Katz, M., Waskow, I., and Olsson, J. Characterizing the psychological state produced by LSD. J. Ab. Psychol., 1968, *73*:1–14.

54. Kislak, J., and Beach, F. Inhibition of aggressiveness by ovarian hormones. Endocrinol. 1955, 56:684–692.
55. Knight, W., Holtz, J., and Sprogis, G. Acetophenazine and fighting behavior in mice. Science, 1963, 141:830–831.
56. Kreiskott, H. Some comments on the killing response behaviour of the rat. In Garattini, S., and Sigg, E. (Eds.) Aggressive Behaviour. New York: John Wiley and Sons, 1969.
57. Lal, H., Defeo, J., and Thut, P. Effect of amphetamine on pain-induced aggression. Comm. Behav. Biol., 1968, 1:333–336.
58. Laties, V. Modification of affect, social behavior and performance by sleep deprivation and drugs. J. Psychiat. Res., 1961, 1:12–25.
59. Lemere, F. The danger of amphetamine dependency. Am. J. Psychiat., 1966, 123:569–572.
60. Levy, I., and King, I. The effects of testosterone propionate on fighting behavior in young male C57B1/10 mice. Anat. Rec., 1953, 117:562.
61. Levy, J. The effects of testosterone propionate on fighting behavior in C57B1/10 young female mice. Proc. West Va. Acad. Sci., 1954, 26:14.
62. Masserman, J. Effects of sodium amytal and other drugs on the reactivity of the hypothalamus of the cat. Arch. Neurol. Psychiat., 1937, 37:617–628.
63. McKenzie, G. Apomorphine-induced aggression in the rat. Brain Res., 1971, 34:323–330.
64. Medina, E. The role of alcohol in accidents and violence. In Popham, R. (Ed.) Alcohol and Alcoholism. Toronto: University of Toronto Press, 1970.
65. Moyer, K. Kinds of aggression and their physiological basis. Comm. Behav. Biol., 1968, 2:65–87.
66. Panksepp, J. Aggression elicited by electrical stimulation of the hypothalamus in albino rats. Physiol. Behav., 1971, 6:321–329.
67. Randrup, A., and Munkvad, I. Relation of brain catecholamines to aggressiveness and other forms of behavioural excitation. In Garattini, S., and Sigg, E. (Eds.) Aggressive Behaviour. New York: John Wiley and Sons, 1969.
68. Reis, D., Moorhead, D., and Merlino, N. Dopa-induced excitement in the cat. Arch. Neurol., 1970, 22:31–39.
69. Resnick, O. The psychoactive properties of diphenylhydantoin: experiences with prisoners and juvenile delinquents. Int. J. Neuropsychiat., 1967, 3: S30–S48.
70. Roberts, W., Steinberg, M., and Means, L. Hypothalamic mechanisms for sexual, aggressive and other motivational behaviors in the opossum, Didelphis virginiana. J. Comp. Physiol. Psychol., 1967, 64:1–15.
71. Rylander, G. Clinical and medico-criminological aspects of addiction to central stimulating drugs. In Sjoqvist, F., and Tottie, M. (Eds.) Abuse of Central Stimulants. New York: Raven Press, 1969.
72. Sands, D. Further studies on endocrine treatment in adolescence and early adult life. J. Ment. Sci., 1954, 100:211–219.
73. Santos, M., Sampaio, M., Fernandes, N., and Carlini, E. Effects of Cannabis sativa (marihuana) on the fighting behavior of mice. Psychopharmacologia, 1966, 8:437–444.
74. Scheckel, C., and Boff, E. Effects of drugs on aggressive behavior in monkeys. Proc. Fifth Int. Cong. Neuropsychopharmacol., 1966, 789–795.
75. Seward, J. Aggressive behavior in the rat. I. General characteristics: age and sex differences. J. Comp. Physiol. Psychol., 1945, 38:175–197.
76. Sheard, M. The effect of p-chlorophenylalanine on behavior in rats: relation to brain serotonin and 5-hydroxyindoleacetic acid. Brain Res., 1969, 15:524–528.
77. Sheard, M. Effect of lithium on foot shock aggression in rats. Nature, 1970, 228: 284–285.
78. Shupe, L. Alcohol and crime. A study of the urine alcohol concentration found in 882 persons arrested during or immediately after the commission of a felony. J. Crim. Law Criminol., 1954, 44:661–664.
79. Silverman, A. Ethological and statistical analysis of drug effects on the social behaviour of laboratory rats. Brit. J. Pharmacol., 1965, 24:579–590.

80. Smith, D. The characteristics of dependence in high-dose methamphetamine abuse. Int. J. Addictions, 1969, 4:453–459.

81. Smith, D., King, M., and Hoebel, B. Lateral hypothalamic control of killing: evidence for a cholinoceptive mechanism. Science, 1970, 167:900–901.

82. Sofia, R. Effects of centrally active drugs on four models of experimentally-induced aggression in rodents. Life Sci., 1969, 8:705–716.

83. Sofia, R. Structural relationship and potency of agents which selectively block mouse killing (muricide) behavior in rats. Life Sci., 1969, 8:1201–1210.

84. Spain, D., Bradess, V., and Eggston, A. Alcohol and violent death. A one-year study of consecutive cases in a representative community. J.A.M.A., 1951, 146:334–335.

85. Stephens, J., and Shaffer, J. A controlled study of the effects of diphenylhydantoin on anxiety, irritability, and anger in neurotic outpatients. Psychopharmacologia, 1970, 17:169–181.

86. Stolk, J., Conner, R., and Barchas, J. Rubidium-induced increase in shock-elicited aggression in rats. Psychopharmacologia, 1971, 22:250–260.

87. Sweet, W., Ervin, F., and Mark, V. The relationship of violent behaviour to focal cerebral disease. In Garattini, S., and Sigg, E. (Eds.) Aggressive Behaviour. New York: John Wiley and Sons, 1969.

88. Tedeschi, D., Fowler, P., Miller, R., and Macko, E. Pharmacological analysis of footshock-induced fighting behaviour. In Garattini, S. and Sigg, E. (Eds.) Aggressive Behaviour. New York: John Wiley and Sons, 1969.

89. Tedeschi, R., Tedeschi, D., Mucha, A., Cook, L., Mattis, P., and Fellows, E. Effects of various centrally acting drugs on fighting behavior of mice. J. Pharmacol. Exp. Ther., 1959, 125:28–34.

90. Tenen, S. The effects of p-chlorophenylalanine, a serotonin depletor, on avoidance acquisition, pain sensitivity and related behavior in the rat. Psychopharmacologia, 1967, 10:204–219.

91. Tepperman, J. Metabolic and Endocrine Physiology. Chicago: Year Book Medical Publishers, 1962.

92. Thoa, N., Eichelman, B., Richardson, J., and Jacobowitz, D. 6-hydroxydopa depletion of brain norepinephrine and the facilitation of aggressive behavior. Science, 1972, 178:75–77.

93. Tinklenberg, J., and Stillman, R. Drug use and violence. In Daniels, D., Gilula, M., and Ochberg, F. Violence and the Struggle for Existence. Boston: Little, Brown and Co., 1970.

94. Turner, W. Anticonvulsive agents in the treatment of aggression. In Garattini, S., and Sigg, E. (Eds.) Aggressive Behaviour. New York: John Wiley and Sons, 1969.

95. Ulrich, R., Hutchinson, R., and Azrin, N. Pain-elicited aggression. Psychol. Rec., 1965, 15:111–126.

96. Valzelli, L. Drugs and aggressiveness. Adv. Pharmacol., 1967, 5:79–108.

97. Valzelli, L., Giacolone, E., and Garattini, S. Pharmacological control of aggressive behavior in mice. Europ. J. Pharmacol., 1967, 2:144–146.

98. Vasquez, A., and Toman, J. Some interactions of nicotine with other drugs upon central nervous function. Ann. N.Y. Acad. Sci., 1967, 142:201–215.

99. Vessey, S. Effects of chlorpromazine on aggression in laboratory populations of wild house mice. Ecology, 1967, 48:367–376.

100. Votava, Z. Aggressive behavior evoked by LSD-25 in rats pretreated with reserpine. In Garattini, S., and Sigg, E. (Eds.) Aggressive Behaviour. New York: John Wiley and Sons, 1969.

101. Welch, B., and Welch, A. Aggression and the biogenic amine neurohumors. In Garattini, S., and Sigg, E. (Eds.) Aggressive Behaviour. New York: John Wiley and Sons, 1969.

102. Wolfgang, M. Patterns in Criminal Homicide. Philadelphia: University of Pennsylvania Press, 1958.

103. Yen, C., Stanger, R., and Millman, N. Ataractic suppression of isolation-induced aggressive behavior. Arch. Int. Pharmacodyn., 1959, 123:179–185.

104. Zimmerman, F. Explosive behavior anomalies in children on an epileptic basis. N.Y.J. Med., 1956, 56:2537–2543.

CHAPTER 15

SLEEP
AND DREAMS

Research on drug-induced modifications of sleep and dreams has been motivated by four largely independent aims. One goal is the development of drugs which promote sound, restful sleep. Its achievement would be most welcome, as evidenced by the fact that despite the shortcomings of barbiturates (to be discussed), approximately 33 60mg barbiturate capsules are manufactured annually for every person in the United States (79, p. 123). Conversely, many drugs are promoted because of their ability to fend off sleep. A third goal is the identification of commonly used drugs which influence nocturnal sleep patterns, in order that physicians and their patients can be apprised of possible symptoms. Should a therapeutically useful drug be found disturbing to sleep, research can be initiated toward the development of less toxic congeners. Finally, drugs are used as tools in basic research to clarify the normal physiological regulators of the sleep-dream cycle.

HYPNOTIC DRUGS

Despite their name, the effects produced by hypnotic drugs are in no way related to hypnotic trance phenomena. The most important property of hypnotic drugs (also called soporifics or somnifacients) is the induction of sleep. Unfortunately, there is no single criterion which is universally successful in determining the value of a night's sleep. The EEG is usually a reliable indicator of the depth and amount of sleep (see Chap. 2), but dissociations between EEG and behavior have been reported after drug administration. For instance, animals treated with atropine often become hyperactive despite having EEG patterns which resemble those seen during sleep, whereas animals given physostigmine behave quietly while displaying activated EEG patterns (8, 88). People's own subjective estimates of the quality and quantity of their sleep, which would appear to be an important datum, often fail to correspond to their EEG records (54). Moreover, the claim to have enjoyed profound sleep may be made even when the health-maintaining qualities of a good night's sleep have not been realized; this may be reflected in deterioration of performance on the following day.

In addition to promoting sleep, the ideal hypnotic should be free of side effects, including addiction potential. It should be inexpensive and effective when taken orally. Ease of awakening should be no different after drug-induced sleep, as compared with normal sleep. Lastly, there should be no hangover.

Barbiturates

Barbituric acid, which does not itself have hypnotic properties, is the parent compound from which the barbiturates are derived. Its chemical formula is given in Figure 15–1. Barbiturates are obtained by replacing the two hydrogens on the carbon atom in position 5 of barbituric acid with alkyl or aryl groups. There are more than 2500 synthetic barbiturates, of which only a few are widely used. Table 15.1 lists some of the more common ones. Some of the barbiturates are prescribed for relief of anxiety, while others, e.g., phenobarbital and mephobarbital, are valuable in the treatment of epilepsy. However, barbiturates are most frequently used to induce sleep. Most barbiturates and other hypnotics as well are capable of producing anesthesia when administered in sufficiently large doses.

The barbiturates are inexpensive. They are effective when taken orally. They are versatile: short-acting barbiturates are prescribed to overcome difficulty in falling asleep; long-acting ones are preferable when the primary complaint is waking during the night and

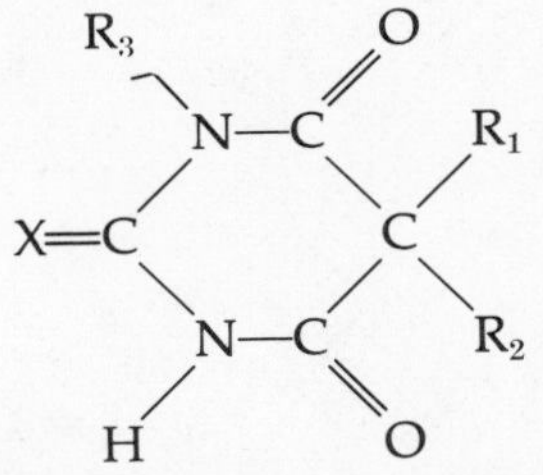

Figure 15–1   General formula of barbiturates.

**TABLE 15.1   Barbiturates Available in the United States:
Names and Structures***

Barbiturate	Trade Name	R_1**	R_2	R_3	X
Allobarbital	Dial	allyl	allyl	H	O
Amobarbital	Amytal	ethyl	isopentyl	H	O
Aprobarbital	Alurate	allyl	isopropyl	H	O
Barbital	Veronal	ethyl	ethyl	H	O
Butabarbital	Butisol	ethyl	sec-butyl	H	O
Butalbital	Sandoptal	allyl	isobutyl	H	O
Butallylonal	Pernoston	sec-butyl	2-bromoallyl	H	O
Butethal	Neonal	ethyl	butyl	H	O
Cyclobarbital	Phanodorn	ethyl	cyclohexen-1-yl	H	O
Cyclopentyl allylbarbituric acid	Cyclopal	allyl	2-cyclopenten-1-yl	H	O
Heptabarbital	Medomin	ethyl	1-cyclohepten-1-yl	H	O
Hexethal	Ortal	ethyl	n-hexyl	H	O
Hexobarbital	Evipal	methyl	1-cyclohexen-1-yl	CH_3	O
Mephobarbital	Mebaral	ethyl	phenyl	CH_3	O
Metharbital	Gemonil	ethyl	ethyl	CH_3	O
Methitural	Neraval	2-methylthioethyl	1-methylbutyl	H	S
Methohexital	Brevital	allyl	1-methyl-2-pentynyl	CH_3	O
Pentobarbital	Nembutal	ethyl	1-methylbutyl	H	O
Phenobarbital	Luminal	ethyl	phenyl	H	O
Probarbital	Ipral	ethyl	isopropyl	H	O
Secobarbital	Seconal	allyl	1-methylbutyl	H	O
Talbutal	Lotusate	allyl	sec-butyl	H	O
Thiamylal	Surital	allyl	1-methylbutyl	H	S
Thiopental	Pentothal	ethyl	1-methylbutyl	H	S
Vinbarbital	Delvinal	ethyl	1-methyl-1-butenyl	H	O

*From "Hypnotics and Sedatives I. The Barbiturates" by Seth K. Sharpless, p. 100, in *The Pharmacological Basis of Therapeutics,* Fourth Edition, L. S. Goodman and A. Gilman (Eds.). The Macmillan Publishing Co., Inc., New York, 1970.
**See Figure 15–1 for placement of R and X on barbituric acid.

inability to return to sleep.(The distinction between short- and long-acting barbiturates has been questioned in recent years.) Their margin of safety is adequate—severe poisoning occurs at about 10 times the hypnotic dose—and they are relatively free of side effects. Nevertheless, several features combine to make the barbiturates less than ideal hypnotic drugs.

Unnatural Sleep

The transition from waking to sleeping is marked by profound changes in many bodily functions: activity of the CNS reflexes, size of pupils, digestion, metabolism, heart rate, blood pressure, composition of blood, respiration, and body temperature. The extent to which these and other changes account for the health-maintaining properties of sleep is unknown. Therefore, sleep which differs from normal may not be as valuable as normal sleep. Barbiturate-induced sleep is abnormal in several respects. Many of the differences are detected by electroencephalography.

Researchers use the EEG to evaluate depth of sleep and to determine when a sleeper is dreaming. They have found that an activated EEG and rapid eye movements (REM's) accompany the dream. Barbiturates delay the first dream period of the night and reduce total dream time and the duration of individual dream episodes (37). There are fewer dreams and fewer rapid eye movements per minute (2, 67). The effect is confined to the first half of the night, during which time slow wave (nondream) sleep occurs with greater than normal frequency. During barbiturate slow wave sleep there is more fast activity than normal, less slow activity, and more spindling (waves of greater than 14 cycles per second superimposed upon the slow waves). Upon withdrawal from the barbiturates, dream time increases, dreams are often very vivid, and nightmares are common (68).

The reticular formation, an area of the brain which is involved in the regulation of sleep and waking, is depressed during barbiturate sleep (81). In addition, stimulation of the reticular formation produces a smaller alerting response than occurs normally. Muscle tonus is reduced, and there are fewer bodily movements (33, 51, 81). Sleeping is subjectively felt to be abnormal, and wakening is achieved only with difficulty (21). There is an aftereffect of drowsiness lasting for 12 to 24 hours (46).

Adverse Side Effects

Barbiturates are relatively free from severe side effects. Most users become euphoric, but some become severely depressed or hostile. Disorders of memory and thought are frequent concomitants of chronic usage. Other symptoms of barbiturate intoxication are slurred speech, impaired vision, vertigo, ataxic gait, and hallucinations. Cardiovascular and respiratory problems are rare at hypnotic doses. Skin eruptions are fairly common.

Overdosage

In New York City, between the years 1957 and 1963, there were 1165 fatalities from barbiturate overdosage (79, p. 123). Each year, over 15,000 people are admitted to United States hospitals suffering from acute intoxication (79, p. 126). Current estimates are that about half of the victims have attempted suicide, but in many cases the overdose is attributed to "drug automatism": a given dose fails to promote sleep but does disorient the patient, who then takes additional pills while failing to remember the earlier ones. Death is usually caused by respiratory depression or circulatory collapse.

Addiction

Jaffe (23, p. 296) offered the opinion that the abuse of barbiturates and related hypnotic drugs probably exceeds that of the opiates. Dependence can be produced in man after a daily dose of 0.4 gm for three months, or of 0.6 gm for as little as one month (19). Withdrawal may be severe.

Evaluation of Barbiturates

The negative aspects of the barbiturates have been emphasized in order to make clear the need for additional research on hypnotic drugs. Nevertheless, they do offer relief to people suffering from an inability to sleep, and the nonbarbiturate hypnotics offer no significant advantages—in fact, one major disadvantage is that their pharmacology is less thoroughly understood. The tragedy of several years ago involving the drug thalidomide illustrates the dangers of ignorance on the part of physicians of the totality of a drug's effects. Thalidomide was prescribed to pregnant women for the purpose of inducing sleep, but use of the drug resulted in the birth of many babies with phocomelia (a congenital deformity in which the hands or feet are attached to the trunk by single, very short bones).

Nonbarbiturates

Bromides

Bromide depresses the CNS and is occasionally found in preparations for inducing sleep or relieving headache pain. Because it has a very slow excretion rate, chronic administration frequently leads to cumulation. Toxic effects include mental clouding, emotional disturbances, and bromide rash.

Chloral Hydrate

Chloral hydrate is a derivative of ethyl alcohol. It is a safe, reliable hypnotic, but is unpleasant to the taste and irritating to the stomach. It is useful with elderly patients, who often suffer confusion from barbiturates. Unlike other hypnotics, it does not depress REM (23). It is dangerous to patients suffering from heart disease or peptic ulcer. Addiction is uncommon, but may occur; the poet Dante Gabriel Rossetti is reputed to have taken about 10 times the hypnotic dose nightly (23, p. 133).

Alcohol

Alcohol depresses the CNS. In low doses, it depresses cortical areas which normally act to restrain behavior. Therefore, the initial effect may be one of apparent stimulation. The reticular formation is very sensitive to alcohol, which partially justifies the occasional use of alcohol as a hypnotic. Alcohol may be useful in cases of insomnia caused by anxiety. However, the sleep which is induced is abnormal—for example, dream time is reduced—and tolerance develops to its effects.

Nonprescription Drugs

Table 15.2 is a list of sleeping preparations which are commonly sold without prescription in one well-stocked pharmacy in San Francisco. The active ingredients of the mixtures are given on the right hand side of the table. They clearly do not differ greatly from each other, despite advertising claims to the contrary. The active principle in all cases is methapyrilene, alone or in combination with scopolamine and/or salicylamide. (Many nonprescription preparations for sedation have the same active principles. As a general rule, most nonprescription drugs which are promoted for treatment of a particular symptom are virtually identical.)

There is often justification for administering two or more drugs concurrently, but the procedure is not without its risks. Indeed, the task of a physician in rapidly identifying the causative agent when there are toxic effects is complicated by multiple drug therapy. An-

TABLE 15.2   Ingredients of Popular Sleep Preparations

Brand Name	Active Ingredients*
Asper-Sleep	M, Sc, aspirin
Dormeez	M
Dormin	M
McKesson	M, Sc, Sa
Nytol	M, Sa
Pro-Sleep	M, Sa, Sc
Restine	M, glyceryl guaiacolate (an expectorant)
Sleep-Eze	M, Sc
Sominex	M, Sc, Sa
Sure Sleep	M, Sa, Sc
S.W.T.	M, Sa
Twilite	M, Sa

*M = methapyrilene; Sc = scopolamine; Sa = salicylamide.

other problem arises with *fixed dose* drug mixtures. These are almost always inadvisable; the use of terms like LD_{50} and ED_{50} should serve as a reminder that individuals vary in responsiveness. Moreover, a patient may be resistant to one drug and susceptible to another. Therefore, whereas dosages of individual drugs are often adjusted in accordance with the patients' reactions, such flexibility is lost in fixed dose mixtures. A final objection to over-the-counter preparations is that they are generally more expensive than the comparable prescription drugs.

With that for preamble, the pharmacology of the three major drugs listed in Table 15.2 shall be briefly described.

METHAPYRILENE. Histamine, which is found in virtually all mammalian tissues, is a substance with important physiological functions. It has been implicated in the genesis of headaches, and injection of histamine produces bronchial constriction and allergic reactions. Antihistamines, of which methapyrilene is an example, antagonize most of the pharmacological actions of histamine and are used clinically in the treatment of allergy and motion sickness. They elicit many unpleasant side effects, the most frequent of which is sedation. Other occasional untoward reactions include dizziness, ringing in the ears, fatigue, blurred vision, loss of appetite, nausea, constipation, diarrhea, dryness of the mouth, palpitation, hypotension, and weakness of the hands. The gastrointestinal tract is particularly sensitive to methapyrilene. Methapyrilene is neither as powerful nor as effective a hypnotic as the barbiturates, especially when it is given in the recommended doses (23, p. 640). Moreover, there is no simple relation between dose and hypnotic effect, and excitatory effects may appear at high doses (23, p. 140). Tolerance rapidly develops to the hypnotic effect. Most antihistamines reduce dream time (37). A final undesirable property of the antihistamines is that people vary greatly in their degree of responsiveness to them.

SCOPOLAMINE. Scopolamine is an antimuscarinic agent which is used primarily in the treatment of parkinsonism, motion sickness, and in preanesthetic medication to inhibit salivation and respiratory tract secretion. Therapeutic doses normally cause drowsiness and dreamless sleep, but restlessness or delirium may be produced instead, especially in the presence of pain or anxiety. Reference to Tables 1.4 and 1.5 indicates the widespread effects of antimuscarinic drugs. Therefore, it is not surprising that hypnotic doses of scopolamine produce many side effects. The most common are dry mouth, blurred vision, sensitivity to light (because of pupillary dilation) and rapid beating of the heart.

SALICYLAMIDE. Salicylamide is related to acetylsalicylic acid (aspirin). Both drugs alleviate certain types of pain, but salicylamide is not effective against moderate to severe pain. Aspirin rapidly and effectively lowers body temperature in febrile individuals, while the antipyretic effect of salicylamide is much less powerful. High doses of aspirin initially stimulate and then depress the CNS. The depression is often accompanied by confusion, dizziness, a ringing sensation in the ears, and delirium. Salicylamide is a more selective CNS depressant; drowsiness occurs in about 10 percent of users. The percentage hardly justifies the use of salicylamide as a hypnotic, since dizziness occurs in 20 percent and gastrointestinal irritation in 10 percent (23, p. 330). Woodbury (23, p. 326) made the claim that the toxicity of aspirin is seriously underestimated

DRUGS FOR MAINTAINING ALERTNESS

Caffeine

Caffeine is one of three important derivatives of xanthine. The other two are theophylline and theobromine. Caffeine is the most

TABLE 15.3   Caffeine Content of Popular Beverages and Nonprescription Drugs

BEVERAGE	CAFFEINE
Cup of coffee	100–150 mg
Cup of decaffeinated coffee	30–70
Cup of tea	100–150
Cup of cocoa	50
12 oz. cola drink	50–80
DRUG	
1 No-Doz tablet	100
1 Vivarin tablet	200

powerful CNS and skeletal muscle stimulant of the three. The approximate therapeutic dose is 100 mg. Theophylline is most active with respect to cardiac stimulation and smooth muscle relaxation, including relaxation of the smooth muscle of the bronchi. As such, it is a valuable agent in the treatment of bronchial asthma and congestive heart failure. The approximate amounts of caffeine in popular beverages and nonprescription preparations are given in Table 15.3.

CNS Effects

Caffeine stimulates the CNS at all levels. It shifts the EEG to a higher frequency (22). Stimulation of the cortex by caffeine enhances mental clarity and allays fatigue. Children are especially sensitive to the excitant effects. Caffeine alleviates some types of headache pain by virtue of its constriction of cerebral arterioles. It is used, therefore, as an ingredient in many headache remedies. Abrupt withdrawal by habitual users commonly results in headaches. Little tolerance develops to the CNS effects of caffeine. See Chapter 4 for some of the deleterious effects of caffeine.

Caffeine delays the onset of sleep (78). During the night, small body movements increase, and rectal temperature is elevated above normal. Since the extent to which rectal temperature falls during sleep correlates highly with subjective estimates of the excellence of sleep (60), it would appear that caffeine not only delays sleep onset but also impairs its quality. Caffeine does not greatly affect dream time (25).

Amphetamines

The amphetamines are a family of sympathomimetic drugs which have powerful CNS actions and are effective when taken orally. Amphetamine may occur as either the D or the L isomer, or as a racemic mixture of DL. The three compounds are qualitatively similar in their actions, but D-amphetamine (dextroamphetamine) acts about twice as powerfully on the CNS as does the DL mixture, and is four times as powerful as the L isomer. They are equipotent in peripheral effects such as dry mouth and increased blood pressure and heart rate. Methamphetamine is similar to D-amphetamine, with a very high ratio of central to peripheral effects.

CNS Effects

Amphetamine depresses appetite; the anorexic effect is extremely marked in dogs, which may starve if given amphetamine each day one hour before the daily meal (35). In man, tolerance develops to the anorexic effects after about four to six weeks of treatment.

Amphetamine shifts the EEG to a higher frequency (22). Psychic effects include wakefulness, alertness, and an improvement in ability to concentrate. Mood is elevated and there is often a feeling of euphoria. Fatigue is diminished, and performance of dull, fatiguing tasks which nevertheless require attentiveness is often improved. When sleep comes, dream time is reduced and bodily movements increase (74). Less time is spent in the deepest stage of sleep (2).

Therapeutic Uses

Amphetamine has been used widely, but perhaps not wisely, for its anorexic and mood-elevating effects; Clement et al. (10) reported the case of a pharmacist who, upon being presented with a signed prescription for 1000 Desoxyn (methamphetamine) tablets, called the physician to find out if the patient had altered the original prescription by adding one or two zeroes to it. The physician reassured the pharmacist that the prescription was correct, then asked, "By the way, what is Desoxyn?"

Amphetamine has been used for many years in the treatment of narcolepsy, and patients do not develop tolerance. Several other uses derive from its capacity to obtund the need for sleep. For instance, it is often prescribed concurrently with drugs such as imipramine, which produce sedation as a side effect. The degree to which sleep deprivation causes impairment on various tasks is reduced by D-amphetamine (44). Laties (48) found that a combination of 10 mg amphetamine plus 100 mg secobarbital reduced feelings of sleepiness in men who had been deprived of sleep for 37 hours. When Kleitman and his subjects were given 10 mg amphetamine every 4 to 8 hours, they were able to withstand much greater periods of sleep deprivation than they were capable of without the drug (40, p. 301).

Eneuresis has been effectively treated with amphetamine when its cause is very deep sleep and consequent inability to attend to sensations of pressure from the bladder. Amphetamine lessens the depth of sleep and consequently facilitates arousal. Amphetamine is also used in the treatment of hyperkinetic children (see Chap. 7).

Dependency

The addiction potential of amphetamines is a subject of dispute. Jaffe (in 23) has argued that addiction is relatively uncommon, but he acknowledged that there have been sprees of heavy usage. For example, Noda (64) reported in 1950 that 1.1 percent of the population of Japan was dependent upon amphetamine. Connell (11) published a monograph on psychoses resulting from chronic amphetamine use which indicated that such reactions were much more common than generally realized. As has been pointed out in an earlier chapter, cause-effect relationships are not established by such studies; it is quite reasonable to argue that individuals who are predisposed to psychosis are likely to abuse amphetamine. Nevertheless, the association between chronic high dose amphetamine usage and psychosis is compelling, and there is additional evidence of permanent organic brain damage (50).

Smith (80) has described high dose methamphetamine toxicity. Intravenous injections, of which there are typically about 10 per day, produce "full body orgasms." Between injections the user is euphoric, hyperactive, and hyperexcitable, and has little need for sleep or food. This phase eventually terminates and is followed by extreme exhaustion and then profound depression. If relief cannot be obtained through supportive therapy, the methamphetamine is often readministered.

The contrast between high (usually intravenous) and low (oral) dose usage must be emphasized. Occasional use of low doses to allay fatigue is not likely to lead to dependence in initially stable individuals (23). There is a withdrawal syndrome of altered sleep EEG patterns after large doses (69), but withdrawal is never life threatening and is, in fact, without major sequelae (23).

Comparison of Amphetamine with Caffeine

Nash (63) summarized his extensive researches on caffeine and amphetamine by concluding that the latter has more positive effects and produces more consistent stimulation. Both drugs improve mood and performance, but amphetamine does so to a greater extent. Caffeine impairs hand steadiness, while amphetamine improves it.

Innes and Nickerson (35) concluded their discussion of amphetamine with the following statement: "Because the beneficial effects of the drug have to be repaid in the coin of fatigue and often depression, and because of the variable reactions in patients, amphetamine should not be used indiscriminately. (See the review by Weiss and Laties, 1962.)" Their comments indicate a misreading of the paper by Weiss and Laties (87), who concluded their review by asking whether or not there is a cost to the enhancement of performance by amphetamine. The answer ". . . is mostly negative. Both from the standpoint of physiological and psychological cost, amphetamines and caffeine are rather benign agents. Except for reports of insomnia, the subjective effects of the amphetamines in normal doses are usually favorable. . . . Caffeine seems somewhat less benign. . . . Caffeine also produces a significant increase in tremor. At dose levels that clearly enhance performance, the amphetamines seem not only more effective than caffeine, but less costly in terms of side effects."

Nicotine

Nicotine stimulates many bodily processes. It increases metabolic rate, heart rate, and blood pressure. It also constricts blood vessels and lowers skin temperature. In addition, nicotine improves hand steadiness (18). Heimstra et al. (30) reported that when the subjects in their study were asked what action they took to alleviate or counteract fatigue during long driving sessions, a large percentage of them indicated that they increased their smoking. Smoking has a stimulant effect upon the quantitative EEG (62), and heavy smokers have less alpha activity than do non-smokers (7).

Domino and his colleagues have conducted an extensive series of investigations on the effects of nicotine, in doses comparable to those obtained in smoking, on sleep mechanisms (15, 16, 42, 90). One of their early interests was whether the EEG action of nicotine is the result of direct action upon the CNS, or whether it is secondary to the peripheral effects on blood pressure and heart rate. They noted that the EEG activation occurs only when the state of the organism prior to injection is one of mild CNS depression or sleep. By cutting the brainstem just anterior to the pons, Domino and his associates were able to produce EEG's in rabbits, cats, dogs, and monkeys that permanently resembled those seen in natural sleep. In all four species, an intravenous dose of 20 μg/kg consistently produced activation within one minute. The compounds epinephrine, serotonin, and vasopressin are released peripherally by nicotine, and the possibility existed that the EEG effects could be secondary to their release. However, when these compounds were administered, their actions were much different from those of nicotine. They did not produce activation in all species tested. Moreover, reserpine, which depletes the CNS of epinephrine, norepinephrine, and serotonin, did not affect the EEG arousal produced by nicotine.

Additional evidence for a direct action of nicotine on the CNS was provided by the use of antagonists. Hexamethonium and mecamylamine both block the peripheral actions of nicotine, but mecamylamine penetrates the blood-brain barrier much more readily, and it alone blocked the EEG activation.

The above studies were conducted upon animals with permanent sleep EEG's. It was also deemed useful to study normal animals, for which purpose electrodes were permanently implanted within the brains of cats. The cats also had indwelling cannulae in the jugular vein, in order that intravenous injections could be administered quickly, precisely, and with no inconvenience. When the cats were sleeping, they were injected with either saline or nicotine. There was no reaction to the saline. The cats showed rapid and brief (3 minutes) EEG and behavioral arousal in response to the nicotine but then returned to sleep, often deeper than before. After 15 to 25 minutes the EEG and behavioral pattern was that of dream sleep.

Domino also tested men. He used both non-smokers and light smokers, and gave intramuscular injections of nicotine at bedtime. There were no significant changes in onset, duration, or pattern of sleep.

Iproniazid

Iproniazid is an antidepressant drug. In 1958 Kline (41) reported that his patients who were treated with iproniazid required only three to four hours of sleep each night. Kline tried the drug himself for several months, with similar results. Others have been unable to replicate his findings, but Kline maintains (in a personal communication) that the original effects remain the same.

CHANGES IN SLEEP PATTERNS OF MAN PRODUCED BY FREQUENTLY USED DRUGS

Table 15.4 is a summary of the effects of a few clinically popular drugs—and some which are used illicitly—on sleep in man. Several points should be borne in mind:

1. The subjects of the studies have not been randomly selected. Many have been either patients in mental hospitals or drug addicts.

2. The studies have been conducted almost exclusively in hospitals. The hospital setting, by creating anxiety or boredom, or because of excessive noise or quiet, may drastically affect sleep patterns. The influence of setting on the response of mice to drugs was seen in a study by Baumel et al. (5). Following injections of any of four hypnotic drugs, mice deprived of social interactions had reduced durations of hypnosis compared with those of nonisolates.

3. Few dose-response curves have been obtained.

4. There have been only a few studies in which repeated administrations were given. Yet sleep disturbances which occur after acute use often disappear with chronic use.

Most clinically used drugs suppress dreaming. Two different mechanisms have been proposed. On the one hand, some drugs may reduce the physiological or psychological need to dream. On the other hand, the need may remain, but its expression may be blocked. The two alternatives can be distinguished by the simple expedient of withdrawing the drug. If there is a rebound increase in dreaming, expression was probably blocked rather than the need reduced. An alternative explanation of rebound increases has been proposed by Oswald (65) and discussed by King (39). They noted that the procedures used to produce REM deprivation are often very stressful. They might possibly produce CNS damage. In that case, REM rebound may not be indicative of a need to make up something which has been lost but may simply be a sign of healing. Oswald believes that the purpose of REM sleep is brain repair.

Oswald (66) theorized that all addicting drugs cause rebound increases of REM. During chronic administration, they reduce the frequency of rapid eye movements per minute, thus probably reducing the vividness of dream episodes. Eye movements are much more profuse on withdrawal nights, during which time nightmares are common. Because nightmares serve to raise anxiety level, relief may be sought in the drugs. Thus, a vicious circle of dependence is created. This, of course, is still highly speculative.

THE PHARMACOLOGY OF SLEEP AND DREAMING

Throughout the central core of the brain stem, extending from the medulla to the thalamus (see Fig. 15–2), is a complex network of neurons which is collectively called the reticular formation (RF). The reticular formation regulates many bodily functions, such as gastrointestinal secretions, vasomotor tonus, and respiration. It also regulates the sleep-wake cycle.

In 1949, Moruzzi and Magoun (61) made the important discovery that electrical stimulation of the RF of anesthetized cats immediately converts the EEG from a sleeping to an aroused pattern. Lindsley et al. (56) extended research on the RF. They made lesions in cats of either the sensory pathways or the RF. Animals in the first group showed normal EEG patterns, while those in the second became permanently stuporous.

Individual neurons within the RF are rarely influenced by all types of stimuli, but different neurons respond to stimulation from every sense modality (76). RF neuronal activity varies with the state of arousal; activity of most neurons is greatest either when the organism is awake or when it is dreaming, and is least in nondream sleep. (Some neurons show the reverse pattern.)

As a result of these and other studies, the role of the RF in controlling the sleep-wake cycle appeared to be straightforward. The conception was of a homogeneous system, with the system's level

TABLE 15.4 Changes in Sleep Patterns of Man which are Induced by a few Selected Drugs

DRUG	LATENCY TO SLEEP ONSET*	TOTAL SLEEP	TOTAL DEEP SLEEP	REM LATENCY	% REM	REM DURING RECOVERY	MISCELLANEOUS EFFECTS	REPRESENTATIVE REFERENCES
Antipsychotics								
chlorpromazine	N		I	D	N, L, D	I	hangover; fewer brief arousals during sleep	52, 86
reserpine			D	D	I	I	more brief arousals	13
lithium					D			47
Antidepressants								
tranylcypromine		N		I	D	I	nightmares during withdrawal	14, 49
nialamide	N	I	N	I	D	N		14
imipramine		N		I	D	N	increased hostility in dreams	45, 75, 86
amitriptyline	I	N			D	N		26, 27
Antianxiety Agents								
diazepam					I	I	dependence and decreased motility in dreams	84
meprobamate					N, D			20, 45
chlordiazepoxide	D	I		N, I	N, L, D			9, 26, 27, 84

						Comments	Ref.
Illicit Drugs							
LSD			D				
marijuana	D	N, I / I, D			I	REM rebound during chronic usage, while total deep sleep remains low; users report ease in falling asleep	3, 34, 73, 83 24
opiates	D	I	D		I	frequent awakenings; disturbed sleep	38, 55
Sex Hormones							
estrogen					I	women in midcycle (when estrogen levels are highest) report dreams involving greatest amount of heterosexual striving	6, 28
progesterone	D	I	N	D		the majority of women dream most when progesterone levels are highest	6, 28

*I = increase; D = decrease; N = no change.

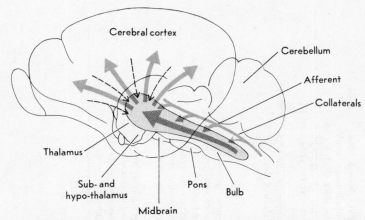

Figure 15–2 Outline of brain of cat showing the extent of the medially placed ascending reticular-activating system of the brain stem (shaded area) and the distribution of collaterals to it from the laterally situated ascending sensory pathways. (From Philip Teitelbaum, *Physiological Psychology*, Englewood Cliffs, New Jersey, Prentice-Hall, Inc., p. 73; taken from material in Starzl, T. E., Taylor, C. W., and Magoun, H. W.: J. Neurophysiol., 1951, *14*: pp. 479–496.)

of activity reflected in the organism's level of arousal. However, further exploration destroyed the apparent simplicity. For example, Feldman and Waller (17) found that lesions of the posterior hypothalamus of cats produced permanent behavioral somnolence without abolishing the EEG arousal response. Lesions of the midbrain RF eliminated the EEG arousal response, but the animals were capable of being behaviorally aroused. Adametz (1) showed that animals with extensive RF lesions may nevertheless have fairly normal sleep-wake patterns. In his study, the lesions were made in two stages, with ample recovery time between them.

An important revision in thinking was necessitated by studies which demonstrated that the RF is not a unitary system but is instead comprised of two antagonistic systems, one activating and the other sleep-promoting. Evidence for a sleep-promoting system is based on observations that electrical or chemical stimulation may induce sleep, and that selective lesions may block sleep. Small doses of depressant substances placed directly into the caudal pons are followed by activation (12). Lesions of the same area produce insomnia (4), as would be expected to occur upon removal of a system which normally inhibits the activating system. The work of Michel Jouvet (which follows) has convincingly demonstrated the existence of antagonistic systems.

Approaches to the Study of Sleep

Jouvet (36) has discussed the relative merits of establishing an electrophysiology or a neuropharmacology of sleep. He believes the latter approach to be more fruitful because (a) the time constant of the electric potentials of the brain is of the order of milliseconds, which is far too short to account for the circadian rhythm of sleep states; and (b) animals which are selectively deprived of dreaming show long-lasting quantitative rebound dreaming, which can most readily be explained by conceiving of accumulation or depletion of substances in the brain or elsewhere. (There is an alternative explanation proposed by Oswald, discussed earlier).

Hypnotoxins

The search for a naturally occurring "hypnotoxin" — that is, a naturally occurring substance that produces sleep when released into the blood — predates Pieron (72), who in 1913 reviewed the then current theories. Some recent work has been encouraging. Monnier and Hosli (59) prepared pairs of rabbits so that they shared a common blood supply. Then, when both rabbits were asleep, they electrically stimulated the reticular activating system of one of them; and when both were awake, they stimulated the sleep system (within the thalamus) of one of the rabbits. In both situations, both rabbits responded. The findings indicate that some blood-borne substance controls sleep and waking. Monnier also extracted substances from the blood of sleeping or awake rabbits. Extracts from sleeping donors induced sleep when injected into awake recipients, and extracts from rabbits which were awake awakened sleeping rabbits. Pappenheimer et al. (70) removed cerebrospinal fluid from sleep-deprived goats and injected it into the brains of rats. The rats curled up and appeared to sleep naturally. Similarly, Henry et al. (31) reported that cerebrospinal fluid from dream-deprived cats induced dreaming when it was injected into normal cats. Although work on hypnotoxins is suggestive, it will be seen that the pharmacology of sleeping and waking is exceedingly complex.

Monoamines and Sleep

Perhaps because of the well-known stimulant effect of amphetamine, which is a monoamine, and because the monoamines serotonin and norepinephrine are heavily concentrated in the RF, the French physiologist Michel Jouvet organized a research program to test the role of monoamines in the succession of sleep states. (See Appendix 1 for an explanation of the term monoamine). Cats have been his most frequent experimental subjects. Cats normally spend about 50 percent of each day in slow wave sleep, 20 percent in REM sleep, and 30 percent waking.

The effects of serotonin and norepinephrine cannot be tested directly because they do not readily cross the blood-brain barrier. Instead, drugs which are precursors, depletors, or inhibitors of the two monoamines, and which do penetrate the blood-brain barrier, are used. Jouvet also destroyed anatomical sites in which serotonin and norepinephrine are normally found in high concentration.

SEROTONIN. The penultimate step in the synthesis of serotonin is the formation of 5-hydroxytryptophan (5-HTP). Injections of 5-HTP result in the appearance of slow wave sleep and the suppression of REM sleep. Reserpine depletes serotonin, norepinephrine, and dopamine from the brain. It suppresses slow wave sleep for about 12 hours and REM sleep for about 24 hours. Secondary injection of 5-HTP restores serotonin levels to normal and produces slow wave sleep.

Serotonin levels can also be reduced by administration of the drugs p-chlorophenylalanine or p-chloromethamphetamine. Both drugs produce insomnia which, in the case of p-chlorophenylalanine, has been correlated with the decrease in cerebral levels of serotonin. Secondary injection of 5-HTP restores normal sleep.

Serotonin is found in heavy concentration in neurons of the raphe system, which are near the midline of the brain and extend from the medulla up through the mesencephalon. Jouvet lesioned the raphe system in cats, then monitored their EEG's during the 10 to 13 days in which the serotonin terminals were being voided. The cats showed varying degrees of insomnia, depending on the extent of the lesion. Those which received large lesions (greater than 80 percent of the raphe system destroyed) slept less than 15 percent of the time and had no REM sleep at all. At the end of 13 days, the cats were killed and their brains analyzed for serotonin. The smallest quantities of serotonin were found in those cats with the largest lesions. The cumulative evidence thus implicates serotonin in the control of slow wave sleep. In addition, since REM sleep appeared only after some minimum level of slow wave sleep was reached, Jouvet theorized that one of the products of the metabolism of serotonin is necessary to act as a priming mechanism for REM sleep. This conjecture gains additional support from the observation that the monoamine oxidase inhibitors, which inhibit the metabolic breakdown of serotonin, also strongly suppress REM sleep.

There are other favorable data for the idea that serotonin promotes slow wave sleep. When L-tryptophan, a serotonin precursor, is administered to humans, slow wave sleep increases (89). Spooner and Winters (82) injected serotonin into baby chicks, which have permeable blood-brain barriers, and induced sleep. Koella (43) injected serotonin directly into the brains of cats and observed sleep. The brain concentration of serotonin in rats, which are nocturnal, is higher during the day than at night (77).

NOREPINEPHRINE. Jouvet's strategy with norepinephrine paralleled that with serotonin. Dihydroxyphenylalanine (DOPA) is a precursor of both norepinephrine and dopamine. Injections produced waking. On the other hand, dihydroxyphenylserine is a direct precursor of norepinephrine, and it increases both slow wave and REM sleep. The injection of reserpine reduces both stages of sleep. The effect is countered by DOPA, which restores the levels of dopamine and norepinephrine and is attended by the reappearance of REM.

Both α-methyl-p-tyrosine and disulfiram inhibit the synthesis of norepinephrine, and both suppress REM. Two substances which may act as false transmitters — that is, they may accumulate at nerve endings which normally release norepinephrine and may ineffectually replace it — are α-methyl-m-tyrosine and α-methylDOPA. REM is reduced by both drugs.

Brain structures which control REM are located outside the raphe system in the heavily pigmented locus coeruleus of the dorsal pons. Destruction of the locus coeruleus suppresses REM without affecting slow wave sleep. Destruction of the locus coeruleus also reduces the concentration of norepinephrine in the brain. It thus appears that REM sleep is controlled, in part, by norepinephrine.

ACETYLCHOLINE. Hernandez-Peon (32) mapped brain circuits in the cat that were cholinergic and that induced sleep when stimulated. The work of Domino, summarized earlier, also points toward a role for ACh in the control of sleep. Atropine reduces amount of REM sleep, while ACh or carbachol, when placed within the brain near the locus coeruleus, increases it. Jouvet has suggested that the release of ACh may trigger the norepinephrine mechanism for the induction of paradoxical sleep.

Torda's Theory

After an extensive series of studies (summarized in Ref. 85) with rats as subjects, Torda offered several modifications to Jouvet's theory. She used p-chlorophenylalanine, α-methyl-p-tyrosine, and disulfiram to deplete brain stores of serotonin and/or norepinephrine. She performed chemical assays on the brains of 75 rats in order to ensure that her procedures were effective. She combined the depletion procedure with microinjections of serotonin and/or norepinephrine directly into the brains. She found that depletion of serotonin produced insomnia, which was reversed in less than

a second by the microinjection of serotonin. Depletion of norepinephrine increased the proportion of slow wave sleep, while reducing
the proportion of the other two stages. Injections of norepinephrine
restored the pattern to normal. Depletion of both amines produced
insomnia. Serotonin restored sleep. When norepinephrine was injected during the sleep, low doses reduced the depth of sleep and
higher doses induced REM. When rats depleted of both amines received norepinephrine before serotonin, they showed arousal. Small
doses of serotonin shortened the period of arousal, and large doses induced REM. Torda concluded that the balance between serotonin
and norepinephrine is critical in determining sleep stage. An excess
of serotonin is associated with sleep, an excess of norepinephrine
with arousal, and some critical balance between them is associated
with REM.

Evaluation of Jouvet's Theory

Jouvet has made an important contribution toward our understanding of the neuropharmacology of sleep. He has been unable
to test the direct effects of the monoamines upon the stages of sleep
but has brilliantly combined several indirect methods. However,
he is not without his critics. Mandell et al. (57) feel that there is a
norepinephrine and a serotonin "bandwagon." They pointed out
that these substances have been invoked to explain drive, mood,
schizophrenia, depression, mental deficiency, neuroendocrine regulation, and, not surprisingly, sleep and dreams. However, there are
more than 20 amino acids in the human brain (71), and their role
in controlling various behaviors has been neglected. Mandell et
al. tested the effects of 25 amino acids on sleep and arousal in young
chickens. Only 8 were without effect; 6 were behaviorally activating,
and 11 produced depression. Therefore, they argued that attempts
to specify the particular sleep neurotransmitter are certainly premature.

In 1966, Marley (58) summarized the results of studies on the
central effects of epinephrine, norepinephrine and dopamine. Excitant and depressant effects were reported in almost equal numbers
in the 87 references he listed.

The extent of the difficulty of trying to ascertain the neurotransmitters involved in sleep is evident from inspection of Table 15.4.
Most drugs which have any psychoactive properties modify REM
sleep. The totality of their actions on catecholamines and serotonin is
not presently known.

Perhaps the most trenchant critic of the neurotransmitter approach has been King. In an excellent review (39), he suggested many
reasons for exercising caution in interpreting data. For one thing,

REM is easily disrupted by stress, pain, disease, or other unusual conditions. Therefore, just because a drug reduces REM, there is no reason to conclude that it affects specific neurotransmitter mechanisms. That nonspecific factors may be acting to reduce REM is especially likely when high, even toxic, doses of drugs are used, as in some of the studies with reserpine, disulfiram, phenoxybenzamine and Dibenamine.

Species differences, which are commonly found in sleep research, are largely ignored by Jouvet. He cites findings with other species when they are favorable to his theory but ignores unfavorable data. The species he works with — cats — is atypical. Thus, although reserpine abolishes REM in cats, it increases it in primates and possibly in rabbits. On the other hand, α-methyltyrosine increases REM in cats, but not in monkeys or rats.

Jouvet's criterion for the states of sleep and arousal has been the EEG record, but King claimed that p-chlorophenylalanine, like atropine and physostigmine, may cause a dissociation between EEG and behavior. In the event of a behavior/EEG dissociation, e.g., when an animal which is obviously awake has a sleep EEG record, the behavioral datum must take precedence.

King doubted that the drugs were acting by the mechanisms proposed by Jouvet. For example, reserpine, which depletes the brain of norepinephrine, abolished REM in cats. DOPA, a precursor of norepinephrine, returned REM to baseline levels. Jouvet's interpretation — that DOPA acted by restoring levels of norepinephrine — is incorrect; DOPA does not have that action in reserpinized animals. Loading an animal with precursors of neurotransmitters, which was a substantial part of Jouvet's strategy, generally produces many nonspecific effects. King also criticized the interpretations of the p-chlorophenylalanine data. Its hypothesized mechanism of action was to change brain levels of serotonin, but the correlation between brain serotonin levels and EEG changes was very poor.

Finally, King cited the work of Henley and Morrison. They found that lesions of the locus coeruleus had only one direct effect on REM: skeletal muscle tone, which is normally lost, was retained. As a result, the animals moved around and twitched violently, behaviors which might easily have served to awaken them from sleep. Clearly, the disruption of REM in that case would be a secondary one.

SLEEP THERAPY

Sleep therapy is used in many parts of the world to treat various behavioral disorders. Hypnotic and tranquilizing drugs are used to keep the patient in a state of sleep for 12 to 22 hours each day for three days to four weeks. Recently, the practice was revived in the United States. Hartmann (29) described the results with four schizophrenic female patients. They were treated for 70 to 96 hours. Sleep was maintained with chlorpromazine and amobarbital. Patients were awakened for about 20 minutes every four hours in order that they might eat and use the bathroom.

The patients spent no more time in the deepest stage of sleep than they otherwise would have. They dreamed excessively. The treatment was judged by Hartmann to be about as effective as other forms of treatment, but may have reduced the period of hospitalization. It did relieve acute symptomatology.

REFERENCES

1. Adametz, J. Rate of recovery of functioning in cats with rostral reticular lesions. J. Neurosurg., 1959, 16:85–98.
2. Baekeland, F. Pentobarbital and dextroamphetamine sulfate: effects on the sleep cycle in man. Psychopharmacologia, 1967, 11:388–396.
3. Barratt, E., Beaver, W., White, R., Blakeney, P., and Adams, P. The effects of the chronic use of marijuana on sleep and perceptual-motor performance in humans. Presented at Symposium on Aeromed. Aspects of Marihuana, FAA, June, 1972.
4. Batini, C., Moruzzi, G., Palestini, M., Rossi, G., and Zanchetti, A. Effects of complete pontine transactions on the sleep-wakefulness rhythm: the midpontine pretrigeminal preparation. Arch. Ital. Biol., 1959, 97:1–12.
5. Baumel, I., DeFeo, J., and Lal, H. Decreased potency of CNS depressants after prolonged social isolation in mice. Psychopharmacologia, 1969, 15:153–158.
6. Benedek, T. Psychosexual Functions in Women. Studies in Psychosomatic Medicine, Vol. II. New York: Ronald Publishing Co., 1952.
7. Brown, B. Some characteristic EEG differences between heavy smoker and non-smoker subjects. Neuropsychologia, 1968, 6:381–388.
8. Bures, J., Buresova, O., Bohdanecky, Z., and Weiss, T. The effect of physostigmine and atropine on the mechanisms of learning. In Steinberg, H., de Reuck, A., and Knight, J. (Eds.) Animal Behaviour and Drug Action. Boston: Little, Brown and Co., 1964.
9. Cherpillod, C., Bovet, J., Krassoievitch, M., and Tissot, R. Action de quelques tranquillisants sur la motilité pendant le sommeil. Psychopharmacologia, 1965, 8:302–308.
10. Clement, W., Solursh, L., and Van Ast, W. Abuse of amphetamine and amphetamine-like drugs. Psychol. Rep., 1970, 26:343–354.
11. Connell, P. Amphetamine Psychosis. London: Chapman and Hall Ltd., 1958.
12. Cordeau, J. Functional organization of the brain stem reticular formation in relation to sleep and wakefulness. Rev. Canad. Biol., 1962, 21:113–125.
13. Coulter, J., Lester, B., and Williams, H. Reserpine and sleep. Psychopharmacologia, 1971, 19:134–147.
14. Cramer, H., and Kuhlo, W. Effets des inhibiteurs de la mono-aminoxydase sur le sommeil et l'electroencephalogramme chez l'homme. Acta Neurol. Psychiat. Belg., 1967, 67:658–669.
15. Domino, E., and Yamamoto, K. Nicotine: effect on the sleep cycle of the cat. Science, 1965, 150:637–638.
16. Domino, E., Yamamoto, K., and Dren, A. Role of cholinergic mechanisms in states of wakefulness and sleep. Prog. Brain Res., 1968, 28:113–133.

17. Feldman, S., and Waller, H. Dissociation of electrocortical activation and behavioral arousal. Nature, 1962, *196*:320–322.
18. Frankenhaeuser, M., Myrsten, A., Waszak, M., Neri, A., and Post, B. Dosage and time effects of cigarette smoking. Psychopharmacologia, 1968, *13*:311–319.
19. Fraser, H., Wikler, A., Essig, C., and Isbell, H. Degree of physical dependence induced by secobarbital or pentobarbital. J.A.M.A., 1958, *166*:126–129.
20. Freeman, F., Agnew, H., and Williams, R. An electroencephalographic study of the effects of meprobamate on human sleep. Clin. Pharmacol. Ther., 1965, 6:172–176.
21. Galeano Munoz, J. Hypnotics and euhypnics. Prog. Brain Res., 1965, *18*: 227–228.
22. Gibbs, F., and Maltby, G. Effect on the electrical activity of the cortex of certain depressant and stimulant drugs—barbiturates, morphine, caffeine, benzedrine, and adrenalin. J. Pharmacol. Exp. Ther., 1943, *78*:1–10.
23. Goodman, L., and Gilman, A. *The Pharmacological Basis of Therapeutics*. New York: The Macmillan Publishing Co., 1965.
24. Green, W. The effect of LSD on the sleep-dream cycle. J. Nerv. Ment. Dis., 1965, *140*:417–426.
25. Gresham, S., Webb, W., and Williams, R. Alcohol and caffeine: effect on inferred visual dreaming. Science, 1963, *140*:1226–1227.
26. Hartmann, E. Pharmacological studies in man: pentobarbital (Nembutal), amitriptyline (Elavil), chlordiazepoxide (Librium) and RO5-6901 (Dalmane). Report to Assoc. for Psychophysiol. Study Sleep, 1963. Abst. Psychophysiol. 4:391.
27. Hartmann, E. The effect of four drugs on sleep patterns in man. Psychopharmacologia, 1966, 9:346–353.
28. Hartmann, E. The D-state (dreaming sleep) and the menstrual cycle. Rec. Adv. Biol. Psychiat., 1966, 8:34–35.
29. Hartmann, E. Dauerschlaf. Arch. Gen. Psychiat., 1968, *18*:99–111.
30. Heimstra, N., Bancroft, N., and DeKock, A. Effects of smoking upon sustained performance in a simulated driving task. Ann. N.Y. Acad. Sci., 1967, *142*: 295–307.
31. Henry, P., Cohen, H., Stadel, B., Stulce, J., Ferguson, J., Wagner, T., and Dement, W. CSF transfer from REM-deprived cats to non-deprived recipients. Report to Assoc. for Psychophysiol. Study of Sleep, 1965.
32. Hernandez-Peon, R. Central neuro-humoral transmission in sleep and wakefulness. Prog. Brain Res., 1965, *18*:96–117.
33. Hinton, J. Comparison of the effects of six barbiturates and a placebo on insomnia and motility in psychiatric patients. Brit. J. Pharmacol., 1963, *20*:319–325.
34. Hollister, L., Richers, R., and Gillespie, H. Comparison of tetrahydrocannabinol and synhexyl in man. Clin. Pharmacol. Ther., 1968, 9:783–791.
35. Innes, I., and Nickerson, M. Drugs acting on postganglionic adrenergic nerve endings and structures innervated by them (sympathomimetic drugs). *In* Goodman, L., and Gilman, A. (Eds.) *The Pharmacological Basis of Therapeutics*. New York: The Macmillan Publishing Co., 1965.
36. Jouvet, M. Biogenic amines and the states of sleep. Science, 1969, *163*:32–41.
37. Kales, A., Jacobson, A., Kales, J., Marusak, C., and Hanley, J. Effects of drugs on sleep (Noludar, Doriden, Nembutal, chloral hydrate, Benadryl). Psychophysiology, 1968, 4:391–392.
38. Kay, D., Eisenstein, R., and Jasinski, D. Morphine effects on human REM state, waking state, and NREM sleep. Psychophysiology, 1968, 5:204.
39. King, C. The pharmacology of rapid eye movement sleep. Adv. Pharmacol. Chem., 1971, 9:1–91.
40. Kleitman, N. *Sleep and Wakefulness*. Chicago: University of Chicago Press, 1963.
41. Kline, N. Clinical experience with iproniazid (Marsilid). J. Clin. Exp. Psychopath., 1958, *19*:72–78.
42. Knapp, D., and Domino, E. Action of nicotine on the ascending reticular activating system. Int. J. Neuropharmacol., 1962, *1*:333–351.
43. Koella, W. Neurohumoral aspects of sleep control. Biol. Psychiat., 1969, *1*:161–177.
44. Kornetsky, C., Mirsky, A., Kessler, E., and Dorff, J. The effects of dextroamphetamine on behavioural deficits produced by sleep loss in humans. J. Pharmacol. Exp. Ther., 1959, *127*:46–50.

45. Kramer, M., Whitman, R., Baldridge, B., and Ornstein, P. The pharmacology of dreaming. *In* Martin, G., and Kisch, B. (Eds.) *Enzymes in Mental Health.* Philadelphia: J. B. Lippincott Co., 1966.

46. Kugler, J., and Doenicke, A. Amplitudes and evoked responses in the EEG in humans during sleep and anesthesia. Prog. Brain Res., 1965, *18*:178–182.

47. Kupfer, D., Wyatt, R., Greenspan, K., Scott, J., and Snyder, F. Lithium carbonate and sleep in affective illness. Arch. Gen. Psychiat., 1970, *23*:35–40.

48. Laties, V. Modification of affect, social behavior and performance by sleep deprivation and drugs. J. Psychiat. Res., 1961, *1*:12–25.

49. LeGassicke, J., Ashcroft, G., Eccleston, D., Evans, J., Oswald, I., and Ritson, E. The clinical state, sleep and amine metabolism of a tranylcypromine ("Parnate") addict. Brit. J. Psychiat., 1965, *111*:357–364.

50. Lemere, F. The danger of amphetamine dependency. Am. J. Psychiat., 1966, *123*: 569–572.

51. Lester, B., Coulter, J., Cowden, L., and Williams, H. Secobarbital and nocturnal physiological patterns. Psychopharmacologia, 1968, *13*:275–286.

52. Lester, B., Coulter, J., Cowden, L., and Williams, H. Chlorpromazine and human sleep. Psychopharmacologia, 1971, *20*:280–287.

53. Lester, B., and Guerrero-Figueroa, R. Effects of some drugs on electroencephalographic fast activity and dream time. Psychophysiology, 1966, *2*:224–236.

54. Lewis, S. Subjective estimates of sleep: an EEG evaluation. Brit. J. Psychol., 1969, *60*:203–208.

55. Lewis, S., Oswald, I., Evans, J., and Akindele, M. Heroin and human sleep. EEG, 1970, *28*:374–381.

56. Lindsley, D., Schreiner, L., Knowles, W., and Magoun, H. Behavioral and EEG changes following chronic brainstem lesions in the cat. EEG, 1950, *2*:483–498.

57. Mandell, A., Spooner, C., and Brunet, D. Whither the "sleep transmitter"? Biol. Psychiat., 1969, *1*:13–30.

58. Marley, E. Behavioral and electrophysiological effects of catecholamines. Pharmacol. Rev., 1966, *18*:753–768.

59. Monnier, M., and Hosli, L. Humoral regulation of sleep and wakefulness by hypnogenic and activating dialysable factors. Prog. Brain Res., 1965, *18*:118–123.

60. Monroe, L. Psychological and physiological differences between good and poor sleepers. J. Abnorm. Psychol., 1967, *72*:255–264.

61. Moruzzi, G. and Magoun, H. Brain stem reticular formation and activation of the EEG. EEG, 1949, *1*:455–473.

62. Murphree, H., Pfeiffer, C., and Price, L. Electroencephalographic changes in man following smoking. Ann. N.Y. Acad. Sci., 1967, *142*:245–260.

63. Nash, H. *Alcohol and Caffeine: A Study of Their Psychological Effects.* Springfield, Ill.: Charles C Thomas, Publisher, 1962.

64. Noda, H. Concerning wake-amine intoxication. Kurume ligakkai Zasski, 1950, *13*:294–298.

65. Oswald, I. Human brain protein, drugs and dreams. Nature, 1969, *223*:893–897.

66. Oswald, I. Sleep and dependence on amphetamine and other drugs. *In* Kales, A. (Ed.) *Sleep Physiology and Pathology.* Philadelphia: J. B. Lippincott Co., 1969.

67. Oswald, I., Berger, R., Jaramillo, R., Keddie, K., Olley, P., and Plunkett, G. Melancholia and barbiturates: a controlled EEG, body, and eye-movement study of sleep. Brit. J. Psychiat., 1963, *109*:66–78.

68. Oswald, I., and Priest, R. Five weeks to escape the sleeping pill habit. Brit. J. Med., 1965, *2*:1093–1099.

69. Oswald, I., and Thacore, V. Amphetamine and phenmetrazine addiction. Physiological abnormalities in the abstinence syndrome. Brit. Med. J., 1963, *2*: 427–431.

70. Pappenheimer, J., Miller, T., and Goodrich, C. Sleep-promoting effects of cerebrospinal fluid from sleep-deprived goats. Proc. Nat. Acad. Sci., 1967, *58*: 513–517.

71. Perry, T., Hansen, S., MacDougall, L., and Schwarz, C. Studies of amines in normal and schizophrenic subjects. *In* Himwich, H., Kety, S., and Smythies, J. (Eds.) *Amines and Schizophrenia.* New York: Pergamon Press, 1967.

72. Pieron, H. *Le Probleme Physiologique du Sommeil*. Paris: Masson and Cle, 1913.
73. Pivik, R., Zarcone, V., Dement, W., and Hollister, L. Delta-9-tetrahydrocannabinol and synhexyl: effects on human sleep patterns. Clin. Pharmacol. Ther., 1972, 13:426–435.
74. Rechtschaffen, A., and Maron, L. The effect of amphetamine on the sleep cycle. EEG, 1964, 16:438–445.
75. Ritvo, E., Ornitz, E., LaFranchi, S., and Walter, R. Effects of imipramine on the sleep-dream cycle: an EEG study in boys. EEG, 1967, 22:465–468.
76. Scheibel, M., Scheibel, A., Mollica, A., and Moruzzi, G. Convergence and interaction of afferent impulses on single units of reticular formation. J. Neurophysiol., 1955, 18:309–331.
77. Scheving, L., Harrison, W., Gordon, P., and Pauly, J. Daily fluctuation (circadian and ultradian) in biogenic amines of the rat brain. Am. J. Physiol., 1968, 214: 166–173.
78. Schwertz, M., and Marbach, G. Effets physiologiques de la cafeine et du meprobamate au cours du sommeil chez l'homme. Arch. Sci. Physiol., 1965, 19: 425–479.
79. Sharpless, S. Hypnotics and sedatives I. The barbiturates. *In* Goodman, L., and Gilman, A. (Eds.) *The Pharmacological Basis of Therapeutics*. New York: The Macmillan Publishing Co., 1965.
80. Smith, D. The characteristics of dependence in high-dose methamphetamine abuse. Int. J. Addictions, 1969, 4:453–459.
81. Soulairac, A., Cahn, J., Gottesmann, C., and Alano, J. Neuropharmacological aspects of the action of hypnogenic substances on the central nervous system. Prog. Brain Res., 1965, 18:194–220.
82. Spooner, C., and Winters, W. Neuropharmacological profile of the young chick. Int. J. Neuropharmacol., 1966, 5:217–236.
83. Tart, C. *On Being Stoned*. Palo Alto: Science and Behavior Books, 1971.
84. Tissot, R. The effects of certain drugs on the sleep cycle in man. Prog. Brain Res., 1965, 18:175–177.
85. Torda, C. Biochemical and bioelectric processes related to sleep, paradoxical sleep, and arousal. Psychol. Rep., 1969, 24:807–824.
86. Toyoda, J. The effects of chlorpromazine and imipramine on the human nocturnal electroencephalogram. Folia Psychiat. Neurol. Jap., 1964, 18:198–221.
87. Weiss, B., and Laties, V. Enhancement of human performance by caffeine and the amphetamines. Pharmacol. Rev., 1962, 14:1–36.
88. Wikler, A. Pharmacological dissociation of behavior and EEG "sleep patterns" in dogs: morphine, N-allyl-normorphine and atropine. Proc. Soc. Exp. Biol. Med., 1952, 79:261–265.
89. Williams, H., Lester, B., and Coulter, J. Monoamines and the EEG stages of sleep. Activ. Nervosa. Sup., 1969, 11:188–192.
90. Yamamoto, K., and Domino, E. Nicotine-induced EEG and behavioral arousal. Int. J. Neuropharmacol., 1965, 4:359–373.

CHAPTER 16

ELECTRICAL STIMULATION OF THE BRAIN

One of the most exciting and important scientific findings of the last 20 years has been the discovery by Olds and Milner (29) that animals with electrodes implanted in certain areas of their brains learn responses which produce small trains of electrical stimulation through the electrodes. The required response is predesignated by the experimenter; with some electrode placements, it soon begins to be emitted at the maximal rate the animal is capable of. Psychologists say that an event is positively reinforcing, i.e., rewarding, if an organism learns to repeat responses which produce the event. By this definition, electrical stimulation of the brain (ESB) can be an extremely potent positive reinforcer; most researchers feel that ESB functions like normal rewards. Its significance is that it points the way to an understanding of the neural bases of pleasure.

ESB is not a behavior as, for example, sexuality, social interactions, and the emission of learned responses are behaviors. Rather, it is a technique for eliciting behaviors. As such, it perhaps does not warrant a separate chapter in a book on psychopharmacology. However, because of its enormous impact on the scientific community, as judged by the many hundreds of papers which have been concerned with it, ESB shall be accorded a brief synoptic treatment.

370

PROCEDURAL ASPECTS OF ESB

Methods of Measurement

In the earliest experiments, current was applied whenever rats walked into a particular part of the test chamber (24). They began staying in the appropriate places at far greater than chance level. They also learned to run mazes for ESB. The most popular piece of apparatus for testing ESB is the Skinner box. When a rat is placed into a small box with a protruding lever, the animal explores, and occasionally presses upon the lever. A typical response rate is 50 bar presses per hour. When each press is followed by ESB, responses are emitted at incredibly high rates, often as many as 10,000 per hour. Moreover, the animals do not satiate easily. When rats had continuous access to a lever for 20 days, they averaged 29.2 responses per minute (53). Despite the power of the effects, ESB probably does not produce unalloyed pleasure. For example, cats which readily learn to run to one place to obtain stimulation also learn to run to another place to turn it off (40).

Species

The bulk of ESB work has been with rats as subjects, but many other species show good self-stimulation behavior. Among those which have been successfully tested are fish, chickens, rabbits, cats, dogs, goats, monkeys, dolphins, and man. Heath and his colleagues at Tulane have implanted electrodes for self-stimulation into many psychiatric and a few nonpsychiatric patients (discussed later in this chapter). The patients responded as though the stimulation were extremely pleasurable, and in several instances there were dramatic remissions of symptoms (3).

ESB AS REWARD

Comparison with Conventional Rewards

Animals work for ESB as they work for food. The similarity was emphasized by Olds (25), in regard to the performance of rats during both the acquisition and extinction phases of maze-running. However, ESB is more powerful than are conventional rewards. Falk (8) reported that thirsty rats given a choice of water or ESB bar press for the latter except under conditions of extreme deprivation. Routtenberg and Lindy (42) allowed rats one hour daily access to food, which was sufficient for them to maintain body weight. When they were then given a choice between ESB and food, they began working for ESB and would have starved to death had not the experiment been terminated. Similarly, when rats which had been deprived of food for as long as 10 days were offered a choice in a T-maze between food and ESB, they chose the latter (44). Olds (26) used still another method for comparing the reward value of food and ESB. Rats which had been deprived of food were required to cross an electrified grid in order to gain access to food. They were stopped when the current level was raised to 180 μa; with ESB as reward, rats tolerated 425 μa.

Anatomical Substrate of the Reward System

Rewarding effects of stimulation are obtained from about 35 percent of electrode placements. Stimulation of some brain sites — surprisingly, only about five percent — is aversive. Stimulation of the bulk of the brain, including the entire neocortex, is motivationally neutral, so far as lever pressing for ESB is concerned.

The reward system is anatomically diffuse. Approximately half of the points stimulated within the rhinencephalon (see Fig. 16–1) are positive. The most intense positive effects are obtained from the posterior hypothalamus. The medial forebrain bundle is similar in shape to a long tube which extends from the olfactory bulb and rhinencephalon, and it passes along the lateral hypothalamus and

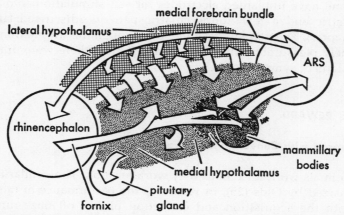

Figure 16–1 Schematic diagram showing the major connections of the lateral and medial portions of the hypothalamus. The medial forebrain bundle interconnects the ascending reticular system (ARS), the lateral hypothalamus, and the rhinencephalon. (From Robert A. McLeary and Robert Y. Moore, *Subcortical Mechanisms of Behavior: The Physiological Functions of Primitive Parts of the Brain,* New York, Basic Books, 1965.)

into the ventrolateral midbrain. It appears to be the focus of the reward system. The reward pathway is probably bidirectional, since reduction of activity in areas either above or below the medial forebrain bundle, by lesions or administration of xylocaine, reduces response rate (47).

ESB and Drive Reduction

It might seem that rewarding events should be associated with satisfaction of some basic drive. A good night's sleep and a full stomach are generally regarded as sources of pleasure. This intuitive notion, which is the basis for many theories of motivation, is almost surely wrong. For example, when a hungry rat is stimulated in a part of the hypothalamus called the ventromedial nucleus, eating is inhibited. The stimulation acts in some respects like food in the stomach and therefore might be expected to be rewarding. Yet rats learn to bar press to avoid ventromedial nucleus stimulation. Glucagon, a hormone which raises blood sugar level and reduces appetite, reduces the rate of responding for ESB (2). By contrast, manipulations which induce hunger appear to be rewarding. Stimulation of the highly rewarding medial forebrain bundle induces such powerful hunger that stimulated rats, despite having been satiated with food immediately prior to testing, cross an electrified grid for food reward—a grid that is too great a barrier for rats which have been deprived of food for up to seven days (19). It is paradoxical but true that ESB can at one and the same time be rewarding and hunger-producing. It should be pointed out that stimulation in a barren environment is not as rewarding as when the animal has access to food (17).

Electrical stimulation of appropriate areas of the brain has been shown to induce drinking, sexual behavior, gnawing, nest building, and aggressiveness. Electrical stimulation of all of these areas is rewarding. The generalization has been made that excitation of any neural system which normally mediates any consummatory response is rewarding (10).

PHARMACOLOGICAL MANIPULATIONS AND ESB

Hormones

Olds (21) implanted electrodes into the lateral hypothalamus of male rats and tested them daily until their self-stimulation rates had stabilized. Then they were all castrated and tested while androgen levels declined. Next they were given testosterone replacement therapy and tested for several more days. The rats were also tested under conditions of high and low hunger drive. Olds found an inverse correlation between the effects of hunger and the effects of testosterone. That is, when hunger augmented responding for stimulation through a given electrode, testosterone tended to decrease responding, and vice versa. In general, testosterone increased responding for stimulation from the more laterally placed electrodes and decreased responding for stimulation from the medially placed ones. The observation that drug effects on self-stimulation are to some extent dependent on electrode placement has been repeatedly confirmed (16, 35, 46). It seems likely that researchers will have to organize effects according to placements before they will be able to develop systematic relationships. For purposes of simplification, this injunction will be largely ignored in what follows.

Hodos and Valenstein (14) used estrogen and progesterone injections in doses which induce sexual receptivity in female rats and measured the effects of the hormonal manipulations on self-stimulation behavior. The hormones did not influence the rate of self-stimulation, although the rats did become receptive. Prescott (38) noted that hormone injections do not completely mimic natural estrus, and accordingly he studied variations in responding throughout the normal course of the estrus cycle in intact rats. Five of the six rats which were tested responded most on the day of estrus, and the sixth responded most on the day following estrus. Rats are more active when in estrus than at other times, but Prescott ensured against the possibility that the increased self-stimulation scores during estrus were artifacts of increased activity. He placed a second bar, which was never reinforced, into the test boxes, and responses on the second bar did not significantly change throughout the estrus cycle.

The Adrenergic System

Positive Data

Stein (49) and Poschel and Ninteman (37) have postulated that norepinephrine is necessary for the maintenance of self-stimulation behavior. The evidence is varied. Fuxe and co-workers (9, 13) developed a technique for identifying catecholamines at the cellular level, and found an ascending system of fibers which overlaps extensively with the reward system as mapped by Olds. Amphetamine, which owes part of its action to the release of norepinephrine, strongly potentiates self-stimulation (48). Reserpine (26) and tetrabenazine

(34), both of which first release and eventually deplete brain stores of catecholamines, suppress self-stimulation. Chlorpromazine and haloperidol block adrenergic transmission and inhibit ESB (49). Amphetamine and norepinephrine are structurally similar — they have in common a phenethylamine molecule — and when the metabolism of phenethylamine is prevented by prior administration of MAOI, it augments ESB (51). The facilitating effect of amphetamine is counteracted by prior treatment with either reserpine or α-methyl-p-tyrosine, both of which reduce levels of brain norepinephrine. The selective depletors disulfiram and diethyldithiocarbamate both suppress self-stimulation. The suppression is reversed by intraventricular injections of L- or DL-norepinephrine, but not by D-norepinephrine, which is biologically inactive, or by dopamine or serotonin (54). During ESB, the synthesis of norepinephrine is increased (55).

Stein and Wise (47) injected radioactive norepinephrine into the brains of rats and then measured radioactivity in the perfusate from various brain areas. When stimulation was applied to rewarding areas of the brain, radioactivity increased. It was unchanged when stimulation was applied to various areas which did not maintain self-stimulation. The implication is that norepinephrine is released upon activation of the reward system.

To summarize the evidence: (1) the reward system and the catecholamine system may be one and the same; (2) drugs which release norepinephrine increase responding for ESB, while drugs which interfere with adrenergic functioning decrease responding; (3) during ESB the synthesis of norepinephrine is increased; and (4) norepinephrine is released when the reward system is stimulated.

Data Incompatible with the Norepinephrine Hypothesis

The evidence just cited is not conclusive, for there are some negative data. Roll (41) argued that the suppression of self-stimulation after the administration of disulfiram may be unrelated to norepinephrine stores, but might instead be a consequence of the behavioral depression produced by the drug. Breese et al. (4) attempted to meet Roll's objection by using the drug 6-hydroxydopamine, which also depletes the brain of norepinephrine, but which had been shown in other studies not to affect locomotor activity. Although self-stimulation was suppressed, the experiment would have been much more convincing if the locomotor activity scores of the test animals had been shown to be unaffected by the particular dose levels used in the experiment. The activity of rats has been depressed by comparable doses of 6-hydroxydopamine (12).

A second challenge to the norepinephrine hypothesis comes from Olds (23), who implanted micropipettes in the reward area of rats. Each bar press by the animals resulted in direct injection of three microliters of drug. Olds found increases in rates of responding when rats worked for carbachol, which is related to acetylcholine, or for testosterone, or for substances which chelate or precipitate calcium. The latter group of chemicals act by withdrawing ionic calcium from the fluid which bathes neurons, which has the effect of causing the cells to discharge. Substances which acted in this manner include sodium EDTA, sodium phosphate, and sodium pyrophosphate. When epinephrine, norepinephrine, or serotonin were combined with sodium pyrophosphate, the latter's effects were countered. On the basis of these results, Olds suggested that the reward area is positively sensitive to ACh and is inhibited by other neurotransmitters. If such is the case, the stimulation seen with adrenergic drugs would be due to their peripheral effects.

Antelman and his colleagues (1) also questioned the norepinephrine hypothesis. They found that the suppression of self-stimulation behavior produced by 6-hydroxydopamine could be reversed. The reversal was accomplished by simply stimulating the rats several times in the test chamber, without requiring that they bar press for the stimulation. The priming stimulation became unnecessary within less than a week. Antelman et al. considered the possibility that bar-pressing was maintained because the depletion of norepinephrine had been less than 100 percent, and the receptors had become supersensitive to stimulation by norepinephrine. (Supersensitivity is a common finding following denervation.) They rejected the idea, because injections of the adrenergic blocking agent phentolamine into rats which had been treated with 6-hydroxydopamine, and whose self-stimulation levels had returned to baseline, produced only small and temporary rate deficits. The phentolamine ensured against the utilization of any norepinephrine which remained after 6-hydroxydopamine treatment.

M. Olds (32) showed that both amphetamine and scopolamine were effective in counteracting chlorpromazine- or tetrabenazine-induced depressions of self-stimulation. Since amphetamine is adrenergic while scopolamine is anticholinergic, the deficits must have resulted from action on more than one neurotransmitter.

Finally, Domino and Olds (7) showed that the effects of amphetamine are dependent both on the dose used and on the initial rate of response of the subjects. High doses reduced self-stimulation in rats, regardless of the initial rate of response. Moderate doses (2 mg/kg, i.p.) increased responding in rats with low levels of response and increased it to an even greater extent in rats with electrodes in the reward area which had not previously shown self-stimulation behavior; however, bar-pressing was reduced in rats which had initially been responding at high rates.

A Theory, and More Negative Data

Although it is clear that peripherally applied adrenergic substances generally augment self-stimulation, there is some doubt that the effect is caused by their action on central norepinephrine transmission. Nonetheless, Wise and Stein (54) have made an explicit formulation of the neurochemical basis of ESB. They believe that norepinephrine is released when neurons within the reward system are fired, and that amphetamine acts not simply by making more norepinephrine available but by potentiating its release from neurons which are already firing. The need for the distinction arose from experiments (their own and those of Olds) which showed that ESB was depressed by injections of norepinephrine into intact rats. Presumably, the depression was caused because the norepinephrine discharged neurons randomly.

In light of the foregoing objections to the general theory concerning the role of norepinephrine in the reward system, the more specific hypothesis of Wise and Stein seems premature. Moreover, although they stated (52, p. 318) that iproniazid does not facilitate ESB, Poschel and Ninteman (35) have shown that it does. The relevance of this finding is that iproniazid, like other MAOI's, acts by retarding the destruction of norepinephrine rather than by promoting its release. Similarly, ESB is augmented by both cocaine (50) and imipramine (15), which promote adrenergic functioning by preventing the reuptake of released norepinephrine, thus producing continuous stimulation at postsynaptic sites.

The Cholinergic System

On the basis of the results obtained from the application of carbachol directly to reward areas (as previously discussed), Olds and Olds (30) raised the possibility of central cholinergic involvement in reward processes. Further evidence was provided by Jung and Boyd's (16) work with rats and Stark and Boyd's work with dogs. They showed that ESB was decreased by physostigmine but not by neostigmine; the latter does not enter the brain. Methylatropine, which does not enter the brain, did not block the physostigmine effect, but atropine did. Domino and Olds (6) and Olds and Domino (33, 34) showed that nicotine and arecoline, both of which promote cholinergic functioning, depressed ESB. In the case of nicotine there was a reversal of effect—64 minutes after injection, the rats had rates of self-stimulation which were higher than pre-injection levels. The depression was blocked by scopolamine, but not by doses of methylscopolamine which were equivalent in peripheral effects. Mecamylamine, a ganglionic blocking agent which enters the brain, potentiated the physostigmine effect. The effect was not potentiated by trimethidinium, a ganglionic blocker which does not penetrate into the brain. Olds and Domino concluded that drugs which both promote muscarinic cholinergic functioning and penetrate into the brain depress self-stimulation.

The nicotinic drugs have biphasic effects of both central and peripheral origin. The drugs were also tested for their effects on the escape response to stimulation of the midbrain tegmentum, an area of the brain where stimulation has aversive effects. Rats continued to display coordinated escape behavior after doses which greatly suppressed self-stimulation.

For the most part, cholinergic antagonists have produced small effects on ESB. Both increases and decreases in responding have been reported (5, 7, 16). Nevertheless, it appears that the case for cholinergic involvement in reward processes is at least as well established as that for adrenergic involvement.

Miscellaneous Drugs

Olds and Travis (31) showed that drugs act independently on reward and escape mechanisms. He tested rats in a box which contained two levers: during alternating two-minute periods the rats were able to press first one bar, for stimulation of the reward area, and then the second bar, for escape from stimulation of the aversive area. Chlorpromazine reduced self-stimulation at doses which did not affect escape behavior; pentobarbital and meprobamate blocked escape at doses which spared self-stimulation. Morphine depressed both about equally. Olds (27) showed that LSD first depressed and sometimes then augmented self-stimulation at doses which spared escape. Doses of amphetamine which did not affect self-stimulation nevertheless potentiated escape behavior.

The fact that rats choose ESB in preference to food or to water, and the fact that they often stimulate themselves to exhaustion, demonstrates that responding for ESB is maladaptive. On this basis, Olds (22) postulated that there is a similarity between ESB and the maladaptive behavior of psychotic agitation. In both cases, he argued, stimulation of the reward system might increase the rewarding value of the next stimulation, until some maximum level is reached and maintained. This positive feedback mechanism would ensure a steady emission of responses which produce the reward. If the theory is correct, then drugs which calm psychotic agitation should also reduce responding for ESB. Olds administered five different phenothiazine derivatives to test this proposed relationship.

Prochlorperazine, which was rated best at calming psychotic agitation, produced the greatest ESB response decrement. The other drugs—triflupromazine, chlorpromazine, promethazine, and promazine—were identically aligned with respect to antipsychotic effect and reduction in self-stimulation rate.

Reserpine, another antipsychotic drug, also reduces response rate. In high doses, reserpine also produces behavioral depression. Several drugs which reverse the reserpine depression increase ESB responding. Among them are amphetamine, cocaine, caffeine, and methylphenidate (50). Other stimulant drugs, such as picrotoxin, pentylenetetrazole, strychnine, and nicotine, neither counteract reserpine depression nor potentiate self-stimulation (20).

The depressant drug pentobarbital and several anticonvulsant drugs augment self-stimulation under some conditions (18, 39). On the other hand, Domino and Olds (7) found that the anticonvulsant diphenylhydantoin invariably decreased responding for ESB.

EFFECTS OF DRUGS ON ESB IN HUMANS

Heath and his colleagues at Tulane have conducted a series of studies on ESB in humans (summarized in Ref. 11). They used hospital patients, primarily schizophrenics, but also people suffering from epilepsy, intractable pain, and a variety of other ailments. They implanted multiple cannulae in 10 of their patients and stimulated their brains with various chemicals. They got few consistent results: drugs which produced profound changes at one brain site, in one patient, had different effects—or none at all—when tested in other patients or in the same patient at other sites. The brain area from which the most consistent results were obtained was the septal region; large EEG changes were accompanied by feelings of pleasure, usually sexual (indeed, one woman experienced orgasm for the first time, and has since been able to experience it regularly). The most consistently effective drugs were acetylcholine and norepinephrine. They were effective only in nonschizophrenic patients, and only when placed through cannulae which were in the septal region. Stimulation with atropine produced undesirable changes, including irritability and an increase in psychotic symptoms.

DRUG ABUSE AND SELF-STIMULATION

There is no obvious relationship between the effects of drugs on mood and on self-stimulation. Cocaine, amphetamine, methylphenidate, and methamphetamine, all of which are abused because they produce euphoriant effects, augment rates of self-stimulation. Morphine, LSD, and alcohol (43) depress rates. Caffeine increases responding for ESB, while nicotine has complex, biphasic effects. ESB is potentiated by the minor tranquilizers diazepam and chlordiazepoxide and depressed by the major tranquilizers. Thus, the practical significance of drug-induced changes in rates of self-stimulation is still a mystery, although a fascinating one.

REFERENCES

1. Antelman, S., Lippa, A., and Fisher, A. 6-hydroxydopamine, noradrenergic reward, and schizophrenia. Science, 1972, 175:919–920.
2. Balagura, S., and Hoebel, B. Self-stimulation of the lateral hypothalamus modified by insulin and glucagon. Physiol. Behav., 1967, 2:337–340.
3. Bishop, M., Elder, T., and Heath, R. Attempted control of operant behavior in man with intracranial self-stimulation. In Heath, R. (Ed.) The Role of Pleasure in Behavior. New York: Harper and Row, 1964.
4. Breese, G., Howard, J., and Leahy, J. Effect of 6-hydroxydopamine on electrical self-stimulation of the brain. Brit. J. Pharmacol., 1971, 43:255–257.
5. Carlton, P. Cholinergic mechanisms in the control of behavior by the brain. Psychol. Rev., 1963, 70:19–39.
6. Domino, E., and Olds, M. Cholinergic inhibition of self-stimulation behavior. J. Pharmacol. Exp. Ther., 1968, 164:202–211.
7. Domino, E., and Olds, M. Effects of d-amphetamine, scopolamine, chlordiazepoxide, and diphenylhydantoin on self-stimulation behavior and brain acetylcholine. Psychopharmacologia, 1972, 23:1–16.
8. Falk, J. Septal stimulation as a reinforcer of and an alternative to consummatory behavior. J. Exp. Anal. Behav., 1961, 4:213–215.
9. Fuxe, K. Evidence for the existence of monoamine neurons in the central nervous system. IV. The distribution of monoamine terminals in the central nervous system. Acta Physiol. Scand., 1965, 64:37–84.
10. Glickman, S., and Schiff, B. A biological theory of reinforcement. Psychol. Rev., 1967, 74:81–109.
11. Heath, R. Pleasure response of human subjects to direct stimulation of the brain: physiologic and psychodynamic considerations. In Heath, R. (Ed.) The Role of Pleasure in Behavior. New York: Harper and Row, 1964.
12. Herman, Z., Kmieciak-Kolada, K., and Brus, R. Behaviour of rats and biogenic amine level in brain after 6-hydroxy-dopamine. Psychopharmacologia, 1972, 24:407–416.
13. Hillarp, N., Fuxe, K., and Dahlstrom, A. Demonstration and mapping of central neurons containing dopamine, noradrenaline, and 5-hydroxy-tryptamine and their reactions to psychopharmaca. Pharmacol. Rev., 1966, 18:727–741.
14. Hodos, W., and Valenstein, E. Motivational variables affecting the rate of behavior maintained by intracranial stimulation. J. Comp. Physiol. Psychol., 1960, 53:502–508.
15. Horovitz, Z., Chow, M., and Carlton, P. Self-stimulation of the brain by cats: effects of imipramine, amphetamine, and chlorpromazine. Psychopharmacologia, 1962, 3:455–462.
16. Jung, O., and Boyd, E. Effects of cholinergic drugs on self-stimulation response rates in rats. Am. J. Physiol., 1966, 210:432–434.
17. Mendelson, J. Role of hunger in T-maze learning for food by rats. J. Comp. Physiol. Psychol., 1966, 62:341–349.
18. Mogenson, G. Effects of sodium pentobarbital on brain self-stimulation. J. Comp. Physiol. Psychol., 1964, 58:461–462.
19. Morgane, P. Medial forebrain bundle and "feeding centers" of the hypothalamus. J. Comp. Neurol., 1961, 117:1–26.

20. Olds, J. Brain centers and positive reinforcement. Proceedings of the 27th International Congress of Psychology, Washington, D.C., 1963.

21. Olds, J. Effects of hunger and male sex hormones on self-stimulation of the brain. J. Comp. Physiol. Psychol., 1958, 51:320–324.

22. Olds, J. Hypothalamic substrates of reward. Physiol. Rev., 1962, 42:554–604.

23. Olds, J. The induction and suppression of hypothalamic self-stimulation behavior by micro-injection of endogenous substances at the self-stimulation site. Proceedings of the Second International Congress of Endocrinology, London, 1964.

24. Olds, J. Physiological mechanisms of reward. Nebraska Symp. On Motivation, 1955, 3:73–138.

25. Olds, J. Runway and maze behavior controlled by basomedial forebrain stimulation in the rat. J. Comp. Physiol. Psychol., 1956, 49:507–512.

26. Olds, J. Self-stimulation experiments and differentiated reward systems. In Jasper, H. (Ed.) Reticular Formation of the Brain. Boston: Little, Brown and Co., 1958.

27. Olds, J. Studies of neuropharmacologicals by electrical and chemical manipulation of the brain in animals with chronically implanted electrodes. In Bradley, B. (Ed.) Neuro-Psychopharmacology. New York: American Elsevier Publishing Co., 1959.

28. Olds, J., Killam, K., and Bach y Rita, P. Self-stimulation of the brain used as a screening method for tranquilizing drugs. Science, 1956, 124:265–266.

29. Olds, J., and Milner, P. Positive reinforcement produced by electrical stimulation of the septal area and other regions of the rat brain. J. Comp. Physiol. Psychol., 1954, 47:419–427.

30. Olds, J., and Olds, M. Drives, rewards, and the brain. New Directions in Psychology II, 1965, 329–410.

31. Olds, J., and Travis, R. Effects of chlorpromazine, meprobamate, pentobarbital and morphine on self-stimulation. J. Pharmacol. Exp. Ther., 1960, 128:397–404.

32. Olds, M., Alterations by centrally acting drugs of the suppression of self-stimulation behavior in the rat by tetrabenazine, physostigmine, chlorpromazine, and pentobarbital. Psychopharmacologia, 1972, 25:299–314.

33. Olds, M. and Domino, E. Comparison of M and N cholinergic agonists on self-stimulation behavior. J. Pharmacol. Exp. Ther., 1969, 166:189–204.

34. Olds, M., and Domino, E. Differential effects of cholinergic agonists on self-stimulation and escape behavior. J. Pharmacol. Exp. Ther., 1969, 170:157–167.

35. Poschel, P. Mapping of rat brain for self-stimulation under monoamine oxidase blockade. Physiol. Behav., 1969, 4:325–331.

36. Poschel, P., and Ninteman, F. Excitatory (antidepressant?) effects of monoamine oxidase inhibitors on the reward system of the brain. Life Sci., 1964, 3:903–910.

37. Poschel, P., and Ninteman, F. Norepinephrine: a possible excitatory neurohormone of the reward system. Life Sci., 1963, 2:782–788.

38. Prescott, R. Estrous cycle in the rat: effects on self-stimulation behavior. Science, 1966, 152:796–797.

39. Reid, L., Gibson, W., Gledhill, S., and Porter, P. Anticonvulsant drugs and self-stimulating behavior. J. Comp. Physiol. Psychol., 1964, 57:353–356.

40. Roberts, W. Both rewarding and punishing effects from stimulation of posterior hypothalamus of cat with same electrode at same intensity. J. Comp. Physiol. Psychol., 1958, 51:400–407.

41. Roll, S. Intracranial self-stimulation and wakefulness: effect of manipulating ambient brain catecholamines. Science, 1970, 168:1370–1372.

42. Routtenberg, A., and Lindy, J. Effects of the availability of rewarding septal and hypothalamic stimulation on bar-pressing for food under conditions of deprivation. J. Comp. Physiol. Psychol., 1965, 60:158–161.

43. St. Laurent, J., and Olds, J. Alcohol and brain centers of positive reinforcement. In Fox, R. (Ed.) Alcoholism — Behavioral Research, Therapeutic Approaches. New York: Springer Publishing Co., 1967.

44. Spies, G. Food versus intracranial self-stimulation reinforcement in food-deprived rats. J. Comp. Physiol. Psychol., 1965, 60:153–157.

45. Stark, P., and Boyd, E. Effects of cholinergic drugs on hypothalamic self-stimulation response rates in dogs. Am. J. Physiol., 1963, 205:745–748.
46. Stark, P., Turk, J., Redman, C., and Henderson, J. Sensitivity and specificity of positive reinforcing areas to neurosedatives, antidepressants, and stimulants. J. Pharmacol. Exp. Ther., 1969, 166:163–169.
47. Stein, L. Chemistry of purposive behavior. In Tapp, J. (Ed.) Reinforcement and Behavior. New York: Academic Press, 1969.
48. Stein, L. Effects and interactions of imipramine, chlorpromazine, reserpine, and amphetamine on self-stimulation: possible neuro-physiological basis of depression. In Wortis, J. (Ed.) Recent Advances in Biological Psychiatry. New York: Plenum Publishing Corp., 1962.
49. Stein, L. Psychopharmacological substrates of mental depression. In Garattini, S., and Dukes, M. (Eds.) Antidepressant Drugs. Amsterdam: Excerpta Medica Foundation, 1967.
50. Stein, L. Reciprocal action of reward and punishment mechanisms. In Heath, R. (Ed.) The Role of Pleasure in Behavior. New York: Harper and Row, 1964.
51. Stein, L. Self-stimulation of the brain and the central stimulant action of amphetamine. Fed. Proc., 1964, 23:836.
52. Stein, L., and Wise, C. Behavioral pharmacology of central stimulants. In Clark, W., and del Guidice, J. (Eds.) Principles of Psychopharmacology. New York: Academic Press, 1970.
53. Valenstein, E., and Beer, B. Continuous opportunity for reinforcing brain stimulation J. Exp. Anal. Behav., 1964, 7:183–184.
54. Wise, C., and Stein, L. Facilitation of brain self-stimulation by central administration of norepinephrine. Science, 1969, 163:299–301.
55. Wise, C., and Stein, L. Increased biosynthesis and utilization of norepinephrine during self-stimulation of the brain. Fed. Proc., 1970, 29:485.

A BRIEF
INTRODUCTION
TO ORGANIC
CHEMISTRY

The serious student of pharmacology would be wise to take one or more courses in organic chemistry and biochemistry. This section is an exceedingly sketchy introduction to organic chemistry, the chemistry of the compounds of carbon (which far exceed in number the compounds which do not contain carbon). Carbon atoms can combine with other carbon atoms to an extent which far surpasses the ability of any other atom to combine with a like atom. Thus, complex chains and rings, some containing thousands of atoms, can be formed. The simplest organic compound is methane, which consists of a single carbon atom to which is attached four hydrogen atoms. The formula is CH_4, diagrammed below.

$$H-\overset{\displaystyle \overset{H}{|}}{\underset{\displaystyle \underset{H}{|}}{C}}-H$$

methane

Compounds which contain only carbon and hydrogen are called hydrocarbons. If one of the hydrogen atoms is removed from a molecule of methane, there is left a CH_3 group, called a methyl group, which has a spare bond to which can be attached a larger molecule. Thus, the next simplest compound is ethane (C_2H_6), which consists of two methyl groups joined together. Butane, which has the formula C_4H_{10}, can exist in either of two distinct forms.

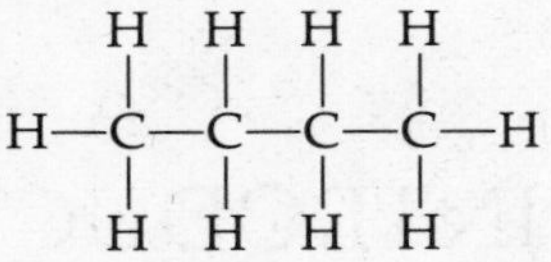

$$
\begin{array}{cccc}
\text{H} & \text{H} & \text{H} & \text{H} \\
| & | & | & | \\
\text{H}-\text{C}-\text{C}-\text{C}-\text{C}-\text{H} \\
| & | & | & | \\
\text{H} & \text{H} & \text{H} & \text{H}
\end{array}
$$

butane

$$
\begin{array}{ccc}
\text{H} & \text{H} & \text{H} \\
| & | & | \\
\text{H}-\text{C}-\text{C}-\text{C}-\text{H} \\
| & | & | \\
\text{H} & | & \text{H} \\
& \text{H}-\text{C}-\text{H} & \\
& | & \\
& \text{H} &
\end{array}
$$

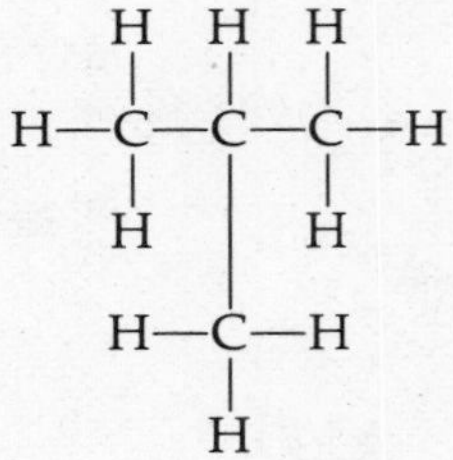

isobutane

Although the chemical formula of the two butanes is the same, the arrangement of the atoms and hence the properties of the compounds differ. Such compounds are called isomers; large molecules often have a great many isomers.

Each carbon atom of methane, ethane, and butane has four bonds, to four different atoms of carbon or hydrogen. These are called saturated hydrocarbons. Compounds which contain less hydrogen per atom of carbon are called unsaturated. Unsaturated compounds are possible because carbon atoms can be joined to each other by a double bond, as is the case with ethylene, or even by a triple bond, as with acetylene.

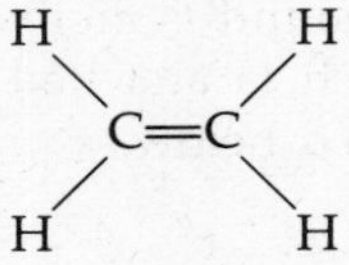

$$
\begin{array}{cc}
\text{H} & \text{H} \\
\diagdown & \diagup \\
\text{C}=\text{C} \\
\diagup & \diagdown \\
\text{H} & \text{H}
\end{array}
\qquad\qquad
\text{H}-\text{C}\equiv\text{C}-\text{H}
$$

ethylene 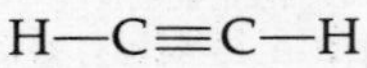   acetylene

Chains of carbon atoms, whether saturated or unsaturated, and whether arranged in a straight line or branching, are called aliphatic hydrocarbons. Carbon atoms which are arranged in the form of a ring are called cyclic hydrocarbons, the most important of which is benzene. The benzene molecule is cyclic and contains three double bonds. Its formula is shown below.

$$
\begin{array}{c}
\text{H} \\
| \\
\text{C} \\
\diagup \diagdown \\
\text{H—C} \qquad \text{C—H} \\
|| \qquad \quad | \\
\text{H—C} \qquad \text{C—H} \\
\diagdown \diagup \\
\text{C} \\
| \\
\text{H}
\end{array}
$$

benzene

Chemists have adopted a shorthand for representing benzene, in which the carbon and hydrogen atoms are omitted. It is understood whenever a geometric structure is used that a carbon atom is present at every angle, and that a hydrogen atom is attached to each angle unless another atom or group is indicated.

benzene: diagrammatic formula

Groups which are derived from aliphatic compounds are called alkyl groups. Some cyclic hydrocarbons have properties similar to aliphatic hydrocarbons and are classed with them. Benzene and compounds which resemble benzene chemically are called aromatic compounds. Groups derived from aromatic compounds are called aryl groups. The symbol R is often used to represent any alkyl or aryl group. Thus, $R—CH_3$ would represent the family of compounds which includes methane, butane, and isobutane. The family of alcohols is symbolized by $R—OH$. The simplest alcohol is methyl alcohol, CH_3OH, which is a highly toxic substance when taken internally. The alcohol found in alcoholic beverages is ethyl alcohol, also called ethanol or just alcohol. The formula is CH_3CH_2OH.

$$
\begin{array}{c}
\text{H} \quad \text{H} \\
| \qquad | \\
\text{H—C—C—OH} \\
| \qquad | \\
\text{H} \quad \text{H}
\end{array}
$$

ethanol

A very important class of alcohols is that in which the —OH group is attached directly to a benzene ring. The simplest member of the group has the formula C_6H_5OH and is called phenol. Other members of the group are called phenols. These include several natural and synthetic sex hormones and contraceptive substances. The oxidation products of phenols are called quinones, the simplest of which is catechol.

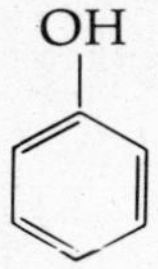

OH

phenol

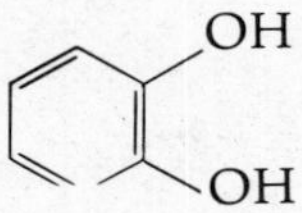

catechol

CATECHOLAMINES

Catecholamines, which include some of the most important substances with which pharmacologists work, are comprised of catechol to which an amine group is attached. Amines are derived from ammonia (formula NH_3) by the replacement of one of the hydrogens with an organic group. Amines are weak bases, i.e., they turn litmus paper blue. Amines are classified as primary (mono), secondary, tertiary, or quaternary, depending on the number of hydrogen atoms which are replaced by organic groups.

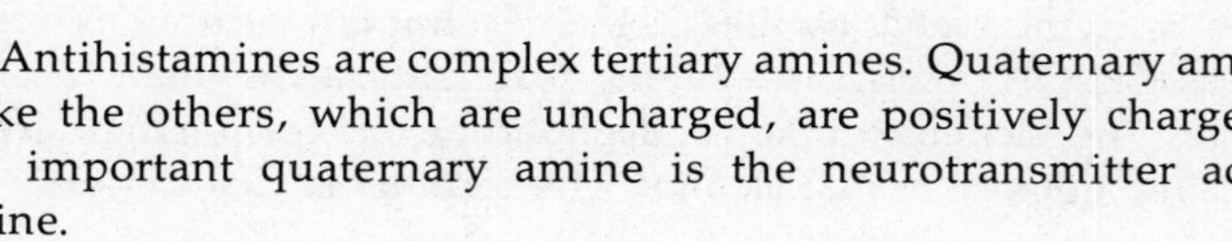

$$R—NH_2 \qquad R—\overset{\displaystyle R'}{\underset{}{N}}—H \qquad R—\overset{\displaystyle R''}{\underset{}{N}}—R' \qquad \left[R—\overset{\displaystyle R''}{\underset{\displaystyle R'''}{N}}—R' \right]^+$$

primary (mono) amine   secondary amine   tertiary amine   quaternary amine

Antihistamines are complex tertiary amines. Quaternary amines, unlike the others, which are uncharged, are positively charged. A very important quaternary amine is the neurotransmitter acetylcholine.

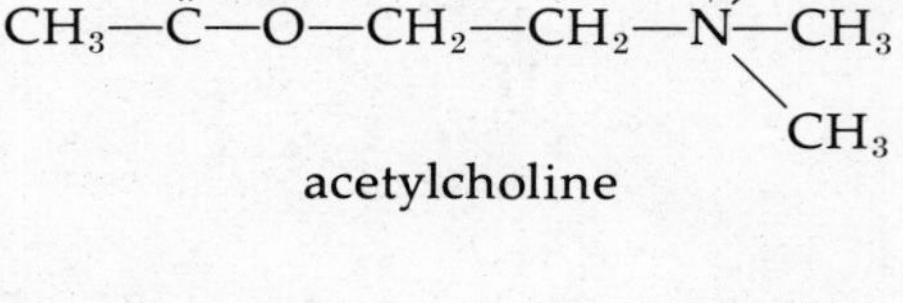

$$CH_3—\overset{\displaystyle O}{\overset{\displaystyle \|}{C}}—O—CH_2—CH_2—\overset{\displaystyle CH_3}{\underset{\displaystyle CH_3}{\overset{+}{N}}}—CH_3$$

acetylcholine

Some Important Catecholamines

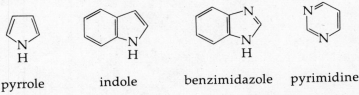

epinephrine   norepinephrine

dopamine

HETEROCYCLIC COMPOUNDS

Some cyclic compounds contain atoms other than carbon in the ring. These are known as heterocyclic compounds. The most important of them contain nitrogen as the heteroatom. These include alkaloids, which are naturally occurring compounds. Many alkaloids exert powerful pharmacological effects.

pyrrole   indole   benzimidazole   pyrimidine

Strychnine and physostigmine both contain the pyrrole ring as part of their molecule. Indole amines include the probable neurotransmitter serotonin and the structurally similar LSD, DMT, DET, psilocin, and harmaline. The benzimidazoles possess some narcotic activity. The barbiturates are derivatives of pyrimidine.

serotonin

LSD

Two other very important nitrogen heterocyclic compounds are isoquinoline and purine. The opium alkaloids are isoquinoline derivatives (see p. 61 for their structural representations); the xanthines, of which caffeine is best known, are purine derivatives.

isoquinoline   purine   caffeine

A GLOSSARY OF PSYCHOACTIVE DRUGS

This table has been adapted from Usdin, E., and Efron, D. (Eds.), *Psychotropic Drugs and Related Compounds.* DHEW Pub. No. (HSM) 72-9074, 1972. The abbreviations used in the table are given below.

AD	antidepressant	mg	milligram
b.i.d.	2 times per day	q.i.d.	4 times per day
g	gram	S	stimulant (psycho)
H	hallucinogen	Sed	sedative
Hyp	hypnotic	T	tranquilizer
i.m.	intramuscular	t.i.d.	3 times per day
i.v.	intravenous	T-Ma	major tranquilizer
kg	kilogram	T-Mi	minor tranquilizer
		μg	microgram

Note: only one brand name is listed for each drug.

Generic Name	Brand Name	Chemical Structure	Prominent Action	Human Oral Dose in mg (Except as Noted)	Pages Where Discussed
acetophenazine	Tindal	phenothiazine	T-Mi	40–80	315, 327
acetylcholine	Arterocholine	amine			269, 318, 363
adiphenine	Tranzetil	diphenylmethane derivative	T	75–150	
amitriptyline	Elavil	phenothiazine analogue	AD	10–50/b.i.d.	153, 164
amobarbital	Amytal	barbiturate	Hyp	100–200	193, 250, 276
amphetamine	Benzedrine	phenylethylamine derivative	S	5–40	83–84, 217–218
arecoline		N-heterocycle	parasympathomimetic		377
atropine		N-heterocycle	antiparasympathetic		59, 163–164
benactyzine	Hyoscyamine	phenylacetic acid derivative	T	40–200	153, 225
2-bromlysergic acid diethylamide	BOL-148	indole (lysergic acid derivative)	antiserotonergic		2
bufotenine		indole derivative	H	2–16 mg/kg/i.v.	58, 229
carisoprodol	Caprodat	carbamate	muscle relaxant	350–1400	198, 240, 349
chloral hydrate	Noctec	aliphatic	Hyp and Sed	0.3–2 g	3–4, 156, 164
chlordiazepoxide	Librium	benzodiazepine	T-Mi	5–20/t.i.d.–q.i.d.	148–149, 172–175
chlorpromazine	Thorazine	phenothiazine	T-Ma	75–500	
chlorprothixene	Taractan	phenothiazine analogue	T-Mi	15–30/t.i.d.	329
clomacran	SKF 14336	phenothiazine analogue	T-Ma	30–400	
cocaine		N-heterocycle	S; euphoriant		44, 87
cyclazocine	UM 407	N-heterocycle	narcotic antagonist	0.25–4	132, 235
D-amphetamine	Dexedrine	phenylethylamine derivative	S	5–50	153, 223
deanol	Deaner	carbinol	S; T	25–400	
desipramine	Pentrofane	phenothiazine analogue	AD	75–200	328
diacetylmorphine (heroin)		N-heterocycle	analgesic; narcotic	450	59–61, 81–83, 138, 142
diazepam	Valium	benzodiazepine	T-Mi	6–60	156, 315
dibenamine		aromatic		4–6 mg/kg/i.v.	
diethyltryptamine		indole derivative	H	14–70 mg/i.m.	54
dimethyltryptamine	DMT	indole derivative	H	14–70 mg/i.m.	54–55
diphenhydramine	Benadryl	diphenylmethane derivative	antihistaminic	25–50	
diphenylhydantoin	Dilantin	N-heterocycle	anticonvulsant	100–600	259–260
disulfiram	Antabuse	amine	used to treat chronic alcoholism	125–500	134–135

Drug	Trade name	Chemical class	Type	Dosage	Pages
DOET		phenylethylamine derivative	euphoriant	0.75–4	–
DOM		phenylethylamine derivative	H	3–5	–
epinephrine	Vasotonin	phenylethylamine derivative	sympathomimetic	0.2–1/s.c.	181–182, 318
ethanol (ethyl alcohol)		carbinol			47–48, 80–81
ethomoxane	Ethlomoxane	benzodioxane derivative	T		332
fluphenazine	Anatensol	phenothiazine	T-Ma	0.5–20	162
gamma-aminobutyric acid (GABA)	Gammalon	amine			252
glutethimide	Doriden	N-heterocycle	T-Mi	125–500	126, 171
guanethidine	Ismelin	N-heterocycle guanidine derivative	antiadrenergic	10–100	314–315
haloperidol	Haldol	butyrophenone	T-Ma	0.5–9	164
harmaline		harmine derivative	H		55, 172
hexobarbital	Evipan	barbiturate	Hyp	0.25–0.5 g	328, 329
heroin (see diacetylmorphine)					
6-hydroxydopa		phenylethylamine derivative	adrenergic blocker	50–400	335
hydroxyzine	Atarax	N-heterocycle	T-Mi	3 mg/kg	–
ibogaine		indole derivative	H		328
imipramine	Tofranil	phenothiazine analogue	AD	30–300	4, 150–152
iproniazid	Marsalid	N-heterocycle	AD	10–150	153, 356
isocarboxazid	Marplan	N-heterocycle	AD	10–90	153, 172
isoniazid	Nidaton	N-heterocycle		3–1000	–
L-DOPA	Pardopa	phenylethylamine derivative	antiparkinsonism	500 mg/b.i.d.–q.i.d.	313
lithium	Eskalith	amine	antimanic	0.02–.05 mg	152, 164
lysergic acid diethylamide	LSD-25	indole (lysergic acid derivative)	H		2, 4, 52–53, 67–68, 75–77, 337, 380
mecamylamine	Inversine	amine	H	25–100	15
meperidine	Demerol	phenylpiperidine derivative	analgesic	100–200/t.i.d.–5 × day	61
mephenesin	Relaxant	aromatic	muscle relaxant	200–2000	50, 191
meprobamate	Miltown	carbamate	T	300–600	155–156, 172–173
mescaline		phenylethylamine derivative	H		53–54, 227–228
methadone	Depridol	diphenylmethane derivative	analgesic	2.5–5/b.i.d.	129–131
methamphetamine	Methedrine	phenylethylamine derivative	S	100–400	45, 354
methaqualone	Quaalude	N-heterocycle	T-Mi; Hyp		48
methohexital	Brevital	barbiturate	Hyp	50–120/i.v.	157
methylpentynol	Dormidin	carbinol	T; Hyp	25–1000	222

A Glossary of Psychoactive Drugs. *Continued*

Generic Name	Brand Name	Chemical Structure	Prominent Action	Human Oral Dose in mg (Except as Noted)	Pages Where Discussed
methylphenidate	Ritalin	N-heterocycle	S	10-60	3, 160, 164
methysergide	Sansert	indole (lysergic acid derivative)	not H, but anti-serotonergic	4-8	328
myristicin (active principle of nutmeg)		non-N-heterocycle	H		50
nalorphine	Nalline	N-heterocycle	narcotic antagonist		132, 235
nialamide	Mygal	N-heterocycle	AD	25-500	153, 172
nitrazepam	Mogadon	benzodiazepine	Hyp; Sed	5-200	328
norepinephrine	Levarterenol	phenylethylamine derivative	sympathomimetic		318, 375
oxazepam	Serax	benzodiazepine	T-Mi	10-30/t.i.d.-q.i.d.	328
parachlorophenylalanine	Fenclonine	phenylethylamine derivative	antiserotonergic		319
paraldehyde	Paral	non-N-heterocycle	Hyp		–
pargyline	Pargiline	aromatic	AD	75-150	316
pemoline	Cylert	N-heterocycle	S	20-40	193
pentazocine	Talwin	N-heterocycle	narcotic antagonist	25-50	132, 235
pentobarbital	Nembutal	barbiturate	Hyp	30-300	126, 258
pentylenetetrazol	Metrazol	N-heterocycle	S	100-300	159-160, 258
perphenazine	Trilafan	phenothiazine	T-Ma	2-24	240
phenelzine	Nardil	phenylethylamine derivative	AD	20-150	153, 172
phenmetrazine	Preludin	N-heterocycle	S	25-75	87, 336-337
phenobarbital	Luminal	barbiturate	Hyp	15-100	4, 155
physostigmine	Eserine	indole derivative	P	1-3	269, 273-274
piperadrol	Meretran	N-heterocycle	AD	3-7.5	4, 155
piperidine	A 1746	N-heterocycle	T-Ma		–
procaine	Novocaine	benzoic acid derivative	analgesic	100-160/i.m.	236
prochlorperazine	Compazine	phenothiazine	T-Ma	25-250	168
promazine	Sparine	phenothiazine	T-Ma	10-209	329, 379
promethazine	Atosil	phenothiazine	Sed; antiemetic	25-50	379
propoxyphene	Darvon	diphenylmethane derivative	analgesic	65 mg/q.i.d.	
psilocybin	CY-39	indole derivative	H	4-8	4, 227-228
reserpine	Serpasil		T-Ma; hypotensive antiparasympathetic	0.1-9	172-174, 315
scopolamine		N-heterocycle	Hyp		59, 270-273
secobarbital	Seconal	barbiturate		50-200	233

serotonin		indole derivative	vasoconstrictor		174, 362
synhexyl	Thrombtonin	cannabis derivative	H	5–200	73
tetrabenazine	Nitoman	N-heterocycle	T-Ma	25–200	319, 329
Δ8-tetrahydrocannabinol		cannabis derivative	H		–
Δ9-tetrahydrocannabinol		cannabis derivative	H	24–50 μg/kg/smoked	64
thiazesim	Altinil	N-heterocycle	AD	1–300	330
thiopental	Pentothal	barbiturate	Hyp	50–75/i.v.	346
thioridazine	Mellaril	phenothiazine	T-Mi	50–800	162
tranylcypromine	Parnate	phenylethylamine derivative	AD	10–60	153, 172
trifluoperazine	Eskazine	phenothiazine	T-Ma	2–40	168
trimethadione	Tridione	N-heterocycle	anticonvulsant	1000–1600	225
tybamate	Solacen	carbamate	T-Mi	250–2000	164
yohimbine	Aphrodine	reserpine derivative	H	0.5 mg/kg/i.v.	311, 315

Index

395